DECISION MAKING IN
Periodontology

DECISION MAKING IN

Periodontology

Walter B. Hall, A.B., D.D.S., M.S.D.

Professor and Chairman
Department of Periodontics
University of the Pacific School of Dentistry
San Francisco, California

SECOND EDITION

Artwork by
Eric Curtis, D.D.S.
Private Practice
Safford, Arizona

B.C. Decker
An Imprint of Mosby–Year Book, Inc.

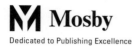

Mosby
Dedicated to Publishing Excellence

Publisher: George Stamathis
Editor: Robert W. Reinhardt
Assistant Editor: Melba Steube
Project Manager: Arofan Gregory

Mosby—Year Book, Inc.
11830 Westline Industrial Drive
St. Louis, Missouri 63146

ISBN 08106-7526-X

92 93 94 95 96 CL/MY 9 8 7 6 5 4 3 2 1

CONTRIBUTORS

DONALD F. ADAMS, D.D.S., M.S.
Professor and Chairman of Periodontology,
University of Oregon School of Dentistry,
Portland, Oregon

EDWARD P. ALLEN, D.D.S., Ph.D.
Department of Periodontics, Baylor
University School of Dentistry,
Dallas, Texas

BURTON E. BECKER, D.D.S.
Private Practice, Periodontics,
Tucson, Arizona

WILLIAM BECKER, D.D.S., M.S.D.
Private Practice, Periodontics,
Tuscon, Arizona

JORDI CAMBRA, M.D., D.D.S., M.E.
Private Practice, Periodontics,
Barcelona, Spain

MIGUEL CARASOL, M.D., D.D.S.
Associate Professor, Department de
Medicina y Cirugia Bucofacial, Facultad de
Odontologia, Ciudad Universitoria,
Madrid, Spain

CARLO CLAUSER, M.D.
Private Practice,
Florence, Italy

PIERPAOLO CORTELLINI, M.D.
Department of Periodontics, University of
Siena School of Dentistry,
Siena, Italy

GERALD J. DeGREGORI, D.D.S., M.S.
Associate Professor, Department of
Periodontics, University of the Pacific
School of Dentistry,
San Francisco, California

LAVIN FLORES-de-JACOBY, D.D.S., DR. MED. DENT.
Professor in Periodontology,
Phillipps-Universitat, Marburg,
Marburg, Germany

CRAIG GAINZA, D.D.S.
Private Practice, Periodontics,
Vallejo, California

TIMOTHY F. GERACI, D.D.S., M.S.D.
Private Practice, Periodontics,
Oakland, California

WALTER B. HALL, A.B., D.D.S., M.S.D.
Professor and Chairman, Department of
Periodontics, University of the Pacific
School of Dentistry,
San Francisco, California

GONSALO HERNANDEZ VALLEJO, M.D., D.D.S.
Professor, Departmento de Medicina y
Cirugia Bucofacial, Facultad de
Odontologia, Ciudad Universitaria,
Madrid, Spain

WILBUR HUGHES, D.M.D.
Associate Professor, Department of
Periodontics, University of the Pacific
School of Dentistry,
San Francisco, California

LUTHER H. HUTCHENS, Jr., D.D.S., M.S.D.
Professor, Department of Periodontics,
University of North Carolina School of
Dentistry,
Chapel Hill, North Carolina

KENNETH W. KARN, D.D.S.
Assistant Professor, Department of
Periodontics, University of the Pacific
School of Dentistry,
San Francisco, California

E. BARRIE KENNEY, B.D.Sc, D.D.S., M.S.
Professor, Department of Periodontics,
University of California, Los Angeles
School of Dentistry,
Los Angeles, California

JOHN KWAN, D.D.S.
Private Practice, Oakland, California,
Adjunct Assistant Professor, Division of
Periodontology, University of California
School of Dentistry,
San Francisco, California

ALAN S. LEIDER, D.D.S., M.A.
Professor, Department of Oral Pathology,
University of the Pacific School of
Dentistry,
San Francisco, California

WILLIAM P. LUNDERGAN, D.D.S.
Assistant Professor, Department of
Periodontics, University of the Pacific
School of Dentistry,
San Francisco, California

FRANCISCO MARTOS MOLINO, M.D., D.D.S.

Private Practice, Periodontics,
San Diego, California

GEORGE K. MERIJOHN, D.D.S.

Private Practice, Periodontics, Assistant
Professor, Department of Periodontics,
University of the Pacific School of
Dentistry,
San Francisco, California

PRESTON D. MILLER, Jr., D.D.S.

Private Practice, Periodontics,
Memphis, Tennessee

KATHY I. MUELLER, M.S., D.M.D.

Assistant Professor, Department of Fixed
Prosthodontics, University of the Pacific
School of Dentistry,
San Francisco, California

W. PETER NORDLAND, D.D.S.

Private Practice, Periodontics
San Diego, California

GIOVAN PAOLO PINI-PRATO, M.D., D.D.S.

Professor and Chairman, Department of
Periodontology, University of Siena School
of Dentistry,
Siena, Italy

PETER B. RAETZKE, D.M.D., M.S.D.

Professor and Chairman, Department of
Periodontology, Zahnartliches Universitats-
Institut der Stiftung Carolinum,
Frankfurt, Germany

CHARLES F. SUMNER III, D.D.S., J.D.

Associate Professor, Department of
Periodontics, University of the Pacific
School of Dentistry,
San Francisco, California

ALBERTO SICILLIA, M.D., D.D.S.

Associate Professor, Section of
Periodontics, School of Stomatology,
University of Oviedo, Oviedo, Spain,
Private Practice, Periodontics,
Oviedo, Spain

HENRY TAKEI, D.D.S., M.S.

Professor, Department of Periodontics,
University of California at Los Angeles
School of Dentistry,
Los Angeles, California

JOSE MARIA TEJERINA, M.D., D.D.S.

Professor, Section of Periodontics, School
of Stomatology, University of Oviedo,
Oviedo, Spain
Private Practice, Periodontics,
Oviedo, Spain

JUAN PI URGELL, M.D., D.D.S.

Private Practice, General Dentistry,
Barcelona and Granollers, Spain

GALEN W. WAGNILD, D.D.S., M.S.

Associate Professor, Department of
Restorative Dentistry, University of
California School of Dentistry,
San Francisco, California

JAMES R. WINKLER, D.D.S., Ph.D.

Assistant Professor, Division of
Periodontology, University of California
School of Dentistry,
San Francisco, California

BORJA ZABELEGUI, M.D., D.D.S.

Visiting Professor, Postgraduate,
Periodontics, School of Dentistry,
University Complutense of Madrid,
Madrid, Spain,
Private Practice, Periodontics,
Bilbao, Spain

JON ZABELEQUI, M.D., D.D.S.

Private Practice, Periodontics,
Bilbao, Spain

MARK ZABLOTSKY, D.D.S.

Private Practice, Sacramento, California,
Adjunct Assistant Professor, Division of
Periodontology, University of California
School of Dentistry
San Francisco, California

AXEL ZIMMERMAN, D.D.S., DR. MED. DENT

Phillipps-Universitat Marburg,
Marburg, Germany

GILIANA ZUCCATI, M.D.

Department of Periodontics, University of
Siena School of Dentistry,
Siena, Italy

To my wife, Francella, and my sons, Scott and Gregory,
for their love, support, and understanding during the
preparation of this text.

PREFACE

This is the second edition of *Decision Making in Periodontology*. Much has changed since the first edition was published in 1988. Large sections of the text have been completely redone. New contributors, experts in particular aspects of the field, have been added. The illustrations are new. The basic concept of "decision-making" has not changed. The preface to the first edition is still pertinent.

Decision Making in Periodontology illustrates the thought processes that determine optimal therapy for an individual patient. The approach entails the use of a decision tree for each clinical problem or situation; this is accompanied by a brief explanation of the basis for each decision. The chapters represent common clinical problems, which allow the reader to find solutions that take much longer to retrieve from traditional texts. In addition, several readily available references are included with each chapter.

Decision Making in Periodontology is intended to serve the needs of several groups in the dental care field. Experienced clinicians may seek answers to specific problems and compare their methods with those outlined. Teachers of periodontology may use this text as a stimulus to rethink modes of presenting information and as a model to test whether students have grasped the concepts they have been taught and are able to use them in a practical manner. Undergraduate students will find it useful in integrating concepts they have been taught in a more pedantic way, and postgraduate students may argue the merits of the decision-making process outlined and rewrite the decision trees. Auxiliary personnel will find it helpful in understanding why specific things happen in certain ways within the dental office. In the rapidly progressing and contentious field of periodontology, some of the decisions presented by our international group of authors may be controversial; however, if the decision trees presented here stimulate thought and discussion, the book will have fulfilled its purpose.

Many thanks to Robert Reinhardt who has edited the second edition for Mosby—Year Book. Repeated thanks go to B.C. Decker who originated the concept of "decision-making" texts in medicine and published the first edition. Thanks also to Bella Endzweig who prepared the text, to Dr. Eric Curtis who prepared the illustrations, and to my wife, Francella, and my sons Scott and Gregory, for their encouragement during the preparation of the text.

Walter B. Hall

CONTENTS

GINGIVAL AUGMENTATION

Pure Mucogingival Surgery

DECISION MAKING IN POSTSURGICAL REEVALUATION

MISCELLANEOUS

OSSEOINTEGRATED IMPLANTS

DECISION MAKING IN
Periodontology

INTRODUCTION

Each two-page chapter in this text consists of an algorithm or decision tree, which appears on the right-hand page, and a brief explanatory text with illustrations and references, which appears on the left-hand page. The decision tree is the focus of each chapter and should be studied first in detail. The letters on the decision tree refer the reader to the text, which provides a brief explanation of the basis for each decision. Boxes have been used on the decision tree to indicate invasive procedures or the use of drugs. A combination of line drawings and half tones were selected to clarify the text. Cross references have been inserted to avoid repeating information given in other chapters. References that are likely to be readily available to the practitioner have been selected.

Chapters have been grouped by general concepts in the order that follows the typical sequence of therapy in periodontal practice. An index is included to guide the reader further in locating specific information.

The decisions outlined here relate to typical situations. Unusual cases may require the clinician to consider alternatives; however, in every case, the clinician must consider all aspects of an individual patient's data. The algorithms presented here are not meant to represent a rigid guideline for thinking but rather a skeleton to be fleshed out by additional factors in each individual patient's case.

MEDICAL HISTORY

Walter B. Hall

Before examining a new patient, the dentist should take a medical history. At each future visit, a simple question such as "How have you been since I saw you last?" may elicit an important response, such as "I found out I'm pregnant," which the patient might think to be unimportant to her dental treatment. At recall visits, before any dental examination, the dentist should question the patient more extensively regarding visits to a physician, any illnesses, and any changes in medications. In the Treatment Record, the dentist should indicate that the medical history was updated by noting "No changes in medical history" or by recording specific changes that have occurred. The medicolegal importance of such notations cannot be overemphasized.

A. A health questionnaire ("yes or no" format) is useful in making the patient responsible for the accuracy of the medical history. Such a questionnaire may be filled out while the patient is waiting to see the dentist. Usually questions are grouped by systems. The dentist follows this form as a guideline in questioning the patient further about positive answers and writes further information in the chart.

B. The new patient's age is important in developing a treatment plan and as a guide to certain age-related diseases. Note the date of, and findings at, the patient's last physical examination. List the names and addresses of any physicians treating the patient. List medications currently being taken by the patient and the reasons for their use. Note important medications in an easily seen place, or use colored stickers to indicate these medications in a standard place on the chart.

C. Note heart attacks, rheumatic heart disease, heart surgery, and replacement parts in the heart so that precautions, such as antibiotic prophylaxis for patients with rheumatic heart disease or artificial valves, can be taken. The patient may even require medication before periodontal probing. Many patients are aware of blood pressure abnormalities, but others are not. Many dentists obtain a baseline blood pressure at this time.

D. Diabetes is a major problem in successful management of periodontal diseases. For a known diabetic, determine whether the disease is controlled, and whether the patient has visited a physician within the last 3 to 6 months. If the patient is unaware of having diabetes, questions regarding a personal history of periodontal abscesses and blood relatives with diabetes may suggest a possible problem that should be evaluated medically.

E. Infectious diseases, such as hepatitis, acquired immunodeficiency syndrome (AIDS), or tuberculosis (TB), should be included in the questionnaire. Establish whether a patient who has had hepatitis B is a carrier.

Encourage the patient to be tested for family safety if for no other reason. The test is simple and inexpensive. Acquired immunodeficiency syndrome often has an associated periodontal problem (see p 58). Questioning regarding this disease must be managed discreetly. Tuberculosis is uncommon among native-born Americans but is quite common among recent immigrants.

F. Hepatitis (see E) and cirrhosis are common problems that affect dental care. Cirrhosis may impair a patient's healing potential. Recurrent kidney infections may require antibiotic prophylaxis before periodontal treatment.

G. Patients with seizure disorders may require additional medication before periodontal treatment. Those taking diphenylhydantoin sodium (Dilantin) often develop a "hyperplastic" gingival response, which is discussed on p 52.

H. Asthma can complicate periodontal treatment, especially when epinephrine-containing anesthetics are used. Sinusitis can complicate the differential diagnosis of periodontal pain in the maxillary posterior area.

I. Avoid nonemergency periodontal treatment of any complexity throughout pregnancy but especially in the first and third trimesters. Pregnancy can modify gingivitis. Such "pregnancy gingivitis" often does not respond to treatment until several months following gestation.

J. Gastric or duodenal ulcers may complicate periodontal healing because of dietary restrictions. Colitis may be accompanied by gingival changes.

K. Various types of cancer present complications in periodontal treatment. Leukemias may be accompanied by gingival enlargement. The prognosis for the more severe or advanced types of cancer can force modification of usual treatment plans. Radiation therapy may make surgical treatment unadvisable.

L. Many medicaments and drugs used in periodontal treatment are significant allergens that may have to be avoided with sensitized patients.

M. Some dermatologic diseases, such as lichen planus, pemphigus, and pemphigoid, have periodontal components.

N. Some types of arthritis can restrict dexterity required for plaque removal. Corticosteroid therapy often delays healing following periodontal treatment.

O. Physical or medical disabilities may help to explain the etiology of inflammatory periodontal disease if the patient is unable to perform adequate oral hygiene procedures. Disabilities may influence prognosis and treatment planning as well.

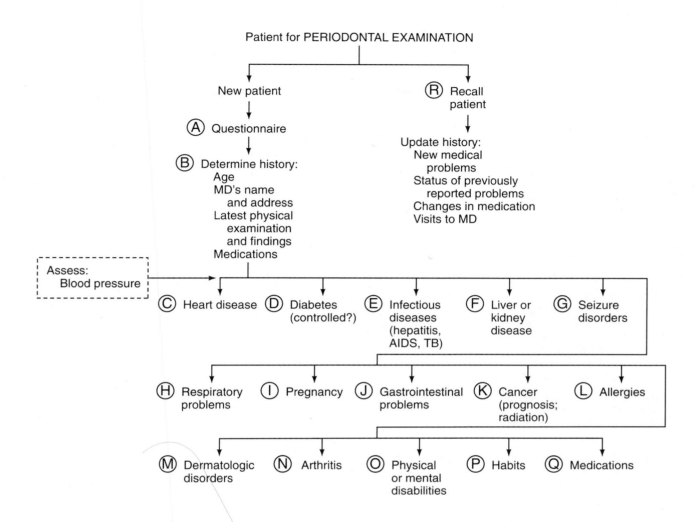

Patient for PERIODONTAL EXAMINATION

New patient

(A) Questionnaire

(B) Determine history:
   Age
   MD's name
      and address
   Latest physical
      examination
      and findings
   Medications

(R) Recall
   patient

Update history:
   New medical
      problems
   Status of previously
      reported problems
   Changes in medication
   Visits to MD

Assess:
   Blood pressure

(C) Heart disease (D) Diabetes
                      (controlled?) (E) Infectious
                                        diseases
                                        (hepatitis,
                                        AIDS, TB) (F) Liver or
                                                      kidney
                                                      disease (G) Seizure
                                                                  disorders

(H) Respiratory
      problems (I) Pregnancy (J) Gastrointestinal
                                   problems (K) Cancer
                                                (prognosis;
                                                radiation) (L) Allergies

(M) Dermatologic
      disorders (N) Arthritis (O) Physical
                                   or mental
                                   disabilities (P) Habits (Q) Medications

P. Heavy smoking or excessive alcohol consumption influence periodontal diagnosis, prognosis, and treatment planning. Vigorous toothbrushing, especially with a hard brush, may explain root exposure. Self-mutilating habits may alter gingival appearance.

Q. Medications used for treatment or management of any medical problem may affect periodontal treatment. Some, such as beta-blockers, may require changes in anesthetics. Others, such as antibiotics, may produce temporary improvements in periodontitis. A dentist must have a recent edition of the *Physicians' Desk Reference* or similar reference to determine possible effects of new medications on the treatment plan.

R. Update the medical history of a recall or continuing patient at every visit. New medical problems, altered status of previously diagnosed medical problems, and changes in medications can affect periodontal treatment.

References

Carranza FA Jr. Glickman's clinical periodontology. 7th ed. Philadelphia: WB Saunders, 1990:476.
Genco RJ, Goldman HM, Cohen DW. Contemporary periodontics. St. Louis: CV Mosby, 1990:203.

DENTAL HISTORY

Walter B. Hall

Taking and recording a dental history is an often-neglected but very important aspect of examination, diagnosis, prognosis, and treatment planning. Because many patients are treated by more than one dentist, this history should be updated regularly. The accuracy and reliability of facts from the dental history are always open to question. The patient's own answers, however, are important to record, because any inaccuracies may influence treatment. If the "facts" don't jibe either with what is seen in the mouth or on radiographs or with the dentist's knowledge of periodontal problems and their treatment, more extensive questioning may be necessary.

A. A questionnaire ("yes or no" format) is useful for gathering data and can be filled out by the patient while waiting to see the dentist. Provide space on the questionnaire for a new patient to indicate the date of the last dental visit and its purpose, the former dentist and reason for changing, and whether radiographs or other materials are available.

B. Further questioning by the dentist is necessary to determine such details as why a certain procedure was done, where in the mouth, and at what time. Space should be available for such annotation in the chart.

C. The patient should note which teeth are missing, and the dentist should ask when they were removed (or if they never appeared) and why.

D. The patient may know that the third molars were extracted or that they are impacted. The dentist should ask about postsurgical problems if the molars were extracted and when the surgery was done. If the molars are present, the dentist should ask whether the patient has ever been told they should be removed, and if so, why surgery was not performed. The dentist should ask about any symptoms (such as pain or swelling) that the patient has had in those areas.

E. Fractures of the jaws or oral tumors that have been removed or noted may be uncovered by asking a general question about other surgery. The dentist must use follow-up questions for details.

F. The dentist should ask about restorations such as crowns, bridges, removable prostheses, and implants. If any are present, he should ask the reason they were placed, when they were placed and by whom, and whether earlier restorations preceded them. A patient's knowledge of these events is likely to be unimpressive.

G. The dentist should ask whether the patient has any endodontically treated teeth. If so, ask when they were treated and, in cases of atypical or inadequate root canal treatments, where they were done. If indicated, ask about other treatments (e.g., apicoectomies and root amputations).

H. The dentist should ask whether the patient has had regular prophylaxes. If so, the dentist should ask when the last one was done, by whom, and the frequency of cleanings.

I. The dentist should ask whether the patient has had "bite" or "jaw pain" problems. If so, a detailed history of the problems, their diagnoses, any treatments, and the dates of these events should be annotated.

J. The dentist should ask whether the patient has had any orthodontic treatment, and if so, should record its nature, the times of treatment, any extractions, and the patient's satisfaction with the outcome.

K. The dentist should ask about clenching and grinding (or bruxism, night grinding), should record the patient's concept of the problem, and should note whether the problem can be related to particular events in life or to any dental events.

L. For a periodontal patient, the periodontal history is most important. An essential question is whether the patient has had a previous periodontal problem diagnosed. If not, questions regarding bleeding, swollen gingiva, pain, or gingival ulcerations may reveal that periodontal problems have existed in the past. If a previous diagnosis had been made, annotate the types of treatment and their times. If no previous treatment has occurred but was suggested, ascertain why no treatment was performed. If previous treatment was performed, determine if there were acute problems, such as necrotizing ulcerative gingivitis (NUG) or periodontitis (see p 46), human immunodeficiency virus (HIV) gingivitis or periodontitis, or a periodontal abscess, and establish when and how they were treated.

M. A recall periodontal patient may have had dental problems or treatment by other dentists since the last visit. Update the dental history, specifically asking whether any problems have occurred, how response has been to earlier treatment, what oral hygiene measures actually have been used, and what dental treatment may have been performed elsewhere.

References

Carranza FA Jr. Glickman's clinical periodontology. 7th ed. Philadelphia: WB Saunders, 1990:477.

Genco RJ, Goldman HM, Cohen DW. Contemporary periodontics. St. Louis: CV Mosby, 1990:331.

Schluger S, Yuodelis R, Page RC, Johnson RH. Periodontal diseases. 2nd ed. Philadelphia: Lea & Febiger, 1990:289.

Patient for PERIODONTAL EXAMINATION

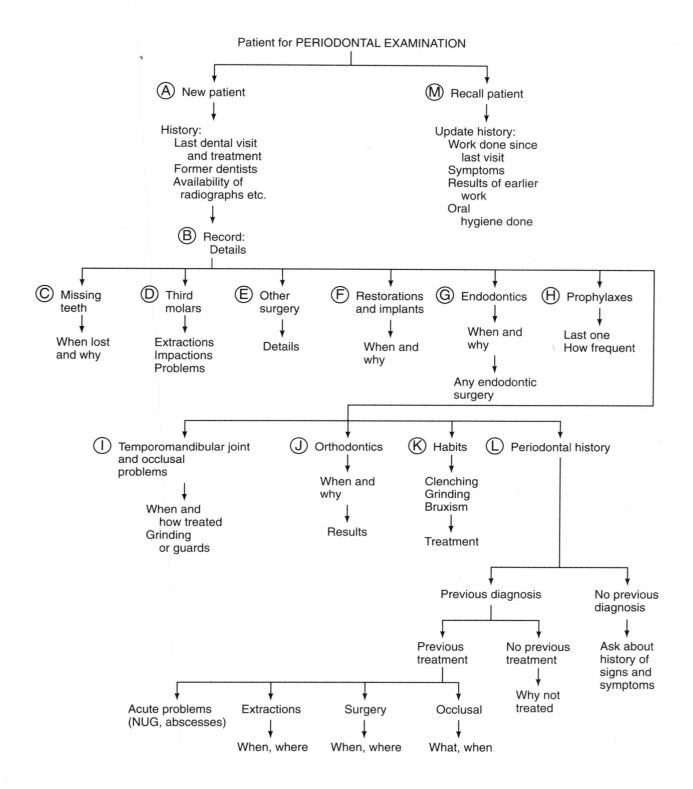

(A) New patient

History:
    Last dental visit
      and treatment
    Former dentists
    Availability of
      radiographs etc.

(B) Record:
    Details

(M) Recall patient

Update history:
    Work done since
      last visit
    Symptoms
    Results of earlier
      work
    Oral
      hygiene done

(C) Missing teeth

When lost and why

(D) Third molars

Extractions
Impactions
Problems

(E) Other surgery

Details

(F) Restorations and implants

When and why

(G) Endodontics

When and why

Any endodontic surgery

(H) Prophylaxes

Last one
How frequent

(I) Temporomandibular joint and occlusal problems

When and how treated
Grinding or guards

(J) Orthodontics

When and why

Results

(K) Habits

Clenching
Grinding
Bruxism

Treatment

(L) Periodontal history

Previous diagnosis

Previous treatment

Acute problems (NUG, abscesses)

Extractions

When, where

Surgery

When, where

Occlusal

What, when

No previous treatment

Why not treated

No previous diagnosis

Ask about history of signs and symptoms

PLAQUE CONTROL HISTORY

Walter B. Hall

A history of plaque control is important to establish during the examination of a new or a recall patient. What the patient is doing, has done, or has been advised to do to control plaque accumulation can explain the current status of plaque control at the time of the examination. Data of a subjective nature also can be collected by the dentist. How patients respond to questions regarding plaque control efforts may be as important to helping them as what they answer. If the tone of the answers is negative, the dentist will have to expend a greater effort or find a new approach to sensitizing the patient to the need for personal effort. If the patient cannot be motivated or is unable to perform adequate plaque control, the dentist's responsibilities will be greater. More frequent visits will be necessary. The patient should be made aware that the cost in money, time, and discomfort will be greater, which may help to motivate him.

A. For a new patient, a history of plaque control regarding past practices as well as current ones is required. Past practices, such as using a hard or medium brush with a scrub stroke, may explain why recession is present. Relating past brushing to techniques currently being used may indicate when recession occurred and whether it is stable or ongoing, which are important factors in deciding whether or not gingival grafting is needed. It is important to ascertain how long the patient has been flossing, how the floss is used, and the concept of what the patient is trying to accomplish. Improper use of floss with a "shoe-shining" motion may explain the origin of floss cuts. If adjuncts such as water spray or irrigation devices, interproximal brushes, wooden interproximal sticks, toothpicks, or a Perio Aide have been used, note the manner of their use and the patient's understanding of their rationale. Damage relating to the misuse of such devices also may be suggested. Note the reasons for discontinuing the use of a device.

Document the patient's current practices in regard to brushing, flossing, and use of adjunctive devices. Note the adequacy of the approaches as satisfactory or needing changes in regard to what is being used and how. If the patient was instructed to do one thing but is doing something different, note and explain this action. At the initial examination, compare the actual results of what is being done with what the patient claims to have been doing and explore discrepancies. Record a plaque index at that time.

B. For a recall patient, ask the patient to demonstrate, at least by motions, his current practices. If the patient has stopped using all recommended devices or has changed the methods of their use, the reason for doing so should be explained and the degree of success with the revised approach should be evaluated. Occasionally, a patient may devise a better means of using a device than the method that was taught. If not harmful, it may be advisable to allow the patient to continue to use the new approach. When the examination is performed, the stated practices can be compared with results and discrepancies explored. Record plaque index at this time as well.

References

Carranza FA Jr. Glickman's clinical periodontology. 7th ed. Philadelphia: WB Saunders, 1990:489.
Schluger S, Yuodelis R, Page RC, Johnson RH. Periodontal diseases. 2nd ed. Philadelphia: Lea & Febiger, 1990:349.

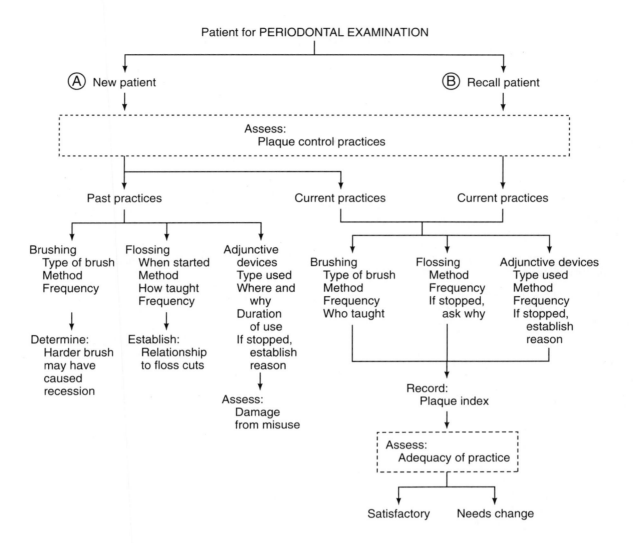

Patient for PERIODONTAL EXAMINATION

(A) New patient   (B) Recall patient

Assess:
Plaque control practices

Past practices   Current practices   Current practices

Brushing
  Type of brush
  Method
  Frequency

Flossing
  When started
  Method
  How taught
  Frequency

Adjunctive
devices
  Type used
  Where and
    why
  Duration
    of use
  If stopped,
    establish
    reason

Brushing
  Type of brush
  Method
  Frequency
  Who taught

Flossing
  Method
  Frequency
  If stopped,
    ask why

Adjunctive devices
  Type used
  Method
  Frequency
  If stopped,
    establish
    reason

Determine:
  Harder brush
  may have
  caused
  recession

Establish:
  Relationship
  to floss cuts

Assess:
  Damage
  from misuse

Record:
  Plaque index

Assess:
  Adequacy of practice

Satisfactory   Needs change

INDICATIONS FOR PERIODONTAL EXAMINATION

George K. Merijohn

Most periodontal diseases are treatable and controllable. Effective periodontal therapy depends upon an accurate and timely diagnosis. A thorough examination is the basis for an accurate diagnosis. When disease is detected and treated earlier in its onset, therapy is more predictable, better tolerated, and more likely to provide lasting results. The vast majority of people can retain their teeth throughout life with thorough treatment, reasonable plaque control, and continuing maintenance care.

On the opposite page is a schematic of the decision-making process that guides patient flow and decisions regarding examination, diagnosis, treatment, and referral.

A. A visual inspection, a clinical attachment level assessment, and evaluation of radiographs are integral parts of a comprehensive periodontal examination. An accurate diagnosis requires all these components. Recent or new radiographs of diagnostic quality are needed to determine the levels of interproximal and interradicular bone support. The purpose of the comprehensive periodontal examination is to record and document all attachment levels, disease activity (bleeding and exudate), mobility, and related occlusal factors. With regard to attachment levels, an accurate assessment of the patient's condition can be made only after the following criteria have been evaluated:

Vertical attachment levels
Pocket/sulcus depth
Soft-tissue recession
Quantity/quality of attached gingiva
Horizontal attachment levels
Furcation involvement

B. The dentist must make a distinction between patients who have previously undergone periodontal surgery and those who have not. For the former, the measurable attachment loss is a result of the disease process and, in many cases, the surgical procedure; therefore, evaluation of disease activity (bleeding or exudate upon probing) and measurement of further attachment loss (periodic comprehensive examinations) become the most important decisive factors in making the diagnosis. Use of the prognosis decision-making process will greatly assist in making treatment decisions (see p 66).

C. After 3 to 6 weeks, evaluate the success of initial therapy with a comprehensive examination or periodontal screening. If the dentist determines that the patient will be referred to the periodontist after initial therapy, then a reevaluation (comprehensive examination) is unnecessary because the periodontist will examine the patient at the first visit. Although it is an optional step, the therapist may choose to do a screening exam before referral for the sake of complete documentation. This can be performed at the last scaling and root-planing appointment or at a separate appointment. An extremely important point, from a documentation and medicolegal standpoint, is that if the patient continues treatment in the general dental office without referral to the periodontist, the patient must have a comprehensive periodontal examination and a diagnosis reestablished by the dentist.

D. A comprehensive examination must always follow advanced therapy in order to determine results and to ensure proper documentation.

E. For patients in maintenance therapy, make routine periodontal assessments at each recall visit and document significant negative changes on the Periodontal Maintenance Record. Comparing these findings to the most recent examination entry on the patient's periodontal exam record will help determine if further attachment loss has occurred. If so, then, the dentist must make another preliminary diagnosis and implement the appropriate therapeutic decisions.

F. The interval between comprehensive examinations is determined by the extent or rate of attachment loss and other presenting factors affecting the prognosis (see p 66). For generally stable periodontiums, a comprehensive examination every 1 to 2 years should suffice as long as the patient is monitored on a periodontal maintenance cycle every 3 months. Additionally, periodic radiographic surveys are important for monitoring bone levels and the results of treatment.

References

Current procedural terminology for periodontics and insurance reporting manual. 6th ed. Chicago: American Academy of Periodontology, 1991.

Guidelines for periodontal therapy. Reprint. Chicago: American Academy of Periodontology, April, 1991.

Merijohn GK. Perio Access periodontal decision making, therapy and record keeping system. 2nd ed. San Francisco: Perio Access, 1988: Chap. 3.

Proceedings of the world workshop in clinical periodontics. Princeton: American Academy of Periodontology, 1989.

Periodontal diseases of children and adolescents. Reprint. Chicago: American Academy of Periodontology, April, 1991.

Periodontal therapy: A summary status report, 1987-88. Reprint. Chicago: American Academy of Periodontology, August, 1987.

Socransky SS, Goodson JM, Lindhe J. New concepts of destructive periodontal disease. J Clin Periodontol 1984; 11:21.

Waerhaug J. The furcation problem: Etiology, pathogenesis, diagnosis, therapy and prognosis. J Clin Periodontol 1980;7:73.

Waerhaug J. The infrabony pocket and its relationship to trauma from occlusion and subgingival plaque. J Periodontol 1979;50:355.

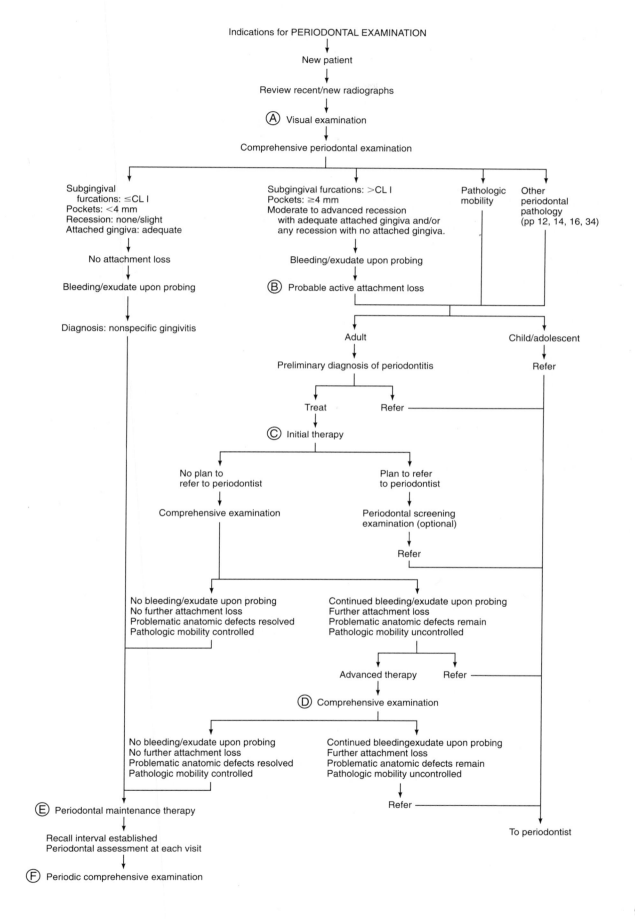

Indications for PERIODONTAL EXAMINATION

↓

New patient

↓

Review recent/new radiographs

↓

Ⓐ Visual examination

↓

Comprehensive periodontal examination

Subgingival furcations: ≤CL I
Pockets: <4 mm
Recession: none/slight
Attached gingiva: adequate

↓

No attachment loss

↓

Bleeding/exudate upon probing

↓

Diagnosis: nonspecific gingivitis

Subgingival furcations: >CL I
Pockets: ≥4 mm
Moderate to advanced recession
  with adequate attached gingiva and/or
  any recession with no attached gingiva.

↓

Bleeding/exudate upon probing

↓

Ⓑ Probable active attachment loss

Pathologic mobility

Other periodontal pathology (pp 12, 14, 16, 34)

Adult

Child/adolescent

↓

Preliminary diagnosis of periodontitis

Refer

Treat   Refer

↓

Ⓒ Initial therapy

No plan to refer to periodontist   Plan to refer to periodontist

↓   ↓

Comprehensive examination   Periodontal screening examination (optional)

↓

Refer

No bleeding/exudate upon probing   Continued bleeding/exudate upon probing
No further attachment loss   Further attachment loss
Problematic anatomic defects resolved   Problematic anatomic defects remain
Pathologic mobility controlled   Pathologic mobility uncontrolled

Advanced therapy   Refer

↓

Ⓓ Comprehensive examination

No bleeding/exudate upon probing   Continued bleedingexudate upon probing
No further attachment loss   Further attachment loss
Problematic anatomic defects resolved   Problematic anatomic defects remain
Pathologic mobility controlled   Pathologic mobility uncontrolled

Refer

Ⓔ Periodontal maintenance therapy

↓

Recall interval established
Periodontal assessment at each visit

↓

Ⓕ Periodic comprehensive examination

To periodontist

INDICATIONS FOR RADIOGRAPHIC EXAMINATION

Walter B. Hall

When a patient comes to the dentist's office seeking treatment, the dentist must decide what radiographs will be needed for diagnosis and for development of a treatment plan. The patient may be a new patient or a patient returning for a recall visit and, thus, already on record. Temporal guidelines for taking new radiographs no longer are regarded as valid. The judgment of the dentist on his need for new or additional films is accepted as valid. He must obtain and evaluate the adequacy of existing radiographs and weigh the potential value to be obtained from new or additional films against the negative effects of cumulative radiation before making the decision.

A. A full series of radiographs is needed for almost all new patients who have teeth. If earlier films exist and are obtained, assess their age in relationship to the patient's current signs and symptoms. If the existing films are recent enough, assess their quality and adequacy in relationship to current problems. Obtain new bite-wing films and new periapical ones necessary to evaluate specific problems. A routine taking of a new full series cannot be justified.

B. If the new patient has no recent radiographs or the existing ones cannot be obtained expediently from the former dentist, take a new full series.

C. When a patient returns for a recall visit, the dentist must decide whether new or additional radiographs are required. If little change has occurred since his preceding visit, as determined by clinical examination and histories, only new bite-wing radiographs and any periapical ones indicated by the examination need to be considered. Annual taking of new bite-wing films no longer is indicated. The dentist's judgment of the value to be obtained from new films suggested by the patient's signs and symptoms must be weighed against the potential danger of cumulative radiation from films that are not critical to diagnosis or treatment planning.

D. If no series has been obtained for many years and a comprehensive radiographic evaluation seems necessary for further treatment planning or definite diagnosis, a new full series is indicated. The decision to take new films is the responsibility of the dentist.

References

Carranza FA Jr. Glickman's clinical periodontology. 7th ed. Philadelphia: WB Saunders, 1990:501.

Prichard JF. The diagnosis and treatment of periodontal disease. Philadelphia: WB Saunders, 1979:67.

Schluger S, Yuodelis R, Page RC, Johnson RH. Periodontal diseases. 2nd ed. Philadelphia: Lea & Febiger, 1990:299.

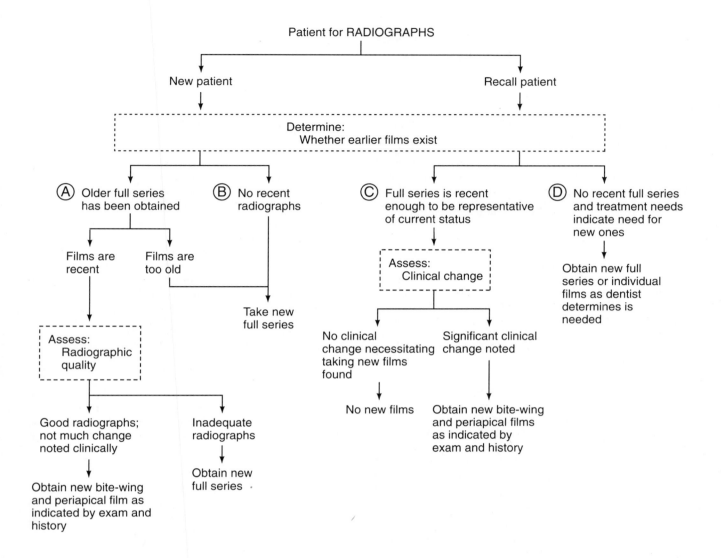

Patient for RADIOGRAPHS

New patient | Recall patient

Determine:
Whether earlier films exist

(A) Older full series has been obtained

(B) No recent radiographs

(C) Full series is recent enough to be representative of current status

(D) No recent full series and treatment needs indicate need for new ones

Films are recent

Films are too old

Take new full series

Assess:
Radiographic quality

Assess:
Clinical change

Obtain new full series or individual films as dentist determines is needed

Good radiographs; not much change noted clinically

Inadequate radiographs

No clinical change necessitating taking new films found

Significant clinical change noted

Obtain new bite-wing and periapical film as indicated by exam and history

Obtain new full series

No new films

Obtain new bite-wing and periapical films as indicated by exam and history

GINGIVAL COLOR CHANGE

Walter B. Hall

Gingival color changes are important visual indications of disease activity. Note and record them in sufficient detail so that further changes can be noted at future examinations. The color changes and their locales are useful in the differential diagnosis of periodontal diseases and other diseases manifested in the gingiva.

A. Gingival color may indicate health or disease. Healthy gingivae vary in color depending upon racial background. American texts often describe healthy gingivae as being salmon pink in color; however, this color is limited to many, but not all, Caucasians. Most of the world's people have some melanin pigmentation to their gingivae in the normal or healthy state. Lighter coffee-colored disseminated melanin pigment is typical of American Indians, Asians, and some Caucasians. Dark tones, sometimes disseminated but more often discretely localized, are characteristic of black people.

B. The effects of disease on the gingiva often are manifested by color changes. If the gingiva becomes whitened, the white may wipe away or it may not. If it wipes off, it is not a true white lesion but probably consists of sloughed cells and debris that have not been wiped away during cleaning. Such debris may accompany painful gingival lesions such as herpetic gingivostomatitis (see p 48) or necrotizing ulcerative gingivitis (see p 46), or human immunodeficiency virus gingivitis or periodontitis (see p 58), in which the patient avoids brushing or eating normally, and the sloughed cell mass and detritus accumulate. Whitened gingiva that is not debridable by wiping often results from smoking. The problem is most often generalized; palatal changes are most common and most extensive, and changes on buccal mucosa or the tongue are often detectable. Trauma, such as occlusal function on an edentulous area, may produce localized areas of gingival whitening. Other whitish changes usually are discrete and localized. They are collectively termed *leukoplakias*. They may be manifestations of serious systemic diseases and merit careful differential diagnosis.

C. The most common color change associated with diseases of the gingiva is redness. Redness is commonly seen with all inflammatory periodontal disease. Marginal and papillary redness is a feature of various types of gingivitis, periodontitis, necrotizing ulcerative gingivitis, herpetic gingivostomatitis, and desquamative gingivitis. In the desquamative gingivitis, the redness usually extends into the attached gingiva. Pale red changes are manifestations of less severe inflammation; brighter red changes indicate a more severe or acute inflammation.

D. Magenta color changes are a manifestation of a chronic inflammatory situation in which stasis of blood flow has occurred as a result of fluid leakage and swelling. Such chronic changes are seen most often in patients with established gingivitis or periodontitis.

References

Carranza FA Jr. Glickman's clinical periodontology. 7th ed. Philadelphia: WB Saunders, 1990:489.

Genco RJ, Goldman HM, Cohen DW. Contemporary Periodontics. St. Louis: CV Mosby, 1990:339.

Grant DA, Stern IB, Listgarten MA. Periodontics. 6th ed. St. Louis: CV Mosby, 1988:533.

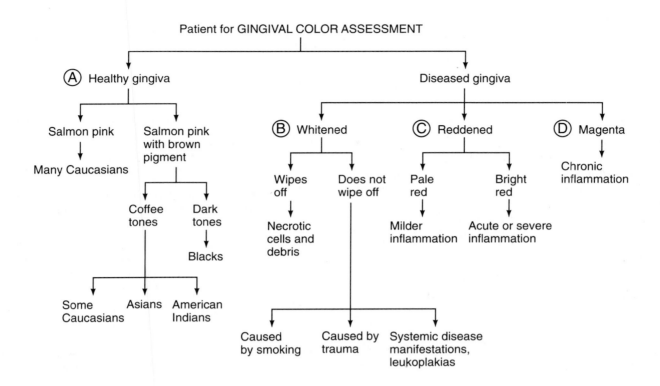

Patient for GINGIVAL COLOR ASSESSMENT

(A) Healthy gingiva

Salmon pink

Many Caucasians

Salmon pink with brown pigment

Coffee tones

Dark tones

Blacks

Some Caucasians

Asians

American Indians

Diseased gingiva

(B) Whitened

Wipes off

Necrotic cells and debris

Does not wipe off

Caused by smoking

Caused by trauma

Systemic disease manifestations, leukoplakias

(C) Reddened

Pale red

Milder inflammation

Bright red

Acute or severe inflammation

(D) Magenta

Chronic inflammation

GINGIVAL BLEEDING

Walter B. Hall

Gingival bleeding during a periodontal examination indicates inflammation. Visual signs of inflammation (swelling, redness, or magenta coloring) may be present at any time. The absence of visual signs of inflammation does not permit a diagnosis of gingival health. The gingiva may be fibrotic as a response to repeated bouts of gingivitis or periodontitis, and the tissue may appear pink and firm. Within the pocket, however, inflammation may be present, but its visual signs are masked from view superficially. A diagnosis of health, therefore, cannot be made with only a visual examination.

A. Upon probing, if no bleeding occurs and crevices are within normal limits, no inflammatory disease is present. If pockets are present but no bleeding occurs, the disease probably is in an inactive state.

B. Bleeding may occur if inflammation is present in pocket areas. If bleeding does occur on probing, inflammatory periodontal disease is present and further examination will permit an accurate diagnosis.

C. When inflammatory signs are present, a short burst of compressed air may elicit "easy" bleeding, especially in interdental areas. "Easy" bleeding of this type is indicative of necrotizing ulcerative gingivitis or periodontitis (see p 46) or of human immunodeficiency virus (HIV) gingivitis or periodontitis (see p 58). Additional aspects of examination and evaluation of

medical and dental history will permit such diagnoses (see pp 2 and 4).

D. If no bleeding occurs upon probing despite the presence of inflammatory signs, the patient may be free of active periodontal disease; however, the absence of bleeding upon probing in the presence of visual signs of inflammation would be a most unusual finding.

E. When bleeding does occur upon probing, active inflammatory periodontal disease is present. Additional evaluation of findings, history, and radiographs would permit definitive diagnosis.

References

Abbas F, VanderValden V, Hart AAM, et al. Bleeding plaque ratio and the development of gingival inflammation. J Clin Periodontol 1986;13:774.

Carranza FA. Clinical periodontology. 7th ed. Philadelphia: WB Saunders, 1990:526.

Grant DA, Stern JB, Listgarten MA. Periodontics. 6th ed. St. Louis: CV Mosby, 1988:342.

Hoffajee AD, Socransky SS, Goodson JM. Clinical parameters as predictors of destructive periodontal activity. J Clin Periodontol 1983;10:257.

Lindhe J. Textbook of clinical periodontology. 2nd ed. Copenhagen: Munksgaard, 1989:362.

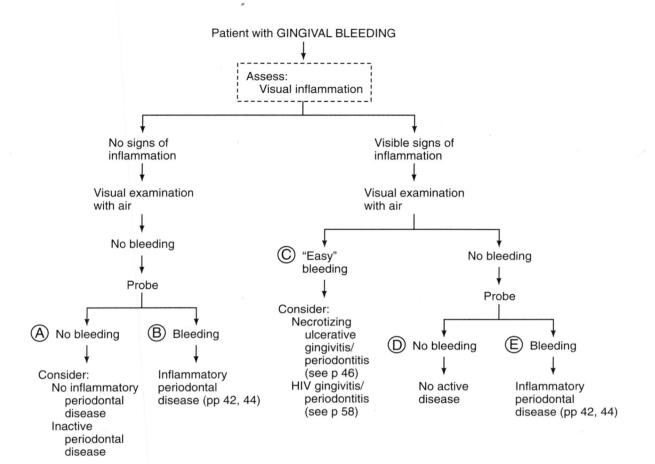

Patient with GINGIVAL BLEEDING

Assess:
Visual inflammation

No signs of inflammation

Visible signs of inflammation

Visual examination with air

Visual examination with air

No bleeding

Ⓒ "Easy" bleeding

No bleeding

Probe

Probe

Ⓐ No bleeding

Ⓑ Bleeding

Consider:
Necrotizing ulcerative gingivitis/ periodontitis (see p 46)
HIV gingivitis/ periodontitis (see p 58)

Ⓓ No bleeding

Ⓔ Bleeding

Consider:
No inflammatory periodontal disease
Inactive periodontal disease

Inflammatory periodontal disease (pp 42, 44)

No active disease

Inflammatory periodontal disease (pp 42, 44)

SPLIT INTERDENTAL PAPILLA

Walter B. Hall

A split interdental papilla is one in which the center of the papilla has been destroyed, leaving a facial and a lingual tab of papillary tissue between which a probe can be moved from one tooth to the other apical to the tips of the remaining portions of the papilla (Figs. 1 and 2). Often a split papilla can be visualized by expressing air between the teeth, deflecting the facial or lingual papillary tabs. Split papillae are most often associated with necrotizing ulcerative gingivitis (NUG) or periodontitis (NUP) or exist following that disease, creating a noncleansable area where adult periodontitis is likely to begin. Necrotizing ulcerative gingivitis or NUP may be a localized or generalized problem. Similar split papillae may occur with human immunodeficiency virus (HIV) periodontitis and can be extremely severe and sudden in occurrence. Orthodontic banding in which bands impinge on papillae or inflammation occurs as a result of difficulties in plaque control and is the second most common cause of generalized or localized split papillae. Injuries caused during restorative procedures may be a cause. Long-term heavy build-up of gross calculus is another common cause of split papillae, especially when the patient has never, or rarely, had dental cleaning. In the last decade, the severe periodontitis associated with acquired immunodeficiency syndrome (AIDS) has been described and has been termed *HIV periodontitis*. It must be differentiated from other lesions associated with split papillae, usually on the basis of history, membership in a high-risk group (recreational drug users, homosexuals and bisexuals, hemophiliacs, dialysis patients, and sexually promiscuous persons), antibody assay for the AIDS virus (HIV), or T-cell lymphocyte assay. These problems and their etiologies are important to note when one is developing a treatment plan. Surgical repair of split papillae can be a significant means of preventing the development or progress of tooth-endangering periodontitis. If the split papillae were caused by a disease with frequent recurrence, such as NUG, NUP, or HIV periodontitis, the dentist must be certain that the patient is no longer highly susceptible to recurrence before a decision is made to proceed with surgery, lest the surgery have to be repeated following a new disease episode. If the split papillae were caused by an injury, however, such as orthodontic banding, a decision can be made to proceed surgically once the movement has been completed.

A. Split papillae can occur as a generalized problem or a localized one. Necrotizing ulcerative gingivitis, NUP, or HIV periodontitis may be localized or generalized in its oral manifestations. Injuries may be localized, especially if related to wounding during restorative procedures, or generalized, especially if related to orthodontic banding or long-term dental neglect.

B. Evidence of an injury may be detected clinically, or its etiology can be elicited by taking appropriate history. In this manner, most injury cases can be diagnosed and appropriate treatment planned. Surgical repair of defects caused by injuries, in which case patient neglect or special susceptibility to disease do not make recurrence likely, is often preferable to repetitive instrumentation at frequent intervals.

C. When no history of injury can be elicited, a differential diagnosis among gingivitis/periodontitis, NUG, NUP,

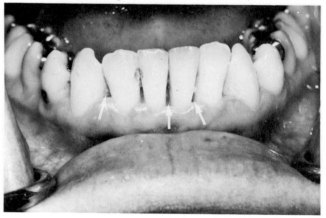

Figure 1. Split interdental papillae.

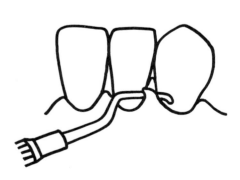

Figure 2. Split interdental papillae.

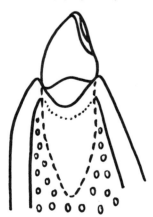

Patient with SPLIT INTERDENTAL PAPILLAE

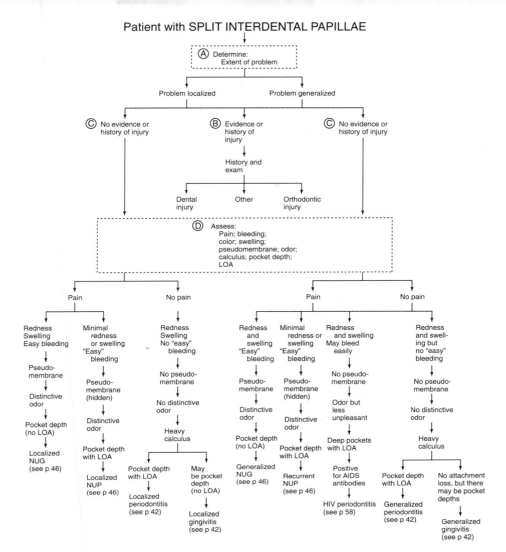

recurrent NUG or NUP, the periodontitis that may follow earlier lesions that caused split papillae that have not been repaired, and HIV periodontitis must be made. Redness and swelling may be signs of any of these lesions. Recurrent NUG or NUP may be masked visually by fibrotic repair following earlier episodes. Human immunodeficiency virus periodontitis usually exhibits marked redness and swelling with spontaneous bleeding and is characterized by sudden, severe episodes that are accompanied by generalized symptoms of illness such as malaise, fever, and gastrointestinal upset.

D. "Easy" bleeding is especially associated with the initial episode of NUG or NUP or their recurrences but must be provoked by brushing or other minor trauma. Bleeding associated with HIV periodontitis may be spontaneous and unprovoked. Neither "easy" bleeding nor spontaneous, unprovoked bleeding is associated with gingivitis/periodontitis. The typical pseudomembrane (i.e., a whitish, tenaciously adherent mass of bacteria, dead cells, and fibrin) that fills the necrosed center of the split papilla is characteristic of NUG, NUP, or HIV periodontitis, but not of gingivitis/periodontitis. A distinctive odor is associated with NUG or NUP, but a different, less unpleasant odor characterizes HIV periodontitis. Pocket depth with loss of attachment (LOA) can occur with any of these lesions, but it may not occur in the initial NUG

episodes. Pain is a symptom especially related to NUG, NUP, and HIV periodontitis, but not to gingivitis/periodontitis. Extremely heavy calculus, heavy enough to fill the embrazure space, that creates the appearance of split papillae may be indicative of gingivitis/periodontitis but may be found with any of these lesions; this necessitates use of the other criteria mentioned to make a differentiation. When AIDS or an AIDS-related syndrome (based especially on patient history) is suspected, an HIV antibody test or a T-cell lymphocyte assay can confirm or rule out this etiology with its sequelae.

References

Carranza FA Jr. Glickman's clinical periodontology. 7th ed. Philadelphia: WB Saunders, 1990:169.

Grant DA, Stern IB, Listgarten MA. Periodontics. 7th ed. St. Louis: CV Mosby, 1988:398.

Grupe HE, Wilder LS. Observations of necrotizing gingivitis in 870 military trainees. J Periodontol 1956;27:255.

Schluger S, Yuodelis R, Page RC, Johnson RH. Periodontal diseases. 2nd ed. Philadelphia: Lea & Febiger, 1990:266.

Winkler JR, Grassi M, Murray PA. Clinical description and etiology of HIV-associated periodontal diseases. In: Robertson RC, Greenspan JS, eds. Perspectives in oral manifestations of AIDS. Littleton, MA: PSG Publishing Co., 1988:49.

LOCALIZED PERIODONTAL PAIN

Walter B. Hall

Localized pain is not a common sign directly associated with most periodontal diseases. Periodontal pain localized to a single tooth or area is usually associated with development of a periodontal abscess, an endodontic problem, cracked tooth syndrome, or any combination of these problems. The differential diagnosis of these problems may be very difficult and requires a careful regimen of testing.

A. Localized swelling and/or redness may or may not be associated with localized periodontal pain. Probing the involved teeth for periodontal pockets is the first step in differential diagnosis. If no pocket depth with attachment loss is found, periodontitis can be ruled out.

B. If pocket depth is detected, inflammatory periodontal disease (most likely an abscess) is present. The next step would be electric pulp testing, testing for reaction to ice and hot gutta-percha applied to the tooth, and, finally, radiographic evaluation for periapical radiolucencies. If no reaction to an electric pulp test occurs, an endodontic problem exists. Hot and cold tests are applied to further clarify whether or not the pulp is vital. A radiograph showing a periapical radiolucency indicates a pulpal problem. The absence of such a radiolucency could indicate that no pulpal problem exists or that the pulpal problem is of insufficient duration to have destroyed enough bone periapically to be visible on the film at the time of the examination. The dentist should evaluate all these findings together to decide whether or not a pulpal problem exists. If the tooth gives a positive pulp test electrically and reacts to hot and cold, and if the radiograph shows no periapical radiolucency, the problem should be treated as a periodontal abscess. If a pulp test is negative, reactions to hot or cold are negative, or a periapical radiolucency is noted on the radiograph, endodontic treatment should be undertaken if the tooth is viewed as salvageable and useful in the overall treatment plan. If the endodontic treatment is successful, periodontal treatment would follow. Whether pocket depth is present or not, endodontic treatment is usually performed before periodontal treatment. If a tooth with pain of periodontal or endodontic origin, or both, is found to be either nonessential to the overall treatment plan or nonsalvageable, it should be extracted.

C. If no pocket depth is detected, the pain may be either endodontic in origin or caused by a crack in the tooth (cracked tooth syndrome), or both. Electric pulp testing, application of ice or hot gutta-percha, and radiographic evaluation may be used, as already described, to determine whether or not the pulp is vital. If no endodontic problem can be diagnosed by these means, one should suspect cracked tooth syndrome (see p 64). Investigate a history of trauma (e.g., an automobile accident, a blow to the mouth). Visual examination for cracks, percussion to elicit sharp pain, and transillumination with fiberoptic light to indicate the depths of cracks assist the diagnosis of cracked tooth syndrome. If the symptoms are not too severe, placing a fixed crown may resolve the problem for some time. More severe cracks may necessitate extraction of the tooth. When a pulpal problem is accompanied by deep cracks extending into the roots of teeth, the prognosis is guarded at best, and the patient should be told that the tooth may be lost.

A vertical or spiral crack extending apically down the root usually is accompanied by deep, narrow pocket formation that is not characteristic in its width of typical periodontitis. Transillumination may disclose the crack extending into the pocket. Meticulous probing may elicit a sharp pain when probing is precisely at the crack position but not immediately on either side of it. If severe, the prognosis is hopeless.

References

Cameron CE. The cracked tooth syndrome: Additional findings. J Am Dent Assoc 1976;93:971.

Cohen S, Burns RC. Pathways of the pulp. 5th ed. St. Louis: Mosby-Year Book, 1991:750.

Hiatt WH. Incomplete crown-root fracture. J Periodontol 1973;44:369.

Pitts DL, Natkin E. Diagnosis and treatment of vertical root fractures. J Endodontics 1983;9:338.

Prichard JF. The diagnoses and treatment of periodontal disease. Philadelphia: WB Saunders, 1979:117.

Patient with LOCALIZED PERIODONTAL PAIN

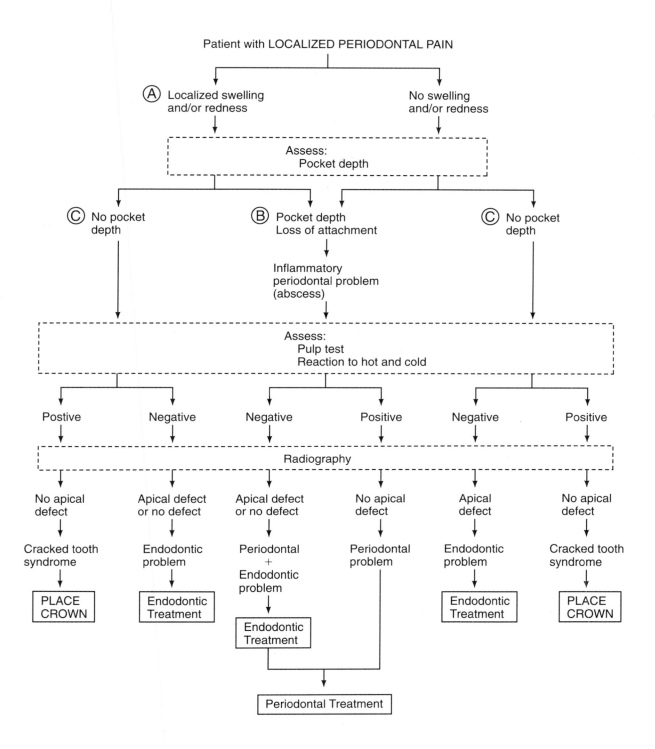

Ⓐ Localized swelling
and/or redness

No swelling
and/or redness

Assess:
Pocket depth

Ⓒ No pocket
depth

Ⓑ Pocket depth
Loss of attachment

Ⓒ No pocket
depth

Inflammatory
periodontal problem
(abscess)

Assess:
Pulp test
Reaction to hot and cold

Postive

Negative

Negative

Positive

Negative

Positive

Radiography

No apical
defect

Apical defect
or no defect

Apical defect
or no defect

No apical
defect

Apical
defect

No apical
defect

Cracked tooth
syndrome

Endodontic
problem

Periodontal
+
Endodontic
problem

Periodontal
problem

Endodontic
problem

Cracked tooth
syndrome

PLACE
CROWN

Endodontic
Treatment

Endodontic
Treatment

Endodontic
Treatment

PLACE
CROWN

Periodontal Treatment

GENERALIZED PERIODONTAL PAIN

Walter B. Hall

Generalized periodontal pain is not a symptom of periodontitis per se. A patient who has generalized periodontitis, however, may experience pain associated with concomitant problems affecting the periodontium, which can make diagnosis difficult. Records and histories of old dental examinations are especially useful in establishing that a patient has a history of nonpainful periodontitis. The development of pain after this time would indicate the onset of a new problem. The most common causes of generalized periodontal pain are necrotizing ulcerative gingivitis or periodontitis (NUG/NUP), human immunodeficiency virus (HIV) periodontitis, herpetic gingivostomatitis, and some systemic infections that may affect the gingiva.

A. Generalized swelling and/or redness of the gingiva are found with most cases of NUG/NUP or HIV periodontitis. With NUG, these changes affect the papillae most severely, but gingival margins often are affected as well. With herpetic gingivostomatitis, these changes are more generalized and not specifically associated with papillae.

B. The absence of pocket depths with attachment loss, as determined by probing, indicates that periodontitis is not involved. If papillary necrosis (destruction of the tips of papillae and pseudomembrane formation) is detected in multiple areas, evaluate the patient's breath for a distinctive, pungent odor. Take the patient's temperature. Question the patient regarding an unusual taste in the mouth (often described as metallic). Evaluate papillae for "easy" bleeding by expressing short bursts of air into each area to determine whether this provocation elicits unusually "easy" bleeding. If papillary necrosis is accompanied by the distinctive odor, a steady, moderately raised temperature, a metallic taste, and "easy" bleeding, the correct diagnosis is NUG. Such patients usually are in the adolescent or young adult age group. Younger persons are rarely affected, but older persons may be affected occasionally.

C. If pocket depths with attachment loss are not present and papillary necrosis is not detected, the pungent odor characteristic of NUG/NUP and the metallic taste should not be present. A high (104–105° F)-to-normal, "spiking" temperature may be detected, but several thermometer readings at 15- to 30-minute intervals may be necessary to detect such changes.

The patient, however, may reveal a history of repetitive sweating and malaise episodes. If tiny, round ulcerations are scattered over the gingiva and occasionally extend onto mucosal surfaces, herpetic gingivostomatitis is indicated. Such patients usually are adolescent, but any age group may be affected.

D. When pocket depths with loss of attachment are present, with or without overt swelling and redness, generalized periodontitis is present, although this problem is rarely associated with periodontal pain. One should seek other causes of generalized periodontal pain. If probing produces more "easy" bleeding than is usual with periodontitis, evaluate abnormal temperature and foul breath. Necrotizing ulcerative periodontitis superimposed on periodontitis may be present. Papillary necrosis may not be obvious in such cases. In an adolescent or young adult, NUP may be an appropriate diagnosis; this diagnosis would be unusual in an older patient. If the patient's history indicates widespread sexual activity, significant drug use (especially intravenous), or membership in a high-risk group for acquired immunodeficiency syndrome (e.g., homosexuals, bisexuals, drug users, Haitians), an evaluation for antibodies to the human immunodeficiency virus (HIV) and T-lymphocyte assay would be helpful in ruling out the severe, rapidly destructive, essentially irreversible periodontitis associated with immunodeficiency.

References

Carranza FA Jr. Glickman's clinical periodontology. 7th ed. Philadelphia: WB Saunders, 1990:149.

Grant DA, Stern IB, Listgarten MA. Periodontics. 6th ed. St. Louis: CV Mosby, 1988:398.

Grassi M, Williams CA, Winkler JR, Murray PA. Management of HIV-associated periodontal diseases. In: Robertson, PG, Greenspan JS, eds. Perspectives in oral manifestations of AIDS. Littleton, MA: PSG Publishing Co., 1988:119.

Schluger S, Yuodelis R, Page RC, Johnson RH. Periodontal diseases. 2nd ed. Philadelphia: Lea & Febiger, 1990:265.

Winkler JR, Grasso M, Murray PA. Clinical description and etiology of HIV-associated periodontal diseases. In: Robertson PG, Greenspan JS, eds. Perspectives in oral manifestations of AIDS. Littleton, MA: PSG Publishing Co., 1988:49.

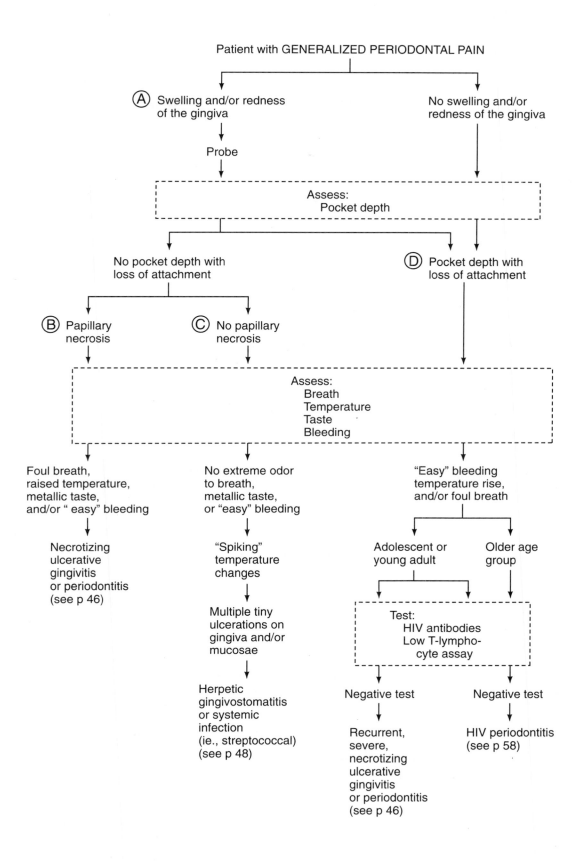

Patient with GENERALIZED PERIODONTAL PAIN

(A) Swelling and/or redness of the gingiva

No swelling and/or redness of the gingiva

Probe

Assess:
Pocket depth

No pocket depth with loss of attachment

(D) Pocket depth with loss of attachment

(B) Papillary necrosis

(C) No papillary necrosis

Assess:
Breath
Temperature
Taste
Bleeding

Foul breath, raised temperature, metallic taste, and/or " easy" bleeding

No extreme odor to breath, metallic taste, or "easy" bleeding

"Easy" bleeding temperature rise, and/or foul breath

Necrotizing ulcerative gingivitis or periodontitis (see p 46)

"Spiking" temperature changes

Adolescent or young adult

Older age group

Multiple tiny ulcerations on gingiva and/or mucosae

Test:
HIV antibodies
Low T-lympho-cyte assay

Herpetic gingivostomatitis or systemic infection (ie., streptococcal) (see p 48)

Negative test

Negative test

Recurrent, severe, necrotizing ulcerative gingivitis or periodontitis (see p 46)

HIV periodontitis (see p 58)

PROBING

Donald F. Adams

Periodontitis is characterized clinically by a loss of attachment (LOA) and the formation of pockets and osseous defects. The documentation of LOA is essential in establishing baseline data, for monitoring treatment results, and for determining periodontal stability. Probes vary in design by length, thickness, and millimeter markings. Characteristics of a good periodontal probe include a thin shaft with a rounded tip, durable markings that are easily read, and ease of sterilization. Commonly, six measurements are recorded per tooth, with each root of the molars treated as a single tooth; therefore, six facial and six lingual recordings are made for each mandibular molar, whereas there are six facial and three palatal recordings for each maxillary molar. The probe is inserted gently into the gingival sulcus and stepped around the tooth at about 1-mm increments (Fig. 1). The probe should be kept as close as possible to the axial direction of the tooth while maintaining contact of the tip with the root surface. Measurements are made from the gingival margin for pocket depth and from the cementoenamel junction (or a similar fixed point) to the gingival margin for recession (Fig. 2).

A. The probing depth and recession measurements added together determine the LOA. Such factors as the health of the surrounding gingiva, the probing force of the operator, and the discomfort tolerance of the patient can make a difference of 1 to 2 mm in probe readings. Bleeding upon probing of minimal pockets accompanied by LOA usually is managed similarly to situations in which no LOA has occurred. If LOA is 5 mm or more, refer the patient to a periodontist for evaluation. When probe depths reach the mucogingival junction (MGJ) or beyond, the dentist should determine the adequacy of the band of keratinized and attached tissue remaining to maintain the health of the periodontium and to resist trauma from the brushing and/or restorative procedures.

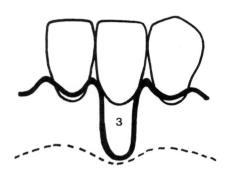

Figure 2. Probing a 6-mm deep mesial pocket.

B. If the probing depth is up to 3 mm with no LOA and no bleeding is noted after gently probing, presume that the gingiva is healthy, and continue regular periodontic maintenance. Bleeding upon probing with minimal crevice depths and no LOA usually means inadequate hygiene by the patient. Review hygiene techniques, scale and polish the teeth, and place the patient on regular maintenance.

C. For patients with pockets that are deeper than 3 mm, evaluate the quality of the patients' plaque control. Inadequate hygiene requires renewed efforts in patient education. Continued noncompliance or lack of patient skills may require referral for management and certainly is a contraindication to more definitive therapy. Bleeding in the presence of adequate hygiene indicates that the disease process is not being con-

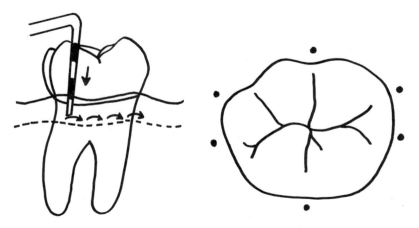

Recording

6	2	5	Li
6	2	4	F

Figure 1. Illustration of technique used in and charting made to record probings.

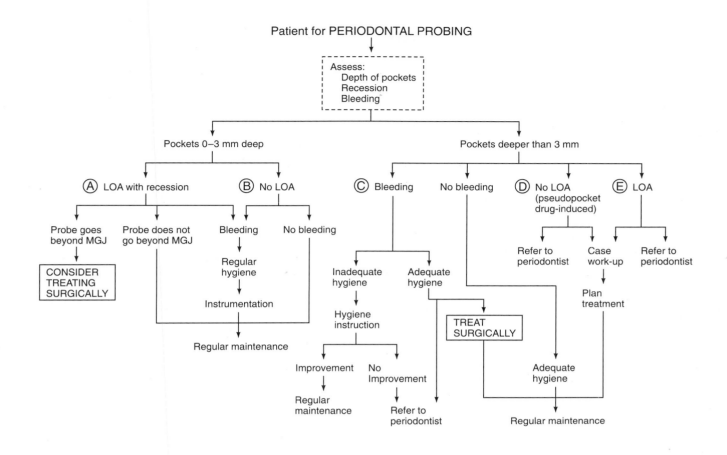

Patient for PERIODONTAL PROBING

Assess:
Depth of pockets
Recession
Bleeding

Pockets 0–3 mm deep

Ⓐ LOA with recession

Probe goes beyond MGJ

CONSIDER TREATING SURGICALLY

Probe does not go beyond MGJ

Ⓑ No LOA

Bleeding

Regular hygiene

Instrumentation

No bleeding

Regular maintenance

Pockets deeper than 3 mm

Ⓒ Bleeding

No bleeding

Inadequate hygiene

Adequate hygiene

Hygiene instruction

Improvement

Regular maintenance

No Improvement

Refer to periodontist

TREAT SURGICALLY

Adequate hygiene

Regular maintenance

Ⓓ No LOA (pseudopocket drug-induced)

Refer to periodontist

Case work-up

Plan treatment

Ⓔ LOA

Refer to periodontist

trolled despite the efforts of the patient. Because a principal goal of periodontal therapy is to create a manageable environment for the patient, the dentist can either treat the affected area or refer the patient to a periodontist. If the choice is to maintain the area by nonsurgical means, it is crucial to monitor the patient regularly and document the treatment properly.

D. Pseudopockets exist when probing depths greater than 3 mm with no LOA are found; they may be drug-induced. A complete case work-up is required if the dentist chooses to manage the patient. Referral to a periodontist is also an option.

E. When LOA is combined with probing depths greater than 3 mm, the options are either referral or a comprehensive periodontal diagnostic work-up and the development of a treatment plan. In all instances,

the patient must be informed of the presence of the problem, the options available for management, and the consequences of each option. Collect and record adequate data, making periodontal probing an integral part of the findings.

References

Listgarten MA. Periodontal probing: What does it mean? J Clin Periodontol 1980;7:165.

Listgarten MA, Mao R, Robertson PJ. Periodontal probing and the relationship of the probe tip to periodontal tissues. J Periodontol 1976;47:511.

Vander Velden U. Influence of periodontal health on probing depth and bleeding tendency. J Clin Periodontol 1980; 7:120.

DIFFERENTIATING TYPES OF FURCATION INVOLVEMENT

Walter B. Hall

Differentiating among three different types of furcation involvements based upon their severity and recording such data are essential parts of record keeping and decision making in treatments involving molar teeth. Furcations, in general, are a common site for recurrence of active bone loss with periodontitis. In some studies, the distal furcations on the maxillary first molars have been shown to be the most common sites of recurrent periodontitis. Difficulty in plaque control in involved furcations may explain this problem. Furcations are difficult for the dentist or hygienist to instrument because of their gothic arch configuration and the internal flutings that are present on many roots. The dentist may be able to get an instrument to the base of a pocket but may be unable to move it effectively without gouging adjacent root surfaces. When maxillary molars exhibit root proximity (roots close together), it may be impossible for the dentist or the patient to clean the distal furcation of the first molar because the roots of the adjacent molars are so close as to prevent an interproximal brush to be fitted between the teeth. In addition, it is impossible to insert an instrument into the furcation from the facial and palatal aspects so as to allow it to cut. The detection and recording of furcation involvements, therefore, are extremely important in developing a treatment plan and a prognosis.

A. As pockets are probed and charted, note and record the involvement of some furcations.

B. Explore all furcations with a no. 3, pig-tailed explorer or similar instrument (termed *furca-finder*). Insert the instrument into the crevice or pocket, rotate it to the interradicular depth of the furcation involvement, and move it laterally and coronally to determine whether a definite catch exists or whether the instrument will slip out of the furcation in any or all directions.

C. An incipient furcation involvement (Class I) exists within the following parameters: a detectable fluting exists where a furcation begins or where the extent is such that a catch in the furcation prevents the instrument's slipping out in one or two directions but not in all three directions (i.e., coronally, mesially, and distally).

D. An incipient furcation involvement (Class I) is recorded on the chart with a $\wedge$ symbol placed in the appropriate furcation with the apex pointing coronally.

E. A definite furcation involvement (Class II) exists when a definite catch of the inserted furca-finder prevents the instrument from slipping out when moved laterally or coronally but definitely stops without going "through and through" to another furcation opening.

F. A definite involvement (Class II) is indicated with a $\triangle$ symbol similarly positioned.

G. A "through-and-through" furcation involvement (Class III) exists *only* when the probe may be inserted in one furca and appears to connect directly with one or more other furcas. (Note: This is a *change* in terminology from the 1988 edition.)

H. A "through-and-through" involvement (Class III) is indicated by placing a $\blacktriangle$ symbol in two or more furcas on a tooth. Whereas Class II furcation involvements may be treated for guided tissue regeneration when they involve 3 mm or more, the technique for guided tissue regeneration in "through-and-through" furcation involvements is still being worked out and is not yet within the standard of care in the United States in 1992, but it may become predictable in the future.

References

Carranza FA. Glickman's clinical periodontology. 7th ed. Philadelphia: WB Saunders, 1990:259.

Easley JF, Drennan GA. Morphological classification of the furca. J Can Dent Assoc 1969;3512.

Genco RJ, Goldman HM, Cohen DW. Contemporary periodontics. St. Louis: CV Mosby, 1990:344.

Grant DA, Stern JB, Listgarten MA. Periodontics. 6th ed. St. Louis: CV Mosby, 1988:921.

Heins PJ, Carter SR. Furca involvement: A classification of bony deformities. Periodontics 1968;6:84.

Schluger S, Yuodelis R, Page RC, Johnson RH. Periodontal diseases. 2nd ed. Philadelphia: Lea & Febiger, 1990:545.

Tarnow D, Fletcher P. Classification of the vertical component of furcation involvement. J Periodontol 1984;55:283.

Patient being examined for FURCATION INVOLVEMENTS

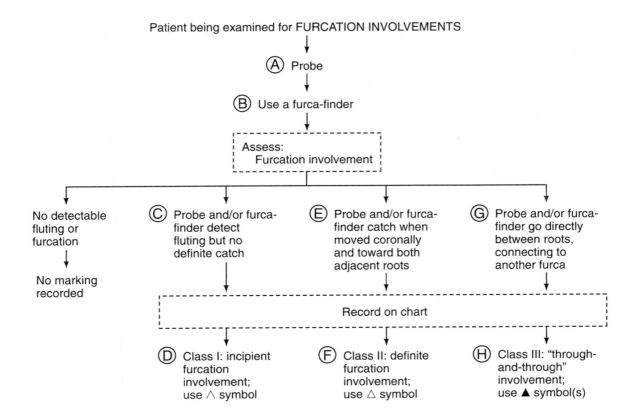

DIFFERENTIATING DEGREES OF MOBILITY

Walter B. Hall

Degrees of mobility may be useful in developing a treatment plan and in making prognoses for periodontally involved teeth. Although single-time measurements of mobility are of limited value (because slight mobilities may represent little more than clenching or pipe-stem chewing the night before the examination), when they are repeated at regular intervals and a change occurs, the change may be quite a significant finding that pinpoints a localized change or indicates a change in parafunctional habits (e.g., bruxism) that may affect the overall prognosis significantly.

A. Mobility is evaluated by placing an instrument on the facial and lingual surfaces of a tooth and applying pressure while rocking the tooth. If the tooth being tested has no tooth adjacent to it, the instruments and pressure should be applied obliquely as well as mesiodistally. A "normal" tooth has a minute amount of "give" to it (i.e., it is not ankylosed). A tooth that moves more than this minute amount but in a total arc of less than 1 mm has Class I mobility. A tooth that moves in an arc of 1 mm or more but less than 2 mm has Class 2 mobility. A tooth that moves in an arc of 2 mm or more and can be depressed into its socket has Class 3 mobility.

B. Mobilities are recorded on the chart within the crown of the tooth at the initial examination. If repeated measurements are made at various intervals, further records may be kept in different colors within the tooth form or in appropriately designated boxes. A marking should be made for each and every tooth, even if it is normal. With an assistant reading the findings, this approach will be more rapid and accurate; also, an empty space has more than one interpretation legally. Arabic numerals (0, 1, 2, 3) may be used to indicate degrees of mobility.

References

Carranza FA Jr. Glickman's clinical periodontology. 7th ed. Philadelphia: WB Saunders, 1990:481.

Hall WB. Clinical practice. In: Steele PF, ed. Dimensions of dental hygiene. 3rd ed. Philadelphia: Lea & Febiger, 1982:153.

Miller SC. Textbook of periodontia. 2nd ed. Philadelphia: Blakiston, 1943:103.

Ramfjord S, Ash MM. Occlusion. 3rd ed. Philadelphia: WB Saunders, 1983:309.

Schluger S, Yuodelis R, Page RC, Johnson RH. Periodontal diseases. 2nd ed. Philadelphia: Lea & Febiger, 1990:322.

Patient being examined for DEGREES OF MOBILITY

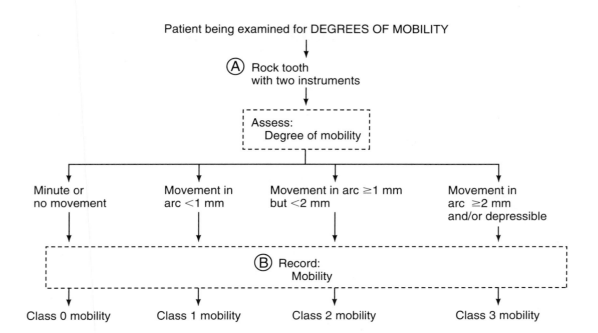

DETERMINING AND RECORDING OCCLUSAL FINDINGS

Walter B. Hall

Occlusal findings should be recorded for all new periodontal patients and should be rerecorded following occlusal adjustment. At recall visits, if the mobility of a tooth changes or the patient develops symptoms of discomfort in a tooth in premature contact, the occlusal examination should be repeated. If mobility, temporomandibular joint symptoms, occlusal pain, furcation involvements, or grossly widened periodontal ligaments are noted or if extensive restorative treatment is planned, occlusal adjustment (see pp 124 and 126) should be considered. There are several approaches to occlusal evaluation, but only one approach is presented here.

A. The rearmost, uppermost, and midmost (RUM) position is obtained by placing the dentist's thumb on the incisal edges of the lower teeth and by tapping the teeth together first, against the thumb several times, and then mandibular against maxillary teeth while exerting gentle posterior and upward pressure against the chin. Alternatively, the dentist can sit behind the patient and grasp the mandible with both hands, gently retracting it and moving it occlusally with the thumbs until two or more teeth can be tapped together. This initial contact is recorded on the chart (Fig. 1). Usually the patient can indicate the area of initial contact. The dentist can check it by placing marking tape between the dried teeth and by tapping them together in the RUM position.

B. Next, the dimensions of the patient's slide from centric relation (CR) contact to centric occlusion (CO), sometimes termed *maximum occlusion* or *acquired centric,* is recorded. The patient is closed to initial contact in the RUM position, and the movement to CO in three planes is recorded. The millimeters of vertical, horizontal, and lateral translation of the jaws and the direction of any lateral deviation of the mandible are recorded (see Fig. 1).

C. Then, the patient is asked to close in CO and to slide the mandible to the right while the teeth are in contact until the facial cusp tip—to—facial cusp tip position is reached. Cross-arch "balancing" (nonworking) side contacts are detected by placing tape on the "balancing" side and having the patient slide the dried teeth from CO to cusp-to-cusp position on the working side. Then, the tape is placed on the right side and the process is repeated indicating working side contacts and "cross-tooth" contacts. These contacts are recorded (see Fig. 1).

D. Left lateral contacts are determined and recorded by repeating the previous procedure, but having the patient slide from CO to left lateral position. These findings are recorded (see Fig. 1).

E. Finally, the patient is asked to close in CO with tape between the dried anterior teeth and to slide anteriorly until the incisal edges of mandibular anterior and maxillary anterior teeth are in contact in the "edge-to-edge" position. If the maxillary anteriors are very mobile, gentle stabilizing pressure may be applied to their facial surfaces with fingers of the left hand so that they move facially, leaving no contact marks from the marking tape to indicate heavy contacts. These contacts should be recorded (see Fig. 1).

F. The occlusal findings are used by the dentist, along with all other examination findings, to determine whether any occlusal adjustment would be beneficial (see p 50).

INITIAL OCCLUSAL FINDINGS

CENTRIC RELATION: Initial tooth contact		EXCURSIVE MOVEMENTS	
1 2 3 4 5 6 7 8 9 10 11 12 13 14 15 16		RIGHT LATERAL	1 2 3 4 5 6 7 8 9 10 11 12 13 14 15 16
32 31 30 29 28 27 26 25 24 23 22 21 20 19 18 17			32 31 30 29 28 27 26 25 24 23 22 21 20 19 18 17
CENTRIC RELATION—CENTRIC OCCLUSION DISCREPANCY:		LEFT LATERAL	1 2 3 4 5 6 7 8 9 10 11 12 13 14 15 16
Forward slide .... mm			32 31 30 29 28 27 26 25 24 23 22 21 20 19 18 17
Vertical slide .... mm		PROTRUSIVE	1 2 3 4 5 6 7 8 9 10 11 12 13 14 15 16
Lateral slide .... R( ) ...... L( ) ...... mm			32 31 30 29 28 27 26 25 24 23 22 21 20 19 18 17
CENTRIC OCCLUSION: Canine classification	Right Side Left Side I II III I II III	MAXIMUM OPENING .... mm	
Vertical overlap (overbite) .... mm		TMJ _____	
Horizontal overlap (overjet) .... mm		MUSCLES _____	

Figure 1. A typical occlusal analysis charting form (courtesy University of Pacific).

Patient for OCCLUSAL EVALUATION

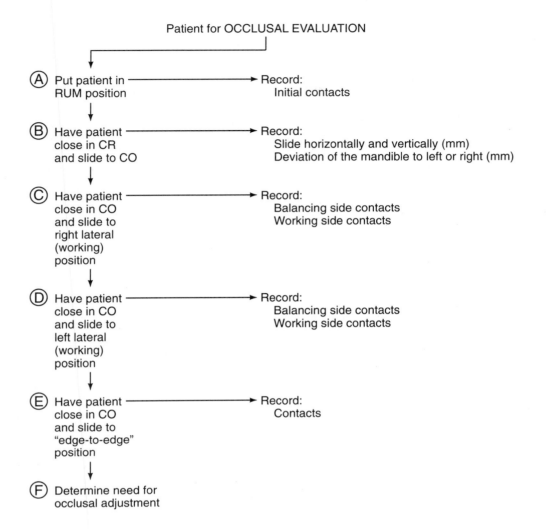

(A) Put patient in ——————→ Record:
RUM position   Initial contacts

(B) Have patient ——————→ Record:
close in CR   Slide horizontally and vertically (mm)
and slide to CO   Deviation of the mandible to left or right (mm)

(C) Have patient ——————→ Record:
close in CO   Balancing side contacts
and slide to   Working side contacts
right lateral
(working)
position

(D) Have patient ——————→ Record:
close in CO   Balancing side contacts
and slide to   Working side contacts
left lateral
(working)
position

(E) Have patient ——————→ Record:
close in CO   Contacts
and slide to
"edge-to-edge"
position

(F) Determine need for
occlusal adjustment

References

Grant DA, Stern IB, Listgarten MA. Periodontics. 6th ed. St. Louis: CV Mosby, 1988:1003.

O'Leary JJ. Tooth mobility. Dent Clin North Am 1969; 13:567.

Ramfjord S, Ash MM. Occlusion. 3rd ed. Philadelphia: WB Saunders, 1983:298.

Schluger S, Yuodelis R, Page RC, Johnson RH. Periodontal diseases. 2nd ed. Philadelphia: Lea & Febiger, 1990:318.

RADIOGRAPHIC EVALUATION

Donald F. Adams

Radiographs are an indispensable aid in identifying the presence of pathology and the conditions that affect prognosis and treatment. As with pocket probing, there are restrictions in interpretation. Exposure guidelines and processing procedures must be followed to achieve adequate contrast. Distortion is minimized by proper angulation of radiograph and x-ray machine head. A properly placed radiograph has few overlapping contact areas, and the entire tooth is visible on periapical views. For periodontal purposes, it is useful to position bite-wing radiographs vertically, so that both maxillary and mandibular bone crests are visible. Individual periapical radiographs are superior in detail to panographic radiographs and are preferred for a more accurate analysis (Fig. 1).

A. The bony crest is usually 1 to 2 mm apical to the cementoenamel junction (CEJ), because of the attachment of collagen fibers immediately below the enamel. Clinical crown-to-root ratios (C:R) are determined by the amount of root remaining in bone compared with the amount of tooth above the bone level. If the level of the bone is essentially equal across an interdental or interradicular area, it is called *horizontal bone loss* and is measured as the percent of bone lost (e.g., 20% of the original bone height is lost). Angular bone loss occurs when one tooth has lost more bone than its neighbor. A line is drawn connecting adjacent CEJs across an interdental space to determine if tipped or extruded teeth have created the illusion of angular bone loss. Some clinicians consider a radiopaque interdental crest as an indication of periodontal stability, whereas active disease results in a crest that appears moth-eaten with loss of

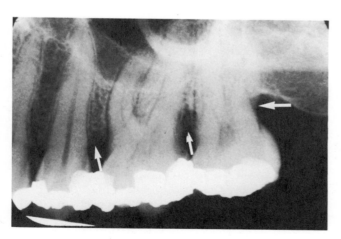

Figure 1. Radiograph suggesting two-walled defects (craters) between the first molar and adjacent teeth, and distal furcation involvement on the second molar.

opacity. This observation is controversial and susceptible to variability in radiographic angulation. Radiographs cannot be used to determine disease activity, only its history. Changes in the continuity of the lamina dura and widening of the apical periodontal ligament indicate a possible involvement. Occlusal trauma can also result in a widened periodontal ligament (PDL) and thickened lamina dura, although the widening is also seen in the PDL along the lateral surfaces of the tooth. Trabeculation can also increase with hyperfunction. In hypofunction, the PDL becomes atrophic and is narrower, along with a diminished lamina dura. Some conditions, such as hyperparathyroidism, may result in the loss of a distinct lamina dura. A variety of nonperiodontal conditions visible on radiographs may affect prognosis and treatment, including the proximity of the maxillary sinuses to the alveolar crest, root proximity, the oblique ridge, and the anatomy of the tuberosity.

B. Radiographs indicate the integrity of restorations that could complicate periodontal maintenance. Marginal ridge discrepancies and open contacts can predispose to food impaction. Improper margins and carious lesions frustrate the plaque control efforts of the patient, whereas calculus and poor crown contours harbor plaque and perpetuate the periodontal problem. Use radiographs to assess tooth position, the presence of caries in the crown or furcation areas and along root surfaces, and the condition of pulp chambers and canals. The size and shape of the anatomic crown are compared with root anatomy and the amount of bone support to determine the stability of the tooth.

C. The number of roots and their shape are closely related to the determination of prognosis and planning treatment. A tooth with the normal complement of roots, adequately spread, can more easily absorb occlusal loads. If the roots are fused or widespread, the maintenance of periodontal health is somewhat easier than if the roots are only slightly separated. On the contrary, widespread roots are often close to adjacent roots, which complicates disease management. A radiolucency in a furcation area may be the result of periodontitis, occlusal trauma, or pulpal necrosis draining through an accessory canal in the chamber floor. Long, bulky roots provide more adequate support in the presence of less bone than spindly, cone-shaped roots. Radiographs show whether a root has hypercementosis or is curved (dilacerated). A smooth blunting of root apices may be the result of orthodontic movement, whereas roughened apices indicate the action of periapical pathology.

Patient for RADIOGRAPHIC EVALUATION

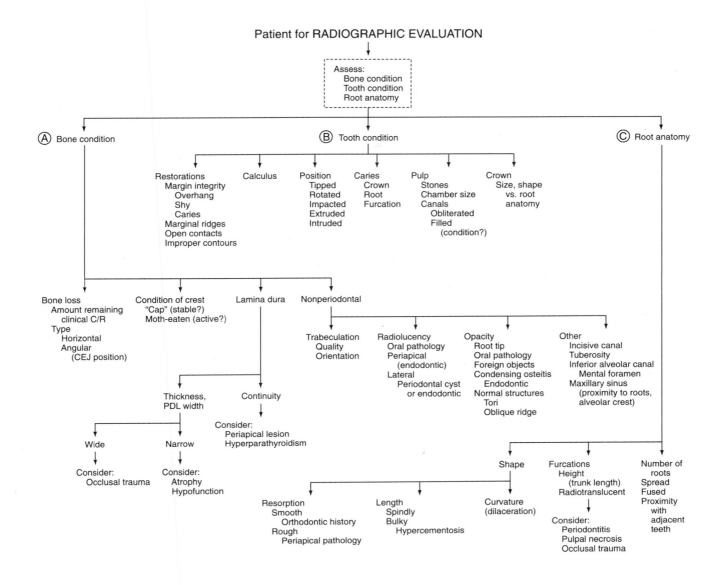

References

Carranza FA Jr. Glickman's clinical periodontology. 6th ed. Philadelphia: WB Saunders, 1984:513.

Prichard JF. Advanced periodontal disease. 2nd ed. Philadelphia: WB Saunders, 1972:142.

INTERPRETING BONE LOSS ON RADIOGRAPHS

Walter B. Hall

A full series of radiographs from a patient should be evaluated first for their ability to be read for diagnostic purposes, although no diagnoses of the status of the bone can be definitive from radiographs alone. Radiographs are only two-dimensional shadow pictures. Angulation, exposure time, and developing time are some factors that may influence suggestions of bone loss when it is not present, not show bone loss when it is present, or accurately portray the existing condition. Facial and lingual bone status is masked by the interposed teeth. Probing is the more definitive means of determining bony contours, and one should always remember that it is more likely to present an accurate picture than the radiograph. The more views that are present, the better the clinician can conceptualize the actual bony status. The angulation of individual films must be sufficiently appropriate so that films can be read. Facial and lingual cusps should be close to being superimposed on the film if it is to be interpreted accurately. Roots should be sufficiently separated so that interproximal bone levels are not masked. If the existing films are inadequate, they should be retaken; however, if one correctly angulated picture is present, the value of retaking other views should be weighed against the dangers of excessive radiation.

A. If the films are adequate, seek evidence of bone loss. If the crest of bone interproximally is more than 1 mm apical to the cementoenamel junction (CEJ), bone loss has occurred. Such a finding does not indicate that periodontal disease is present. Bone loss may be actively occurring or may have occurred earlier and be in a static state at the time the picture was taken. Bone loss also may represent bone removed during osseous surgery.

B. If the bone crest appears to be about 1 mm from the CEJ on the films, no radiographic evidence of bone loss can be described; however, bone loss either may be present facially or lingually and not show or may be masked by existing cortical plates interproximally. Radiographs are only suggestive of existing bone status when the films were taken and are not diagnostic of disease.

C. If bone loss is suggested on the films, it may be "horizontal" or "vertical" in character, as seen on a two-dimensional film. Horizontal bone loss is indicated when the bone loss interproximally on two adjacent teeth is equidistant from the CEJ on each tooth. Vertical bone loss is indicated when the bone crest is more apical to the CEJ adjacent to one tooth than to the other. A two-walled infrabony "crater" also is considered a vertical defect (see p 34). When bone loss has occurred, periodontal disease has been, and may be, present at the time when the film was taken. Use probing and the patient's dental history to determine whether bone loss is truly present and whether it represents existing or quiescent periodontal disease.

References

Grant DA, Stern IB, Listgarten MA. Periodontics. St. Louis: CV Mosby, 1988:552.

Prichard JF. The role of the roentgenogram in the diagnosis and prognosis of periodontal disease. Oral Surg 1961;14:182.

Prichard JF. Advanced periodontal disease. 2nd ed. Philadelphia: WB Saunders, 1972:143.

Suomi JD, Plumbo J, Barbano JP. A comparative study of radiographs and pocket measurements in periodontal disease evaluation. J Periodontol 1968;39:311.

Worth HM. Radiology in diagnosis. Dent Clin North Am 1969;13:731.

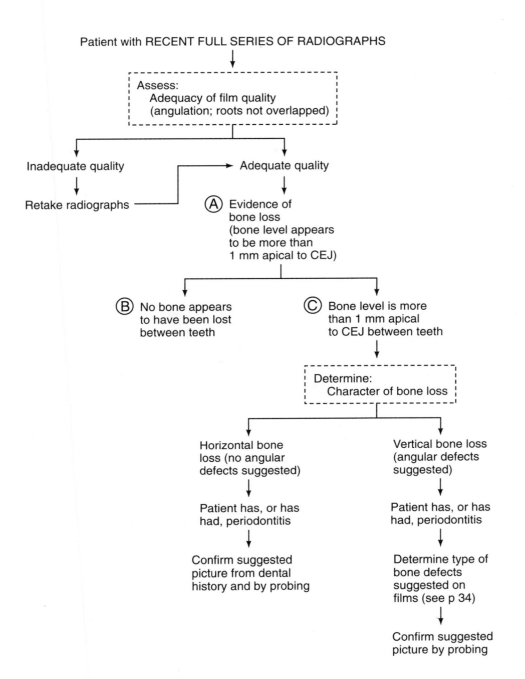

Patient with RECENT FULL SERIES OF RADIOGRAPHS

Assess:
    Adequacy of film quality
    (angulation; roots not overlapped)

Inadequate quality

Retake radiographs

Adequate quality

(A) Evidence of
bone loss
(bone level appears
to be more than
1 mm apical to CEJ)

(B) No bone appears
to have been lost
between teeth

(C) Bone level is more
than 1 mm apical
to CEJ between teeth

Determine:
    Character of bone loss

Horizontal bone
loss (no angular
defects suggested)

Patient has, or has
had, periodontitis

Confirm suggested
picture from dental
history and by probing

Vertical bone loss
(angular defects
suggested)

Patient has, or has
had, periodontitis

Determine type of
bone defects
suggested on
films (see p 34)

Confirm suggested
picture by probing

VERTICAL BONE DEFECTS

Walter B. Hall

When the full series of radiographs of a patient appear to show the presence of vertical bone defects, first evaluate the adequacy of the radiographs to assure that the appearance of these defects is not simply an artifact of poorly angulated films. Roots should not be overlapped, lest existing angular defects be obscured. If the films do not meet these requirements (see p 30), one should obtain additional, adequate films before any conclusions are drawn.

A. Vertical (angular) bone defects are suggested when the bone crest is more apical to the cementoenamel junction adjacent to one tooth than to the other. An infrabony "crater" (a type of two-walled defect) also is considered a vertical defect, although bone loss may not be greater on one tooth than on the other.

B. A typical infrabony crater is present when bone resorption has occurred between two adjacent teeth, with the greatest loss being under the contact area. Facial and lingual control plates remain that extend more coronally. When viewed on a radiograph, one may see two crestal heights separated by a more radiolucent area. Periapical radiographs are more likely to show such crests than are bite-wing radiographs, on which superimposed facial and lingual cortical plates may obscure the radiolucency. With periapical radiographs, angulation of individual radiographs or malalignment of the teeth may result in a two-dimensional picture in which such a defect is suggested but is not present. Confirm the presence of such a defect by probing. When a crater is present, probing will show shallow depths on the line angles of the proximal surfaces of the adjacent teeth with greater depth interproximally. If such findings are not apparent on probing, accept the probing findings rather than the radiographic ones (e.g., no crater is present). If probing confirms the radiographic suggestions, a two-walled infrabony crater most likely is present.

C. When bone loss is greater on one tooth than on the other (adjacent) one, a hemiseptal or one-walled defect may be present. The radiograph will suggest that half of the septum is missing, as seen in Figure 1. No suggestion of a remaining facial or lingual wall coronal to the greatest bone loss will be seen. Probe to confirm the suggested condition. Bone loss will not be more apical under the contact area than at the line angles if a hemiseptal defect is present. Accept the probing findings as correct if they differ from the picture suggested by radiographs.

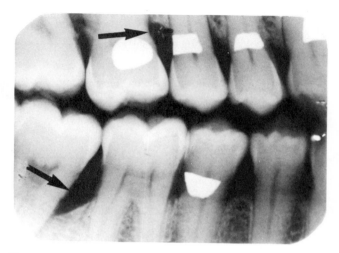

Figure 1. Hemiseptal (one-walled) defects are indicated by the arrows on this radiograph.

D. When additional facial or lingual walls or both are suggested on the film, a two-walled or three-walled infrabony defect may be present. If a third wall is present, two crestal heights may be suggested superimposed over the area of vertical bone loss. The final differentiation of the two types of defects must be made by probing. When pocket depth is less on either the facial or lingual line angle of the affected tooth but the bone loss under the contact area and at the other line angle is deeper and similar, a two-walled defect is present. When the pocket depth at both line angles is less than under the contact area, a three-walled defect is present. Regard the findings on probing as correct if they differ from the suggested radiographic picture.

References

Friedman N. Reattachment and roentgenograms. J Periodontol 1958;29:98.

Prichard JF. Advanced periodontal disease. 2nd ed. Philadelphia: WB Saunders, 1972:175.

Prichard JF. The diagnosis and treatment of periodontal disease in general practice. Philadelphia: WB Saunders, 1979:78.

Schluger S, Yuodelis R, Page RC, Johnson RH. Periodontal diseases. 2nd ed. Philadelphia: Lea & Febiger, 1990:299.

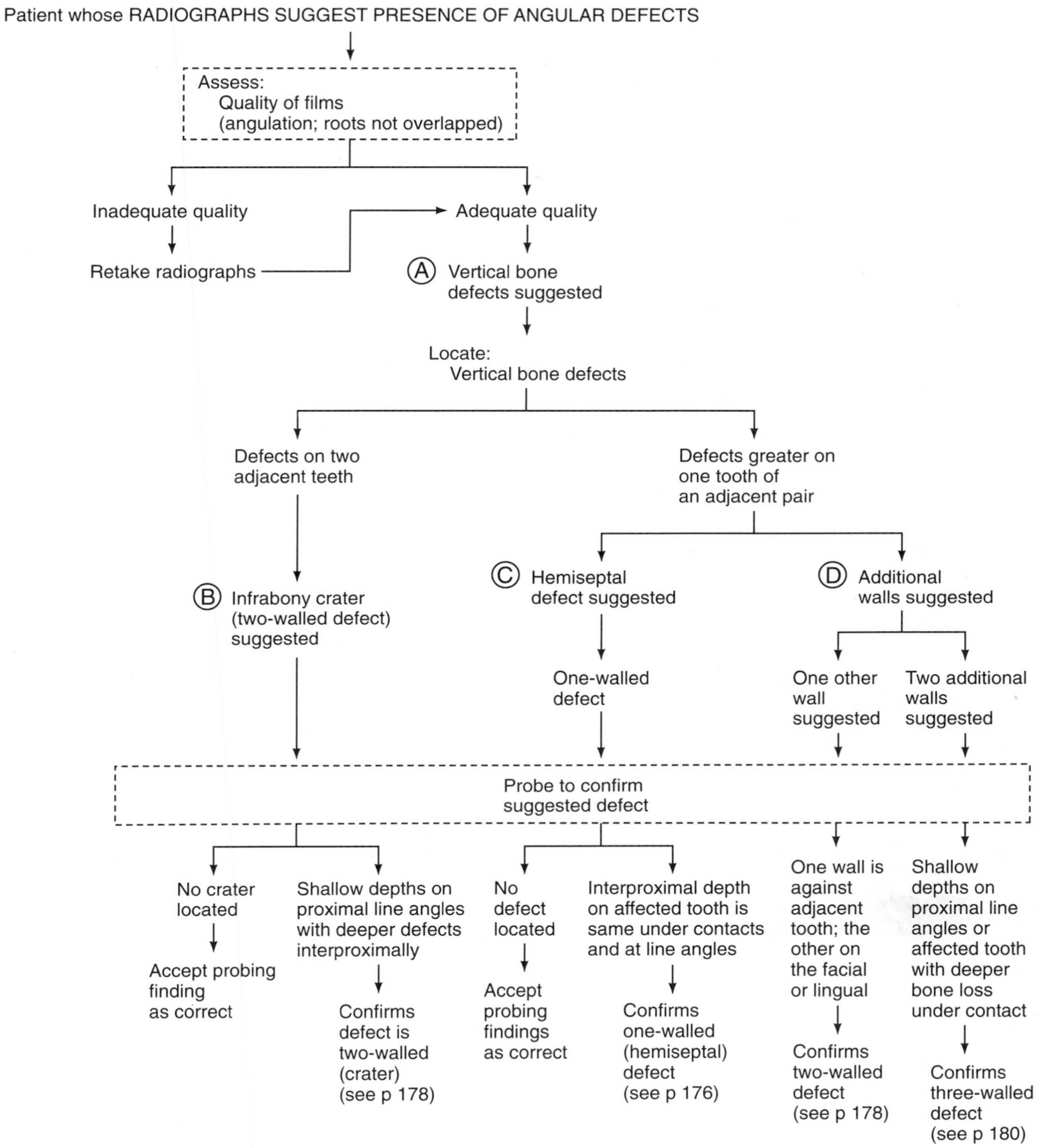

Patient whose RADIOGRAPHS SUGGEST PRESENCE OF ANGULAR DEFECTS

Assess:
Quality of films
(angulation; roots not overlapped)

Inadequate quality

Retake radiographs

Adequate quality

(A) Vertical bone
defects suggested

Locate:
Vertical bone defects

Defects on two
adjacent teeth

Defects greater on
one tooth of
an adjacent pair

(B) Infrabony crater
(two-walled defect)
suggested

(C) Hemiseptal
defect suggested

(D) Additional
walls suggested

One-walled
defect

One other
wall
suggested

Two additional
walls
suggested

Probe to confirm
suggested defect

No crater
located

Shallow depths on
proximal line angles
with deeper defects
interproximally

No
defect
located

Interproximal depth
on affected tooth is
same under contacts
and at line angles

One wall is
against
adjacent
tooth; the
other on
the facial
or lingual

Shallow
depths on
proximal line
angles or
affected tooth
with deeper
bone loss
under contact

Accept probing
finding
as correct

Confirms
defect is
two-walled
(crater)
(see p 178)

Accept
probing
findings
as correct

Confirms
one-walled
(hemiseptal)
defect
(see p 176)

Confirms
two-walled
defect
(see p 178)

Confirms
three-walled
defect
(see p 180)

OVERHANGING MARGIN

Walter B. Hall

An overhanging margin on a periodontically involved tooth makes plaque removal difficult to impossible (Fig. 1). The material of which the restoration was constructed is crucial in deciding how best to resolve this type of problem. Generally, replacement of the defective restoration is the best approach; however, if the overhang is minimal and accessible, less-expensive alternatives, such as smoothing out the overhang or marginal repairs, may be acceptable options.

A. If the defective restoration is an amalgam that is basically adequate and no new caries are involved, smoothing out the overhang would be the approach of choice. If the restoration is grossly defective, involves new caries, or is inaccessible for repair, it should be replaced.

B. If the restoration is a composite and the defect is minimal, it may be smoothed out and polished. If there is a gross defect or new caries, it should be replaced because of the difficulty in doing acceptable repairs to existing composites.

C. If the restoration is a gold inlay or onlay, it will have been cast in relatively soft gold. This type of gold will "pull" or flow when burnished with a rotating stone or polishing bur. If the defect is minimal, the discrepancy can be burnished out; however, if it is a major one, the restoration should be replaced or a repair performed with foil or alloy if the defective area is accessible for preparation and filling.

D. If the overhanging margin is on a gold crown, the gold that has been used will be harder and more difficult to pull. Only minimal discrepancies on gold crown margins are amenable to this approach. If the defect is greater and the area is accessible for preparation and filling, a foil or alloy repair may be performed. Replacement of gold crowns with defective margins is the approach of choice, but it is very expensive.

E. If the overhanging margin is on a gold-alloy crown, this material is even harder and usually cannot be pulled at all. If the defect is accessible, an alloy repair may be adequate. If not, the crown should be replaced.

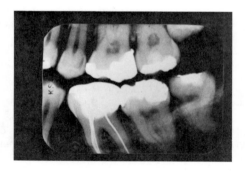

Figure 1. An overhang on the distal surface of the maxillary first molar.

References

Bjorn AL, Bjorn H, Grcovic B. Marginal fit of restorations and its relation to periodontal bone level. Odont Rev 1974;20:311.

Gilmore N, Sheiham A. Overhanging dental restorations and periodontal disease. J Periodontol 1971;42:8.

Renggli HH, Regolati A. Gingival inflammation and plaque accumulation by well-adapted supragingival and subgingival proximal restorations. Helv Odontol Acta 1972;16:99.

Roderiques-Ferrer HJ, Stroham JD, Newman HN. Effect on gingival health of removing overhanging margins of interproximal subgingival amalgam restorations. J Clin Periodontol 1980;7:457.

Schluger S, Yuodelis RA, Page RC. Periodontal disease. Philadelphia: Lea & Febiger, 1977:589.

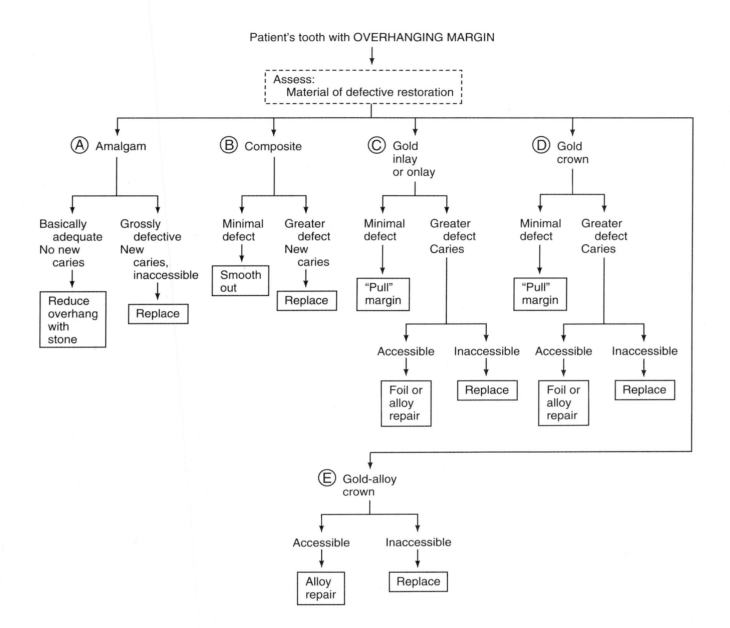

Patient's tooth with OVERHANGING MARGIN

Assess:
Material of defective restoration

Ⓐ Amalgam

Basically
adequate
No new
caries

Reduce
overhang
with
stone

Grossly
defective
New
caries,
inaccessible

Replace

Ⓑ Composite

Minimal
defect

Smooth
out

Greater
defect
New
caries

Replace

Ⓒ Gold
inlay
or onlay

Minimal
defect

"Pull"
margin

Greater
defect
Caries

Accessible

Foil or
alloy
repair

Inaccessible

Replace

Ⓓ Gold
crown

Minimal
defect

"Pull"
margin

Greater
defect
Caries

Accessible

Foil or
alloy
repair

Inaccessible

Replace

Ⓔ Gold-alloy
crown

Accessible

Alloy
repair

Inaccessible

Replace

ROOT EXPOSURE

Walter B. Hall

Root exposure is a common problem. Determining its etiology is essential in deciding whether any reparative or preventive periodontal procedures should be considered in treatment planning. Much difference of opinion about the need for reparative or preventive surgical intervention exists within the profession.

A. Recession may be localized or generalized. The etiologies of the two may be quite different. All teeth should be inspected for recession on both facial and lingual surfaces. A line representing the true position of the free margin of the gingiva in relation to the cementoenamel junction (CEJ) on each tooth should be drawn on the chart (Fig. 1). If recession has occurred, the number of millimeters of recession should be recorded for future reference in determining whether the recession is active or stabilized. This determination often is critical in deciding whether surgical intervention is indicated or not. Some newer charting methods, designed for computerization, do not employ tooth diagrams; instead there is a column in which the position of the margin is described numerically. If the free margin is consistent with the CEJ, it is charted as a 0. If the margin is coronal to the CEJ, it is described as a +1 or +2, for example. If

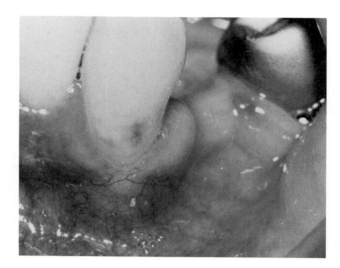

Figure 3. Recession in an area of inadequate attached gingiva has resulted in root exposure.

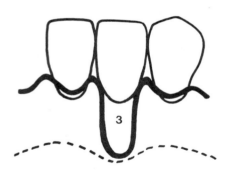

Figure 1. Chart recording an area of recession on a central incisor.

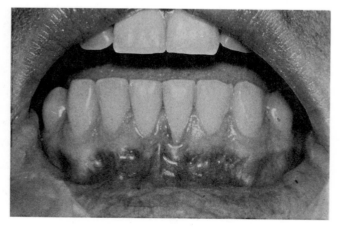

Figure 2. A central incisor with inadequate attached gingiva and recession.

recession has occurred, it would be charted as a −1 or −2, for example (Fig. 2). This determination often is critical in deciding whether surgical intervention is indicated. On those surfaces where a muco-gingival junction is present (both facially and lingually in the lower arch but only facially in the upper arch), its position should be recorded. Where 2 mm or less of total gingiva (free margin to mucogingival junction) is present, a pure mucogingival problem exists, and one should consider the need for surgical intervention in the overall treatment planning process for the patient. In the newer, computer-compatible charts, a line on which total millimeters of gingiva can be entered is utilized for this purpose (Fig. 2).

B. The skill of the dentist in eliciting the facts of a patient's dental history and the temporal placement of those events in that history often are clues to the sequential development of recession. Frequently, a patient's recollection of these events and their temporal sequence must be gleaned by the dentist by repetitive and incisive questioning. The dentist's knowledge of the typical sequencing of events in the process of recession may be used to guide the patient's recollections.

C. Injuries may occur in areas predisposed to recession by the presence of "inadequate attached gingiva" (Fig. 3) or where adequate attached gingiva is present. Such injuries may be the result of a direct wound (e.g., from crusty bread) or repeated bouts of gingivitis. Where inadequate attached gingiva is present, root exposure frequently results. Where an adequate band of attached gingiva is present, unless the wound is very severe, healing usually occurs without much, if any, recession.

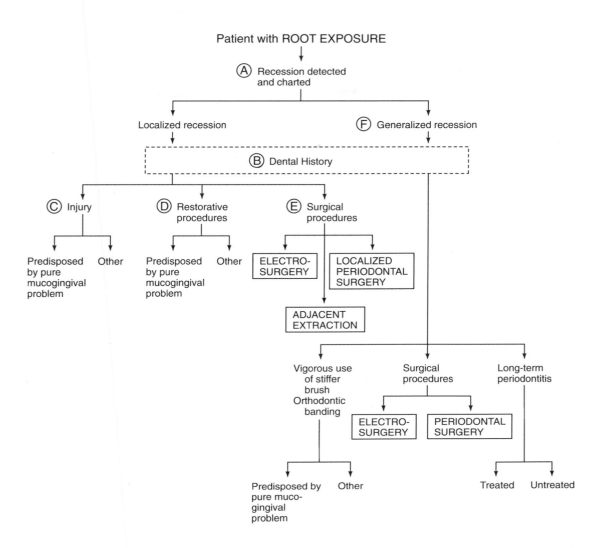

Patient with ROOT EXPOSURE

(A) Recession detected and charted

Localized recession

(F) Generalized recession

(B) Dental History

(C) Injury

(D) Restorative procedures

(E) Surgical procedures

Predisposed by pure mucogingival problem   Other

Predisposed by pure mucogingival problem   Other

ELECTRO-SURGERY

LOCALIZED PERIODONTAL SURGERY

ADJACENT EXTRACTION

Vigorous use of stiffer brush Orthodontic banding

Surgical procedures

Long-term periodontitis

ELECTRO-SURGERY

PERIODONTAL SURGERY

Predisposed by pure muco-gingival problem   Other

Treated   Untreated

D. Restorative procedures, such as subgingival use of a diamond bur, taking an impression subgingivally, or the cementation and polishing of a restoration often result in recession when inadequate attached gingiva is present but far less frequently when a broad band is present.

E. Surgical procedures, such as subgingival root planing, soft-tissue curettage, periodontal flap approaches, or gingivectomy, may produce localized recessions. Electrosurgery often is a direct cause and may even create pure mucogingival problems where none existed before that procedure. The extraction of an adjacent tooth, especially if tissue displacement extends to adjacent teeth, often is followed by localized recession on adjacent teeth. Often it is dramatic when the adjacent tooth had little attached gingiva. The dentist's skills in drawing such information from the patient's dental history are most important here.

F. Generalized root exposure may result not only from events similar to those already described but also from additional factors. Vigorous use of a toothbrush, especially stiffer ones, frequently results in generalized recession, which may be much more extensive on teeth with little attached gingiva (especially canines,

first premolars, and mandibular central incisors). Orthodontic banding and consequent changes in brushing technique may do the same. Most periodontal flap procedures and gingivectomy procedures produce some degree of root exposure with healing. Electrosurgery does the same. Generalized root exposure usually is seen following all pocket-elimination procedures. Repeated root planing and the modified Widman flap also usually result in root exposure. Long-term periodontitis, whether treated or untreated, often results in generalized root exposure as pocket formation progresses apically. The dentist's skill in eliciting these facts and placing them in chronologic sequence are important.

References

Gartrell JR, Mathews DP. Gingival recession: The condition, process and treatment. Dent Clin North Am 1976;20:199.

Gorman WJ. Prevalence and etiology of gingival recession. J Periodontol 1967;38:316.

Hall WB. Pure mucogingival problems. Berlin: Quintessence Publishing, 1984:29.

Moscow BS, Bressman E. Localized gingival recession: Etiology and treatment. Dent Radiogr Photogr 1965;38:3.

INDICATIONS FOR USE OF LABORATORY TESTS

Peter B. Raetzke

The proliferation of microbiologic, biochemical, and immunologic laboratory tests that began in the 1980s has created an increasing problem for practicing dentists. When such tests should be used and how they would influence treatment are subjects of controversy. Can the cost of the test be justified? Can information that would influence treatment be received sufficiently quickly as to be useful? The future of diagnostic laboratory testing seems promising; the present status of available tests is perplexing.

Traditional culturing techniques are too expensive and time consuming for routine use in practice. Dark-field microscopy often gives misleading results. Tests for the presence or activity of apparently significant bacteria such as *P. gingivalis, P. intermedius,* and *Actinobacillus actinomycetemcomitans* (Periogard, Perioscan, Oral B, Periodontal Pathogen) may be misleading. Strong positive readings have been obtained from clinically healthy individuals. Blood serum tests adapted for use with gingival crevice fluid samples may be used to identify enzymes associated with active tissue destruction such as asparate aminotransferase (AST) in an in-office test system (Periogard Periodontal Tissue Monitor, Colgate). It remains to be proven whether an elastase gingival crest fluid test (PrognoStik) to identify enzyme released during polymorphonuclear leukocyte is diagnostic. Many other systems are being developed and evaluated.

The algorithm illustrates certain cases in which commercially available testing may be helpful today.

A. A patient with severe periodontitis and a history suggestive of rapidly progressive periodontitis (RPP), as indicated by successive periods of acute breakdown, may be diagnosed by testing for elevated AST levels (confirming active destruction) and utilizing a pathogen test (certain plaque bacteria, or CPB) to help identify microorganisms involved. Such information is helpful in selecting an appropriate chemotherapeutic regimen and in monitoring the efficacy of treatment.

B. For a patient with a provisional diagnosis of adult periodontitis (AP) wherein initial treatment is followed by acute exacerbations, a similar testing regimen to that in A may elicit a revised diagnosis of RPP.

C. For a patient who has been diagnosed as having AP and is treated in the usual manner (i.e., initial therapy, possible surgery, and so forth) but who has localized recurrences, testing apparently "healthy" areas for AST and specific bacterial activity (CPB) may indicate the need for prompt or more frequent preventive treatment (possibly including chemotherapeutic agents).

D. Following treatment of any periodontitis case, diagnostic tests may be helpful in confirming that health has been achieved. Elevated AST levels may indicate ongoing destruction. Continued significant presence of certain bacterial populations may indicate that a patient is more vulnerable to recurrence of disease activity, necessitating intensified maintenance at more frequent intervals.

CAVEAT

None of the available tests provides definitive diagnostic information upon which treatment can be based. In no way do they replace routine diagnostic procedures in most cases. To date, no "new diagnostic test" can substitute for sound clinical judgment. Currently available tests can only complement the traditional diagnostic regimen.

References

Caton J. Periodontal diagnosis and diagnostic aids. In: Proceedings of the world workshop in clinical periodontics. Chicago: The American Academy of Periodontology, 1989:I1.

Chambers DA, et al. A longitudinal study of aspartate aminotransferase in human gingival crevicular fluid. J Periodont Res1991;26:65.

Curtis MA, et al. Detection of high-risk groups and individuals for periodontal diseases: Laboratory markers from analysis of gingival crevicular fluid. J Clin Periodontol 1989;16:1.

Gmur R, et al. Prevalence of *B. forsythus* and *B. gingivalis* in subgingival plaque of prosthodontally treated patients on short recall. J Periodont Res 1989;24:113.

Listgarten MA, et al. Incidence of periodontitis recurrence in treated patients with and without cultivable *A. actinomycetemcomitans, Prevotella intermedia,* and *Porphyromonas gingivalis:* A prospective study. J Periodontol 1991;62:377.

Muller RF, et al. Bestimmung der Elastase in menschlichen patrodontalen Taschenexsudat und ihre Bedeutung als Entzundungsparameter. Deutsche Zahnarztliche Zeitschrift 1986;41:32.

Omar AA, Newman HN. False results associated with dark-ground microscopy of subgingival plaque. J Clin Periodontol 1986;13:814.

Persson GR, et al. Relationship between gingival crevicular fluid levels of aspartate aminotransferase and active tissue destruction in treated chronic periodontitis patients. J Periodont Res 1990;25:81.

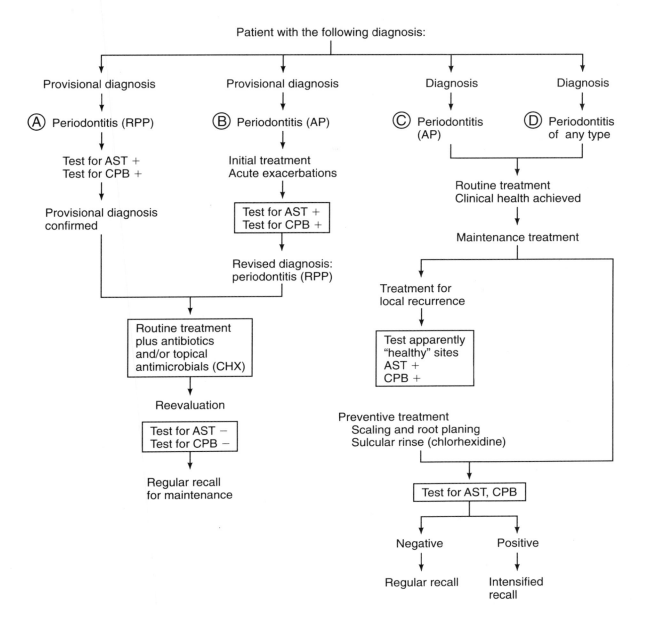

Patient with the following diagnosis:

| Provisional diagnosis | Provisional diagnosis | Diagnosis | Diagnosis |

(A) Periodontitis (RPP)

(B) Periodontitis (AP)

(C) Periodontitis (AP)

(D) Periodontitis of any type

Test for AST +
Test for CPB +

Provisional diagnosis
confirmed

Initial treatment
Acute exacerbations

Test for AST +
Test for CPB +

Revised diagnosis:
periodontitis (RPP)

Routine treatment
Clinical health achieved

Maintenance treatment

Routine treatment
plus antibiotics
and/or topical
antimicrobials (CHX)

Reevaluation

Test for AST −
Test for CPB −

Regular recall
for maintenance

Treatment for
local recurrence

Test apparently
"healthy" sites
AST +
CPB +

Preventive treatment
Scaling and root planing
Sulcular rinse (chlorhexidine)

Test for AST, CPB

Negative

Positive

Regular recall

Intensified
recall

PERIODONTAL HEALTH, GINGIVITIS, AND ADULT PERIODONTITIS

Walter B. Hall

A differential diagnosis among periodontal health, gingivitis, and periodontitis is begun by evaluating medical and dental histories (see pp 2 and 4). Older dental records and radiographs are especially helpful in establishing current disease activity as gingivitis or periodontitis.* Because these diseases are active in spurts, past findings are most helpful.

A. A visual examination usually follows history taking. The gingiva may be inflamed, in which case there will be marginal and papillary swelling and redness, or magenta coloring, or it may appear healthy, appearing pink, firm, and probably stippled. Such an appearance, however, may mask severe periodontitis. Gingiva that has become fibrotic as a result of frequent episodes of inflammation and healing may appear visibly healthy adjacent to deep pockets.

B. Probing should be performed regardless of the visual signs. When the gingiva appears visibly inflamed, probing usually reveals pockets with depths of 3 mm or more and bleeding. Pocket depth alone is insufficient to make a diagnosis between gingivitis and periodontitis. Swelling alone may create pockets of considerable depth that bleed upon probing.

C. A diagnosis of gingivitis can be made when redness and swelling are present without loss of attachment (LOA). If the probe reaches the root, LOA has occurred. When the gingiva is reddish and swollen, pocket depths are present, and LOA has occurred, a diagnosis of chronic adult periodontitis is most likely to be correct; however, when earlier LOA and new localized swelling and redness have occurred, creating pocket depths, gingivitis could be a correct diagnosis. Such situations often apply when patients are recalled following successful treatment. Recurrent inflammation may be present unless ideal oral hygiene efforts have been made by the patient.

D. When radiographs do not suggest active bone loss and pockets are of minimal depth, with evidence of swelling, gingivitis may be an acceptable diagnosis. Fortunately, in cases in which a decision is difficult to make, the differentiation may be more academic than practical, because treatment would be the same anyway.

E. For a diagnosis of chronic adult periodontitis to be made, three concurrent findings must exist. There must be pocket depth, LOA, and active bone loss. Radiographs can be helpful here; however, radiographs are susceptible to aberrations in film placement, machine-head angulation, exposure time, and kilovoltage used in taking the radiograph, and variability in developing technique. Radiographs alone, therefore, are never diagnostic; other findings must be considered. Fuzzy crestal bone may indicate active bone loss, but fuzziness can be created easily on radiographs from healthy patients, as already described. Series of radiographs taken at different times are more likely to yield a correct diagnosis; however, to be diagnostic, they should be taken and prepared in an identical manner. If inflammation, pocket depth, and LOA are present, and radiographs suggest active bone loss, periodontitis is most likely to be the correct diagnosis.

F. In cases with no visible signs of inflammation, periodontal health can be differentiated from chronic adult periodontitis on the basis of the absence of pocket depths greater than 3 mm. If the probe does not extend to the roots and radiographs indicate no bone loss, periodontal health is an appropriate diagnosis. Loss of attachment may result from earlier periodontitis, and radiographic evidence of bone loss may exist, but the combination of no pocket depth and no signs of inflammation suggests periodontal health. Without the visible signs of inflammation, gingivitis would not be a correct diagnosis in this case.

References

Carranza FA. Glickman's clinical periodontology. 7th ed. Philadelphia: WB Saunders, 1990:109.

Parr RW. Examination and diagnosis of periodontal disease. DHEW Publication No. (HRA) 74-36. Washington: US Department of Health, Education and Welfare, 1977.

Prichard JF. Advanced periodontal disease. 2nd ed. Philadelphia: WB Saunders, 1972:116.

World workshop in clinical periodontics. Chicago: American Academy of Periodontology 1989:I-23.

Worth HM. Radiology in diagnosis. Dent Clin North Am 1969;13:731.

---

*Periodontitis occurs in at least six subgroups: adult, prepubertal (mixed dentition), juvenile, rapidly progressive, necrotizing ulcerative periodontitis and human immunodeficiency virus periodontitis.

Patient needing DIFFERENT DIAGNOSIS AMONG PERIODONTAL HEALTH, GINGIVITIS, OR ADULT PERIODONTITIS

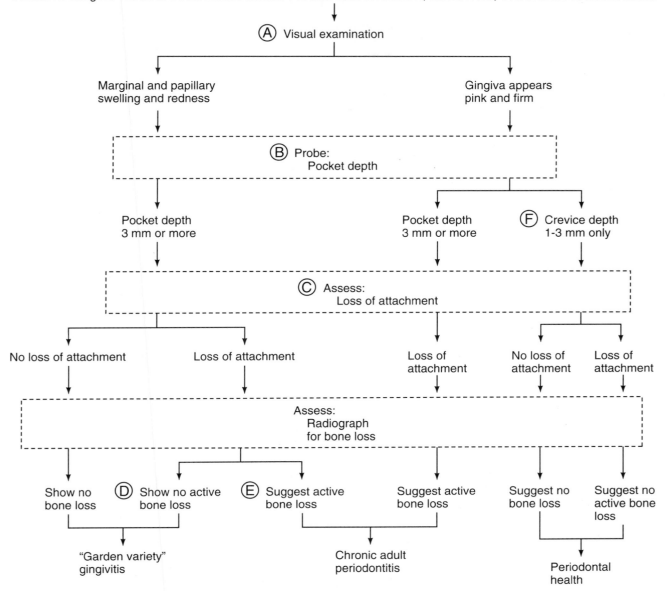

DIFFERENTIAL DIAGNOSIS OF JUVENILE PERIODONTITIS AND RAPIDLY PROGRESSIVE PERIODONTITIS

Francisco Martos Molino

Juvenile periodontitis and rapidly progressive periodontitis share certain common characteristics, such as highly active lesions in specific areas of the mouth and evidence of bone loss in radiographs (Fig. 1). Patients usually present with a family history of periodontitis, but juvenile periodontitis is found in young patients between 11 and 14 years old and affects more women than men. Rapidly progressive periodontitis is found in patients between 20 and 35 and most frequently in patients in their twenties.

A. In juvenile periodontitis, radiographs show bilateral and arch-shaped bone lesions (alveolar bone loss) in incisors and first molars.

B. In rapidly progressive periodontitis, radiographs show severe horizontal and vertical bone loss in most teeth.

C. In juvenile periodontitis, the gums look normal, the loss of periodontal attachment bears no correlation to local factors, and probe depths are 5 mm or more around the incisors and first molars.

In rapidly progressive periodontitis, the symptoms are more obvious during the active phase, with subgingival flora proliferations accompanied by general discomfort, fever, and weight loss. In the inactive phases, probe depths increase, and there is some gum bleeding.

In juvenile periodontitis, the lesions are very active immediately after puberty, although destruction may advance very slowly thereafter or even spontaneously cease altogether. In rapidly progressive periodontitis, the process is cyclic, with periods of exacerbated acute inflammation followed by dormant periods. Both may occur with or without prior history of gingivitis. Rapidly progressive periodontitis may occur spontaneously or after juvenile periodontitis.

D. The bacterial plaque in juvenile periodontitis is not visible; it contains an abundant proliferation of gram-negative species of bacteria, mainly of two types: *Capnocytophaga* and *Haemophilus (Actinobacillus actinomycetemcomitans)*. In rapidly progressive periodontitis, the presence of bacterial plaque can sometimes be seen under clinical observation; gingival bacteroids, however, are always present.

E. In most patients with rapidly progressive periodontitis, the polymorphonuclear leukocytes (PMNs) do not function efficiently (i.e., there is a functional defect in these patients' neutrophils or monocytes). The host response is disturbed by this type of periodontitis, because many patients have defects in their PMNs or monocytes. In patients with juvenile periodontitis, the gram-negative bacterial organisms present produce factors that inhibit the chemotaxis of the PMNs.

Various types of *A. actinomycetemcomitans* produce a leukotoxin that can destroy the PMNs and monocytes. The PMNs of these patients are less efficient in phagocytosis than those of patients with other types of periodontitis. The plasma cells of these

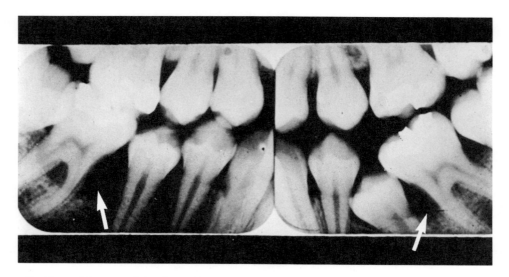

Figure 1. Deep, vertical bone defects mesial to first molars are typical of juvenile periodontitis.

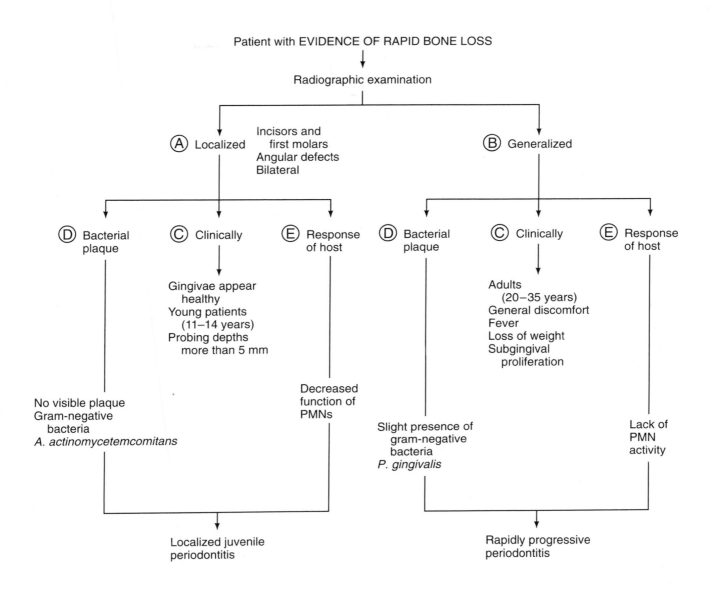

Patient with EVIDENCE OF RAPID BONE LOSS

↓

Radiographic examination

Ⓐ Localized — Incisors and first molars / Angular defects / Bilateral

Ⓑ Generalized

Localized:

Ⓓ Bacterial plaque

Ⓒ Clinically

Gingivae appear healthy
Young patients (11–14 years)
Probing depths more than 5 mm

Ⓔ Response of host

No visible plaque
Gram-negative bacteria
A. actinomycetemcomitans

Decreased function of PMNs

→ Localized juvenile periodontitis

Generalized:

Ⓓ Bacterial plaque

Ⓒ Clinically

Adults (20–35 years)
General discomfort
Fever
Loss of weight
Subgingival proliferation

Ⓔ Response of host

Slight presence of gram-negative bacteria
P. gingivalis

Lack of PMN activity

→ Rapidly progressive periodontitis

---

patients are unable to produce heavy immunoglobulin chains.

Histologically, in juvenile periodontitis, the inflammatory cells infiltrate the patient's connective tissue; 70% of the lesion volume is made up of plasma cells.

The lesions in both these diseases show a fast evolution, although their primary causes are different. The evolution or progression is episodic or cyclic in rapidly progressive periodontitis, whereas it can be very slow or even cease completely in juvenile periodontitis.

Both respond well to treatment by antibiotics after scaling and root planing. Tetracycline is used for juvenile periodontitis, whereas a combination of ampicillin and metronidazole is recommended for rapidly progressive periodontitis. A few patients, however, do not respond to such treatment, even when it is administered according to a correct schedule with correct follow-up.

References

Crawford A, Socransky SS, Bratthall G. Predominant cultivable microbiota of advanced periodontitis [abstract 209]. In: Program and abstracts of the AADR. New York, 1975.

Lavine WS, Page RC, Padgett GA. Host response in chronic periodontal disease. J Periodontol 1976;47:621.

McArthur WP, et al. Leukotoxic effects of *Actinobacillus actinomycetemcomitans*. J Periodont Res 1981;16:159.

Page RC, et al. Rapidly progressive periodontitis: A distinct clinical condition. J Periodontol 1983;54:1973.

Slots J. The predominant cultivable organisms in juvenile periodontitis. Scand J Dent Res 1976;84:1.

NECROTIZING ULCERATIVE GINGIVITIS AND PERIODONTITIS

Gerald J. DeGregori

Necrotizing ulcerative gingivitis is an acute gingival condition that involves primarily the interdental gingival tissues. The patient usually presents for treatment because of "sore and receding gums" (Figs. 1 and 2).

A. Intraoral examination may reveal a reddened gingival margin, the major involvement being the coronal one third of the interdental papilla. This portion of the papilla becomes necrotic and, with subsequent loss of the necrotic portion, assumes the characteristic cra-

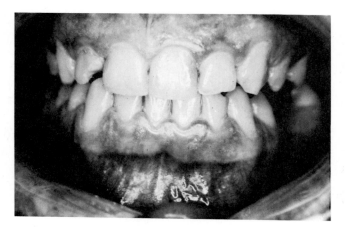

Figure 1. Early necrotizing ulcerative gingivitis.

tered or "punched out" appearance. The disease process may involve only one interdental papilla or all the interdental papillae or any variation thereof. In many cases, the patient's breath has a strong metallic odor.

B. Periodontal probing reveals an essentially intact periodontium, with some additional pocketing resulting from tissue edema. The diagnosis of necrotizing ulcerative gingivitis is based on the clinical appearance of the disease, as the presence of necrotic interdental gingiva or cratered interdental papilla is diagnostic of the disease. Should the disease process affect the underlying alveolar bone, periodontal pocketing will result from loss of attachment. Termed *necrotizing ulcerative periodontitis,* this disease is especially prevalent in areas of extreme root proximity.

C. Because of its similarity to several other acute oral conditions, a differential diagnosis must be made between necrotizing ulcerative gingivitis, acute herpetic gingivostomatitis, and aphthous stomatitis. The main diagnostic feature of necrotizing ulcerative gingivitis is the appearance of gingival necrosis and/or gingival cratering, a feature that is not present in the other acute oral condition mentioned above. Because of the appearance of acquired immunodeficiency syndrome in the last 5 years, recurrent severe cases of necrotizing ulcerative gingivitis should arouse the suspicion of a compromised immune system. Patients

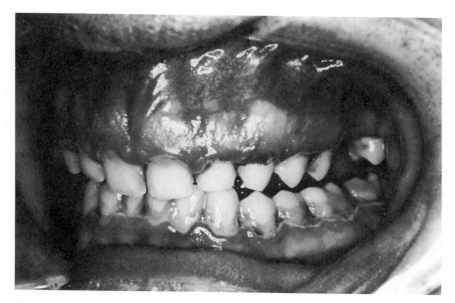

Figure 2. Severe necrotizing ulcerative gingivitis.

Patient with GENERALIZED MOUTH PAIN

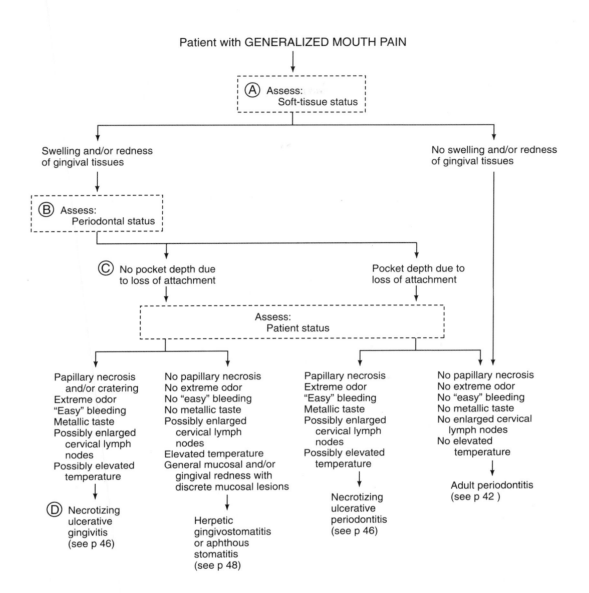

who require repeated treatment should have an immune system competency examination (see p 58).

D. The etiology of necrotizing ulcerative gingivitis is unknown. It is associated with a spirochete, *Borellia vincentii,* and a fusiform bacillus, *Bacillus fusiformis.* These bacteria, however, will not induce necrotizing ulcerative gingivitis if implanted into another mouth, be it laboratory animal or human subject. Stress also may be associated with this disease. When carefully questioned, patients invariably give a history of stress, such as a divorce proceeding, a difficult job, final examinations, or the use of recreational drugs. Research has shown that people susceptible to necrotizing ulcerative gingivitis have white blood cells with lessened chemotactic and phagocytic abilities. Necrotizing ulcerative gingivitis was first described by Plaut and Vincent in the late 1800s. It has been given various names over the years, most notably *trench mouth* because of its prevalence in World War I. It is not contagious, and the patient develops no circulating antibodies to the bacteria involved; thus, the patient may be cured of the disease, only to have it recur within a short period.

Differential diagnosis from HIV gingivitis and HIV periodontitis is discussed on p. 58.

References

Andriolo M, Wolf J, Rosenberg J. AIDS and AIDS-related complex: Oral manifestation and treatment. J Am Dent Assoc 1986;113:586.

Carranza FA, Jr. Glickman's clinical periodontology. 7th ed. Philadelphia: WB Saunders, 1990:149.

Grant D, Stern I, Everett F. Periodontics. 6th ed. St. Louis: CV Mosby, 1988:398.

Grupe HE, and Wilder LS. Observations of necrotizing ulcerative gingivitis in 870 military trainees. J Periodontol 1956;27:255.

Lindhe J. Clinical periodontology. Copenhagen: Munksgaard, 1989:221.

Shannon IL, Kilgore WG, O'Leary TJ. Stress as a predisposing factor in necrotizing ulcerative gingivitis. J Periodontol 1969;40:240.

PRIMARY ACUTE HERPETIC GINGIVOSTOMATITIS

Gerald J. DeGregori

Herpetic gingivostomatitis is an acute oral condition caused by the herpes simplex type I virus. It is contagious to persons who do not have circulating antibodies to the virus. Most adults have developed immunity to herpes simplex type I virus as a result of infection during childhood, which in most instances is subclinical. For this reason, acute herpetic gingivostomatitis is seen most often in infants and children. Recurrence is rare. It usually results from immune system compromise, such as occurs in cytotoxic chemotherapy or acquired immunodeficiency syndrome. Recurrence should prompt thorough medical evaluation of the patient's immune status.

A. The patient usually presents with a complaint of extreme intraoral soreness on chewing and swallowing and shows signs of general debilitation.

B. Intraorally the condition is characterized by multiple greyish-white vesicles that rupture in about 24 hours. Rarely, the patient presents in the vesicular state; rupture of the vesicles, which appear as greyish-white, crater-like lesions surrounded by a red halo (Fig. 1), precipitates the appointment. The lesions may occur anywhere in the oral cavity, including the lips (Fig. 2). The discrete ulcerations are very sore to touch and the pressure of food or the tongue. Differential diagnoses include acute necrotizing ulcerative gingivitis (see p 46) and aphthous stomatitis.

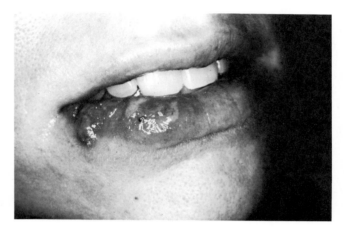

Figure 2. Lip lesion; acute primary herpetic gingivostomatitis.

C. The lesions characteristically remain for 7 to 10 days, and often last for 14 days. During that time, the patient must be encouraged to ingest adequate nourishment despite the intraoral discomfort. Liquid nutritional supplements, "instant breakfast"–type products mixed with milk or ice cream, ensure adequate caloric and liquid intake during the course of the disease. A mixture of 50% Kaopectate and 50% elixir of Benadryl may be used as a mouthwash before meals. It should be swished in the mouth for a period of 2 minutes and then swallowed. Reassuring the patient about the limited course of the disease is important for compliance with this regimen as well as for uneventful recovery. Further, patients should be admonished to observe meticulous hygiene to prevent the spread of the virus to other persons and to other parts of the body, especially the eyes. Recently, Acyclovir has been used in the treatment of severe cases.

References

Carranza FA Jr. Glickman's clinical periodontology. 7th ed. Philadelphia: WB Saunders, 1990:159–162.

Grant D, Stern I, Everett F. Periodontics. 6th ed. St. Louis: CV Mosby, 1988:413.

Lindhe J. Clinical periodontology. 2nd ed. Copenhagen: Munksgaard, 1989:282.

Rateitschak KH, Rateitschak EM, Wolf HF, Hassell JM. Color atlas of periodontology. 1st ed. Stuttgart: Georg Thieme Verlag, 1985:54.

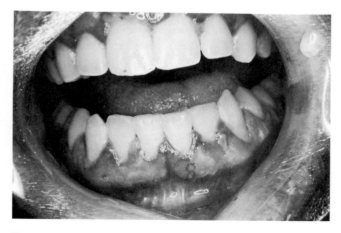

Figure 1. Gingival lesions; acute primary herpetic gingivostomatitis.

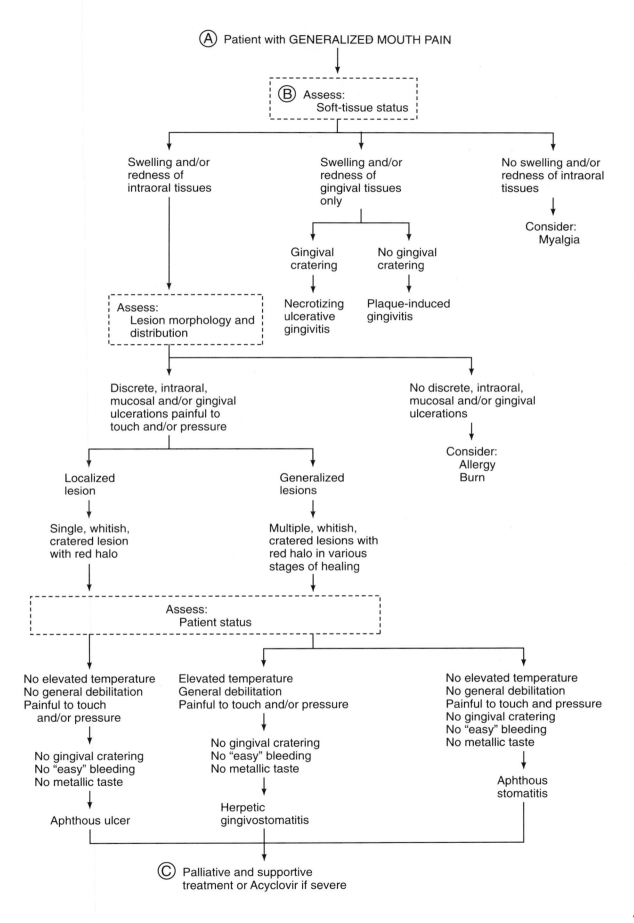

(A) Patient with GENERALIZED MOUTH PAIN

(B) Assess:
Soft-tissue status

Swelling and/or redness of intraoral tissues

Swelling and/or redness of gingival tissues only

No swelling and/or redness of intraoral tissues

Consider: Myalgia

Gingival cratering

No gingival cratering

Necrotizing ulcerative gingivitis

Plaque-induced gingivitis

Assess:
Lesion morphology and distribution

Discrete, intraoral, mucosal and/or gingival ulcerations painful to touch and/or pressure

No discrete, intraoral, mucosal and/or gingival ulcerations

Consider:
Allergy
Burn

Localized lesion

Generalized lesions

Single, whitish, cratered lesion with red halo

Multiple, whitish, cratered lesions with red halo in various stages of healing

Assess:
Patient status

No elevated temperature
No general debilitation
Painful to touch and/or pressure

Elevated temperature
General debilitation
Painful to touch and/or pressure

No elevated temperature
No general debilitation
Painful to touch and pressure
No gingival cratering
No "easy" bleeding
No metallic taste

No gingival cratering
No "easy" bleeding
No metallic taste

No gingival cratering
No "easy" bleeding
No metallic taste

Aphthous stomatitis

Aphthous ulcer

Herpetic gingivostomatitis

(C) Palliative and supportive treatment or Acyclovir if severe

PRIMARY VERSUS SECONDARY OCCLUSAL TRAUMA

Walter B. Hall

Two general types of occlusal trauma must be distinguished before treatment planning. Primary occlusal trauma is diagnosed when a tooth or teeth with "normal" support are overloaded, producing symptoms of looseness or discomfort. Secondary occlusal trauma is diagnosed when a tooth or teeth that have lost support develop symptoms of looseness or discomfort when overloaded or loaded normally (i.e., a load that would not produce symptoms if normal support were present). The treatment differs depending upon the type of occlusal trauma that is diagnosed.

A. Several signs and symptoms are indicative of occlusal trauma. Prime among these is tooth looseness. Others include symptoms of vague to severe pain, especially when faceting of occlusal surfaces is present and muscles of mastication are sensitive to digital manipulation. Generalized tooth sensitivity often relates to clenching and grinding habits (bruxism). Faceting is indicative of hyperfunction; however, once a facet has developed, it remains even if one of the antagonistic teeth is lost.

B. The key means of differentiating between primary and secondary occlusal trauma is determining whether bone loss has occurred (secondary) or not (primary). When root exposure is evident visually, bone loss has occurred. When probing extends to the roots of affected teeth, bone loss has occurred. Radiographically, evidence of bone loss is more speculative unless it is quite advanced, because variations in angulation, development time, kilovoltage, and so on may give misleading impressions of bone loss or its absence. If bone loss has occurred around involved teeth, the correct diagnosis would be secondary occlusal trauma.

C. Other clinical findings at the time of examination may be helpful in the differential diagnosis. If the patient has, or has had, moderate-to-severe periodontitis or is aware of a clenching and grinding habit (bruxism), secondary occlusal trauma is the more likely diagnosis.

D. If a "high" restoration (particularly a new one) is present, a periapical abscess is diagnosed, or the patient admits to a habit such as nail biting or pipe-stem clenching, primary occlusal trauma is the more likely diagnosis.

E. Both types of occlusal trauma may be localized or generalized. Primary occlusal trauma is more likely to be localized; whereas, secondary occlusal trauma is more likely to be generalized. Localized problems can be treated with minimal effort (e.g., selective grinding, splinting). Generalized, moderate-to-severe, secondary occlusal trauma might benefit by occlusal correction, but a bite guard or extensive splinting may be necessary.

References

Carranza FA Jr. Gleckman's clinical periodontology. 7th ed. Philadelphia: WB Saunders, 1990:266.

Genco RJ, Goldman HM, Cohen DW. Contemporary periodontics. St. Louis: CV Mosby, 1990:195.

Grant DA, Stern IB, Listgarten MA. Periodontics. St. Louis: CV Mosby, 1988:500.

Schluger S, Yuodelis R, Page RC, Johnson RH. Periodontal diseases. 2nd ed. Philadelphia: Lea & Febiger, 1990:125.

World workshop in clinical periodontics. Chicago: American Academy of Periodontology, 1989:III-15.

Patient with PRIMARY AND/OR SECONDARY OCCLUSAL TRAUMA

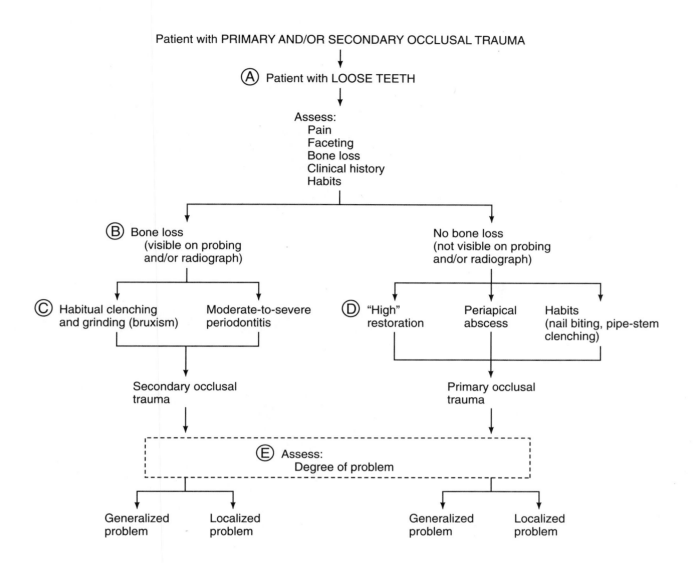

GINGIVAL ENLARGEMENT DIAGNOSIS

William P. Lundergan

Gingival enlargements are a common feature of inflammatory periodontal disease. These enlargements can also represent an endodontic problem, a response either to a medication or to a genetic factor, or a neoplasia. A differential diagnosis requires thorough medical and dental histories, a careful evaluation of the nature of the enlargement (inflammatory vs. fibrotic), and an identification of the etiologic factors. Occasionally, a biopsy may be required to confirm a diagnosis.

A. Inflammatory gingival enlargements are characterized by swelling or edema, redness, and a tendency to bleed with periodontal probing. Long-standing inflammatory enlargements can have a fibrotic component as well. A patient history will help establish the inflammatory enlargement as acute or chronic. Chronic enlargements are generally painless and slow to progress, whereas acute enlargements are characterized by a painful, rapid onset.

B. A localized gingival swelling characterized by acute pain with rapid onset suggests an abscess. One should probe involved teeth for periodontal pocket formation and loss of attachment (LOA). Radiographic evaluation and pulp testing should accompany the periodontal examination. If no pocket formation with LOA is detected, and the tooth is vital, treat the problem as a gingival abscess. If pocket formation with LOA is detected, and the tooth is vital, treat the problem as a periodontal abscess. If the tooth is nonvital, or partially nonvital, an endodontic problem exists. Endodontic therapy is indicated if warranted by the periodontal prognosis and overall treatment plan.

C. A localized or generalized gingival enlargement that is relatively painless and gradual to develop may be classified as a chronic inflammatory gingival enlargement. Chronic inflammatory gingival enlargements

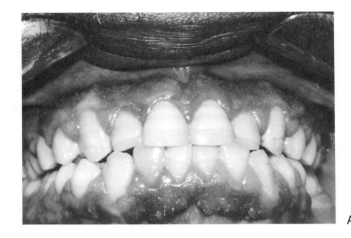

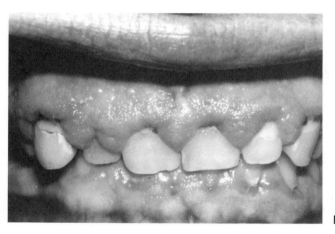

Figure 2. A, Gingival enlargement related to taking Dilantin Sodium. **B**, Gingival enlargement related to taking cyclosporin. Clinically these two gingival enlargements cannot be differentiated. The patient's history permits the diagnosis.

are generally associated with identifiable systemic or local factors. The primary local factor associated with these enlargements is plaque. Secondary local factors can include calculus, poor dental restorations, caries, tooth crowding or misalignment, open contacts with food impaction, orthodontic braces, mouth breathing, and removable appliances. Systemic factors include vitamin C deficiency, leukemia, and the hormonal changes that occur during pregnancy or puberty, or are associated with the use of oral contraceptives. If no local or systemic factors can be identified, the enlargement may be neoplastic, and one should consider a biopsy to establish or confirm a diagnosis.

D. A gingival enlargement that is both inflammatory and fibrotic can represent an enlargement that was initially fibrotic with secondary inflammation, or an enlarge-

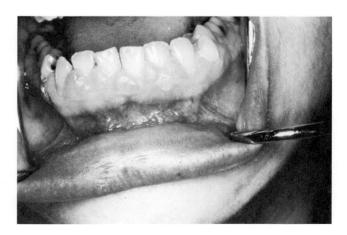

Figure 1. Dilantin sodium hyperplastia.

Patient with GINGIVAL ENLARGEMENT

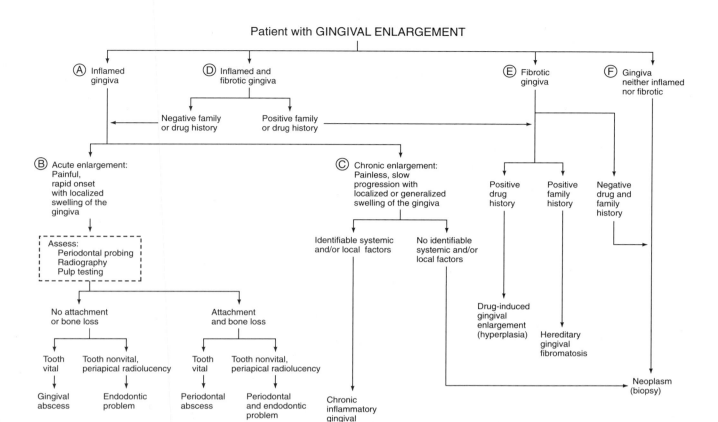

ment that was initially inflammatory but has become secondarily fibrotic. Medical and dental histories should suggest or rule out hereditary and drug-induced fibrotic enlargements. If the family and drug history are negative, the clinician can assume that the enlargement is inflammatory.

E. Fibrotic gingival enlargements are characterized by pink, firm, and lobulated gingivae; however, secondary inflammation can result in a reddish coloration and an increased tendency to bleed. A definitive diagnosis can generally be established with thorough medical and dental histories. Drug-induced gingival enlargements (Figs. 1 and 2) have been associated with phenytoin (Dilantin), cyclosporine (Sandimmune), and nifedipine (Procardia, Adalat). The occurrence of gingival enlargements in association with nifedipine is rare (probably less than 2%). The incidence associated with phenytoin and cyclosporine is much higher (up to 50%). There is evidence that concurrent administration of nifedipine and cyclosporine does have a synergistic effect on the incidence of gingival enlargement. A diagnosis of drug-induced gingival enlargement can be made if the development of the fibrotic enlargement coincided with the administration of one of these medications and the family

history is negative for hereditary gingival fibromatosis. A rare fibrotic gingival enlargement of unknown etiology is hereditary gingival fibromatosis. The diagnosis is suggested by a positive family history of gingival enlargement, which generally begins with the eruption of the primary or permanent dentition. A fibrotic gingival enlargement that does not seem to be drug-induced or familial may be either neoplastic or an inflammatory enlargement that is secondarily fibrotic. If a definitive diagnosis cannot be established from the patient history and clinical examination, a biopsy may be required.

F. An enlarged gingiva that is neither inflammatory nor fibrotic, and does not have identifiable systemic or local etiologic factors, may represent a neoplasm. A biopsy with microscopic evaluation is needed to establish or confirm a diagnosis.

References

Carranza FA Jr. Glickman's clinical periodontology. 6th ed. Philadelphia: WB Saunders, 1984:125–147.
Lundergan WP. Drug-induced gingival enlargements — dilantin hyperplasia and beyond. J Calif Dent Assoc 1989; 17:48.

PURE MUCOGINGIVAL VERSUS MUCOGINGIVAL–OSSEOUS PROBLEMS

Walter B. Hall

Mucogingival problems, which involve the relationships of alveolar mucosa and gingiva, have been divided into pure mucogingival problems and mucogingival–osseous problems. Pure mucogingival problems are those caused by a tooth's erupting in prominence at or near the mucogingival junction so that little or no attached gingiva is present over the prominence of the fully erupted tooth. These problems may be existing ones, where recession has already occurred, or potential ones, where they are predisposed to recession only. Mucogingival–osseous problems are those that are caused by pockets so deepened with periodontitis that little or no attached gingiva remains. Because these problems are of different etiologies, their treatments are different; therefore, properly differentiating between them diagnostically is most important.

A. Determine and record the position of the free margin of the gingiva for all teeth. If the free margin is on the crown of the tooth, no visible recession has occurred, as yet. If the free margin is on the root of the tooth, recession has occurred already. In probing where the free margin is on the crown, the probe may reach only to the cementoenamel junction (CEJ) or may extend to the root surface, in which case loss of attachment has occurred already.

B. Determine and record the location of the mucogingival junction on all facial surfaces and on the lingual surface of mandibular teeth. The distance from the free margin of the gingiva to the mucogingival junction is a measure of the total amount of gingiva on the surface of a tooth. If there is 2 mm or less of total gingiva on a surface, a pure mucogingival problem or a potential one is present, whether the free margin of the gingiva is on the crown or the root of the tooth, because there is always a crevice of at least 1 mm. If more than 2 mm of total gingiva is present, a differential diagnosis cannot be made.

C. For those cases in which more than 2 mm of total gingiva is present, measure pocket depth to differentiate further between pure mucogingival and mucogingival–osseous problems. If the crevice depth is less than 3 mm, arbitrarily (but with reasonable accuracy) diagnose the problem as an existing or potential pure mucogingival problem and treat as such (see p 104). If the pocket depth is 3 mm or greater, diagnose the problem as an inflammatory one and treat it as a mucogingival–osseous problem (see p 78). If more than 2 mm of total gingiva and more than 1 mm of attached gingiva are present and the free margin is still on the crown, the problem is not a mucogingival problem of either type.

Reference

Hall WB. Pure mucogingival problems. Berlin: Quintessence Publishing, 1984:61.

Patient with PURE MUCOGINGIVAL OR MUCOGINGIVAL–OSSEOUS PROBLEMS

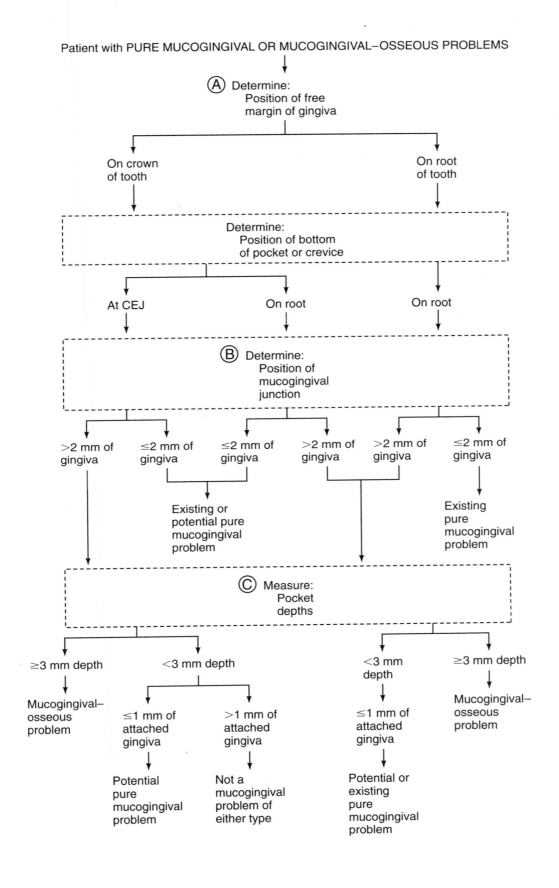

PROBLEMS OF ENDODONTIC AND PERIODONTAL ETIOLOGY

Gerald J. DeGregori

The diagnosis of endodontic problems manifesting as periodontal problems and periodontal problems manifesting as endodontic problems is a clinically demanding discipline. To make a correct diagnosis, clinicians must call upon their entire body of knowledge. Because of the complexity and amount of information necessary to differentiate between endodontic and periodontal etiology, orderly information gathering is essential. One of the most common motivations for patients to seek dental treatment is pain. Inflammatory periodontal disease is seldom symptomatic. Exceptions to this are gingival abscess, periodontal abscess, and necrotizing ulcerative gingivitis, which are the usual causes of soft-tissue pain.

A. Question the patient concerning the presence or absence of tooth pain. If pain is present, locate the area and take a radiograph. If the patient has a history of pain that has since ceased, consider irreversible pulpitis that has progressed to necrosis.

B. Radiographic interpretation may give important diagnostic information concerning the pulpal and periodontal status of the tooth. Evaluate the radiograph for indication of the restorative status of the tooth. If the tooth has a large restoration that could contribute to pulpal degeneration, determine the depth of the base beneath the restoration and possible exposure of a pulp horn. With the advent of improved crown and bridge procedures, more and more teeth are being used as fixed bridgework abutments. Teeth that have been endodontically treated and that contain either a post as part of the tooth reinforcement or have no post present but have lost a great deal of supporting tooth structure to the endodontic treatment should be especially suspect for cracked tooth syndrome (see p 64). Radiographic evaluation of pulp chamber morphology may also give clues to the pulpal status of the tooth. A sclerotic pulp chamber or the presence of pulpal stones in a virgin tooth indicates that the tooth has been subjected to heavy occlusal forces (bruxism/clenching) over a long period. Often, as the secondary dentin or pulp stones are being deposited, the pulpal tissues are strangulated; a resultant abscess may be manifested in the periapical region of the tooth via the main canal or in the furcation area through an auxiliary canal from the pulp chamber into the furcation area. Should the abscess fistulate into the oral cavity through the gingival sulcus, it would be easy to misinterpret the furcation invasion as being periodontal rather than endodontic in origin.

C. Assess periodontal status by periodontal problem. In the examination of the periodontal pocket, consider the case of a periapical lesion present on the mesial or distal root of a maxillary molar tooth that has fistulated out through the gingival sulcus with resultant bone loss and periodontal pocket formation. This situation is especially likely in areas of extreme root proximity. In single-rooted teeth with deep, narrow periodontal pockets, especially on the buccal or lingual of the tooth in a mouth essentially free of periodontal disease, always suspect an endodontic–periodontal involvement. The periodontal pocket may be the manifestation of a fistulous tract from the periapical area. Should the single-rooted tooth be treated endodontically and/or have a large post, the deep periodontal pocket may be the result of root fracture or perforation.

D. Determine pulpal status by a series of tests. First, percuss the tooth in the vertical axis. A positive response by the patient may indicate a periapical abscess. Percussion in the horizontal axis may indicate cracked tooth syndrome (see p 64), in which lateral forces displace the fractured parts, resulting in pain. Second, the application of hot (warm gutta-percha) and cold (ice) stimuli may also indicate pulpal status. Cold sensitivity that does not linger after removal of the cold stimulus indicates reversible pulpitis. Hot and cold sensitivity that lingers after removal of the stimulus indicates irreversible pulpitis. Third, one must be cautious with regard to the interpretation of vitality test results, as a vitalometer reading cannot determine the degree of vitality. In multirooted teeth, the offending root may be nonvital but the vitalometer may give a "normal" response from other roots, thus confusing the operator. Necrotic material within the pulp chamber also is capable of conducting an electrical impulse, resulting in a false "positive" reading. Therefore, vitality readings must be considered along with all other pulpal evaluation tests before a decision is made concerning pulpal status.

E. Prognosis of endodontically and periodontally involved teeth varies with each clinical manifestation. The prognosis of a furcation-involved molar tooth from inflammatory periodontal disease is variable. The prognosis of a furcation-involved molar tooth of endodontic etiology depends on whether the osseous lesion is in communication with the oral cavity. If it cannot be probed, endodontic treatment of the tooth should result in complete resolution of the osseous lesion. If the lesion can be probed, osseous resolution following endodontic therapy cannot be predicted. The tooth with a long-standing lesion nas a poorer prognosis than one with a lesion present for less than 6 months.

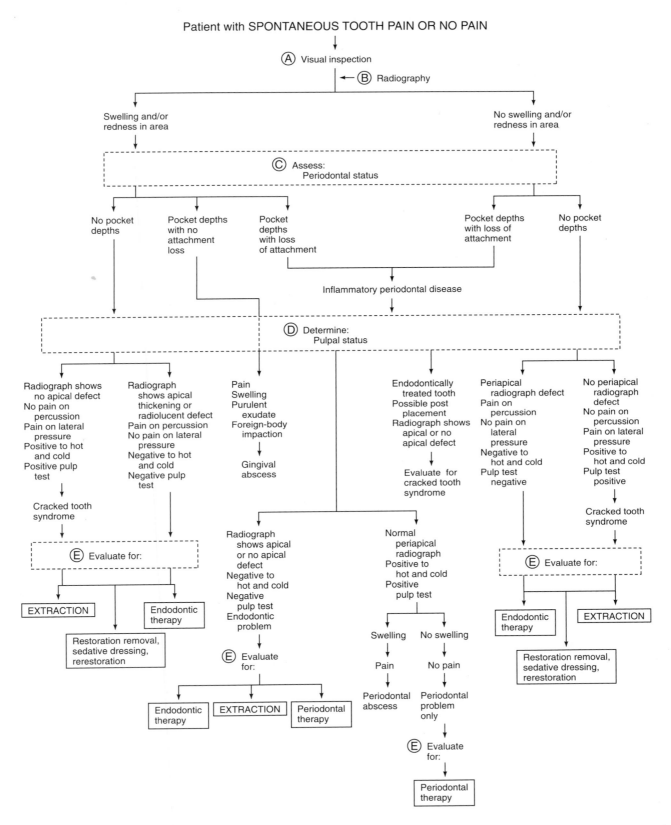

Patient with SPONTANEOUS TOOTH PAIN OR NO PAIN

A. Visual inspection

B. Radiography

Swelling and/or redness in area

No swelling and/or redness in area

C. Assess: Periodontal status

No pocket depths

Pocket depths with no attachment loss

Pocket depths with loss of attachment

Pocket depths with loss of attachment

No pocket depths

Inflammatory periodontal disease

D. Determine: Pulpal status

Radiograph shows no apical defect
No pain on percussion
Pain on lateral pressure
Positive to hot and cold
Positive pulp test

Radiograph shows apical thickening or radiolucent defect
Pain on percussion
No pain on lateral pressure
Negative to hot and cold
Negative pulp test

Pain
Swelling
Purulent exudate
Foreign-body impaction

Gingival abscess

Endodontically treated tooth
Possible post placement
Radiograph shows apical or no apical defect

Evaluate for cracked tooth syndrome

Periapical radiograph defect
Pain on percussion
No pain on lateral pressure
Negative to hot and cold
Pulp test negative

No periapical radiograph defect
No pain on percussion
Pain on lateral pressure
Positive to hot and cold
Pulp test positive

Cracked tooth syndrome

Cracked tooth syndrome

E. Evaluate for:

EXTRACTION

Endodontic therapy

Restoration removal, sedative dressing, rerestoration

Radiograph shows apical or no apical defect
Negative to hot and cold
Negative pulp test
Endodontic problem

E. Evaluate for:

Endodontic therapy

EXTRACTION

Periodontal therapy

Normal periapical radiograph
Positive to hot and cold
Positive pulp test

Swelling

No swelling

Pain

No pain

Periodontal abscess

Periodontal problem only

E. Evaluate for:

Periodontal therapy

E. Evaluate for:

Endodontic therapy

EXTRACTION

Restoration removal, sedative dressing, rerestoration

References

Carranza FA Jr. Glickman's clinical periodontology. 7th ed. Philadelphia: WB Saunders, 1990:870.

Genco RS, Goldman HM, Cohen DW. Contemporary periodontics. St. Louis: CV Mosby, 1990:605.

Luebke G. Vertical crown-root fractures in posterior teeth. Dent Clin North Am 1984;28(4):883.

ACQUIRED IMMUNODEFICIENCY SYNDROME–RELATED PERIODONTITIS

James R. Winkler

Typically, periodontal diseases progress over an extended period with little or no pain and discomfort to the patient. Pain or rapidly appearing signs and symptoms involving the periodontal tissues are conditions that usually require immediate attention. Periodontal lesions that cause generalized pain are rare and include necrotizing ulcerative gingivitis (NUG), herpetic gingivostomatitis, and the recently described lesions associated with acquired immunodeficiency syndrome (AIDS) (Fig. 1). The differential diagnosis between these lesions is not always distinct. The importance of correct diagnosis is based on the need to determine appropriate therapy and to determine whether the disease is self-limiting. Swelling or redness of the papillae and gingival margin is seen in all of these lesions. With NUG, the lesions primarily affect the papillary regions but frequently involve the free gingival margins as well. In the case of herpetic gingivostomatitis, AIDS-related periodontitis, and AIDS-related gingivitis, the redness or swelling is not restricted to the papillae and free margins but can also involve the attached and unattached mucosa.

A. The recent description of a rapidly progressive and severe periodontal lesion associated with infection by the human immunodeficiency virus (HIV) has made it necessary to determine whether or not the disease being observed is related to such infection. Most acute periodontal lesions are self-limiting and respond to conventional therapy. Those associated with HIV infection often do not respond and can cause rapidly progressive periodontal disease. Patients without known relationship to identified risk groups (intravenous drug users, hemophiliacs, blood recipients, homosexuals, and bisexuals) present a challenging differential diagnosis. Difficulty may exist in determining whether an individual has been exposed to HIV infection. A history of exposure to the virus may have important ramifications in determining the treatment, progression, and outcome of periodontal lesions. Often the clinician cannot diagnose HIV infection conclusively based on rapidly progressive periodontal lesions or other intraoral pathologies, such as hairy leukoplakia and candidiasis; however, these findings may be signs of potential infection and are useful in selecting appropriate therapy.

B. Herpetic gingivostomatitis usually is easy to differentiate from typical gingivitis or atypical gingivitis, because it is accompanied by spiking temperature changes, sweating, and malaise along with multiple, tiny, round ulcerations of the oral tissues. It is far more common among children and teenagers, although any age group may be affected.

C. When no tiny ulcerations and little plaque are present, but marginal redness accompanied by multiple petechiae, even in the attached gingiva, and other intraoral signs, such as candidiasis, are present, no response to debridement is likely to occur. One should suspect HIV-associated gingivitis. Evaluate the patient's seropositive status to support the diagnosis.

D. These signs and symptoms may accompany NUG or HIV-associated periodontitis. Necrotizing ulcerative gingivitis most often is seen among teenagers and young adults and may be accompanied by a distinctive foul odor to the breath, a metallic taste in the mouth, a raised temperature, and a general feeling of malaise. The lesions usually are self-limiting and respond promptly to localized debridement, scaling, and root planing and/or antibiotic therapy (usually penicillin). If the disease has occurred only once, its response to this therapy confirms the diagnosis. If the attacks are repetitive over months or years, loss of attachment may occur, making the differential diagnosis more difficult. In severe cases, however, antibiotics are recommended. Metronidazole (250 mg four times a day for 4 days) is the drug of choice. Care should be exercised in individuals with liver disease, and patients should be advised to avoid the use of alcohol while taking this drug. Other antibiotics can be considered on a case-by-case basis. Ideally, the patient's physician should be consulted when antibiotics are used.

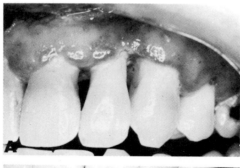

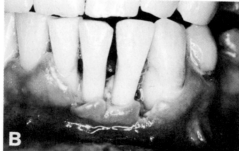

Figure 1. HIV-related periodontitis. **A,** Notice the similarity of necrotic interdental papillae to those seen in necrotizing ulcerative gingivitis (see p 46). **B,** Severe lesions with exposed necrotic bone and "detached" gingiva (courtesy of Cynthia Williams, Dharan, Saudi Arabia).

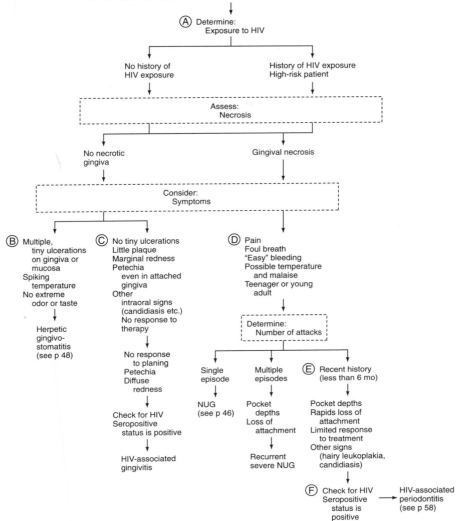

Patient with GINGIVAL REDNESS, SWELLING, AND PAIN

(A) Determine:
Exposure to HIV

No history of HIV exposure

History of HIV exposure
High-risk patient

Assess:
Necrosis

No necrotic gingiva

Gingival necrosis

Consider:
Symptoms

(B) Multiple, tiny ulcerations on gingiva or mucosa
Spiking temperature
No extreme odor or taste

Herpetic gingivo-stomatitis
(see p 48)

(C) No tiny ulcerations
Little plaque
Marginal redness
Petechia even in attached gingiva
Other intraoral signs (candidiasis etc.)
No response to therapy

No response to planing
Petechia
Diffuse redness

Check for HIV Seropositive status is positive

HIV-associated gingivitis

(D) Pain
Foul breath
"Easy" bleeding
Possible temperature and malaise
Teenager or young adult

Determine:
Number of attacks

Single episode

NUG
(see p 46)

Multiple episodes

Pocket depths
Loss of attachment

Recurrent severe NUG

(E) Recent history (less than 6 mo)

Pocket depths
Rapids loss of attachment
Limited response to treatment
Other signs (hairy leukoplakia, candidiasis)

(F) Check for HIV Seropositive status is positive → HIV-associated periodontitis (see p 58)

E. If the patient has a recent history (less than 6 mo) of necrotic gingiva with rapid loss of attachment, a key finding, HIV-associated periodontitis should be suspected. The inflammation in such cases involves both free and attached gingiva. The pain associated with this lesion often is not restricted to the soft tissue but radiates to alveolar and even jaw bone. Some patients report the sensation that their teeth feel as if they hit against the bone on chewing. Some may report waking up with blood on their pillows or blood clots in their mouths. Bare bone may be seen. Other AIDS-related findings, such as hairy leukoplakia or candidiasis, often may be seen. Minimal response to debridement, scaling, and root planing is likely to occur. Indiscriminate use of antibiotics is contraindicated because of the risk of superinfection with *Candida albicans*. Localized adjunctive treatment with Betadine intrasulcular lavage along with debridement may be effective; however, long-term maintenance seems to be difficult without the use of Peridex (chlorhexidine).

F. The rapid rate of attachment loss and lack of response to conventional therapy are the most distinguishing features in the differential diagnosis of this lesion. The HIV seropositive status of the patient should be determined to support the diagnosis.

References

Greenspan JS, Greenspan D, Pindborg JJ, Schiodt M. AIDS and the dental team. Copenhagen: Munksgaard, 1986:8.

Johnson BD, Engle D. Acute necrotizing gingivitis—a review of diagnosis, etiology and treatment. J Periodontal 1986;57:141.

Sabiston CB Jr. A review and proposal for the etiology of acute necrotizing gingivitis. J Clin Periodontal 1986;13:727.

Schiodt M, Pindborg JJ. AIDS and the oral cavity—epidemiology and clinical manifestations of human deficiency virus infection: A review. Int J Oral Maxillofac Surg 1987;16:1.

Winkler JR, Murray PA. Periodontal disease—a potential intraoral expression of AIDS may be rapidly progressive periodontitis. Can Dent Assoc J 1987:15.

PERIODONTAL DISEASES IN DRUG USERS

Miguel Carasol

Periodontal diseases are common in patients addicted to drugs. Typical forms of disease like gingivitis, necrotizing ulcerative gingivitis and periodontitis (NUG/NUP), adult periodontitis, or rapidly progressive periodontitis can be observed, but in many cases, they are diagnosed in advanced stages and are associated with a lot of decayed or missing teeth and a poor oral condition. Moreover, the analgesic effect of these drugs can mask pain derived from caries or periodontal disease. In many cases, extraction is the only solution that dentists can offer. Extraction is one of the most frequent modalities of treatment that this group of patients demands. Toxic effects of drugs on periodontal tissues can lead to particular forms of periodontal diseases; this is the case with cocaine addicts who rub their gingiva with this drug. Finally, the incidence of human immuno-deficiency virus (HIV) infection in intravenous drug users is very high, and specific forms of periodontal disease, like HIV gingivitis and HIV periodontitis, can be found in these patients. A careful medical history and an objective oral interview are recommended for recognizing this problem. Management of drug users can be complicated because of socioeconomic status and irregular habits of these patients. Dental problems have a very low priority for drug addicts, and oral hygiene is frequently neglected by them, so it is very difficult to organize regular appointments, and oral hygiene instructions can be ineffective. Toxicity of drugs must be considered during periodontal treatment. Many organs, like liver, heart, central nervous system, or bone marrow, can be affected, so the dentist has to keep in mind the possibility of an acute hemorrhagic episode, increased anesthetic problems, postoperative infection, and delayed wound healing. Bacterial endocarditis is a potential risk for any intravenous drug abuser, so recommending antibiotic prophylaxis must be considered in any case. Obviously, a strong potential exists for transmission of the hepatitis and acquired immunodeficiency syndrome (AIDS) viruses to the dental team, so infection-control measures are mandatory when handling these patients.

A. Suspect HIV gingivitis in any intravenous drug abuser with bleeding and punctate or diffuse erythema of gingiva and/or alveolar mucosa, especially if it does not respond to conventional therapy or if it is associated with other oral lesions like candidiasis, hairy leukoplakia, and so forth. Human immunodeficiency virus infection is very common in intravenous drug abusers, and serologic study must be completed for diagnosing retrovirus infection.

B. Rubbing cocaine on gingiva is a common procedure in addicts to this drug in order to avoid complications to the nasal mucosa derived from "snorting" the drug. Epithelial and connective necrosis are histologic findings of these lesions, which clinically are very similar to those found in "aspirin burn."

C. Those persons with manic "highs" during cocaine use tend to brush their teeth and gingiva very vigorously, so cervical tooth abrasions and gingival lacerations of these sites are very common. If gingival recession is caused by rubbing cocaine, periodontal treatment with free gingival grafts must be evaluated carefully. Vasoconstriction and vascular damage of gingival connective vessels produced by cocaine can compromise vascularization of gingival graft during healing, so failure of this technique should be considered.

D. Drug addiction should be suspected in any young patient with atypical forms of NUG/NUP. Cocaine users who rub the drug on their gingiva are especially prone to this condition. Necrotic lesions are localized in areas where the drug is applied, and clinical findings include papillary necrosis and/or cratering, which is associated with bone sequestration in some cases. Gingival recession can be observed in those areas. Radiographic findings include interproximal bone loss, but in molars, furcation bone tends to be conserved. Pain, which is one of the cardinal symptoms of NUG/NUP, can be masked in these lesions, probably owing to the anesthetic effect of cocaine.

E. In patients with a history of painful and necrotic lesions in gingiva and rapid and severe loss of attachment, associated to risk factors for AIDS such as drug addiction, suspect HIV periodontitis. To confirm the diagnosis of HIV infection, determine the AIDS seropositive status of the patient. Diagnostic criteria and management of these lesions are discussed in another section of this text (see p 58).

References

Barone R, Ficarra G, Gaglioti D, et al. Prevalence of oral lesions among HIV-infected intravenous drug users and other risk groups. Oral Surg Oral Med Oral Pathol 1990;69:169.

Cook H, Peoples J, Paden M. Management of the oral surgery patient addicted to heroin. J Oral Maxillofac Surg 1989;47:281.

Friedlander ALL, Gorelick DA. Dental management of the cocaine addict. Oral Surg Oral Med Oral Pathol 1988;65:45.

Lee C, Mohammadi H, Dixon RA. Medical and dental implications of cocaine abuse. J Oral Maxillofac Surg 1991;49:290.

Scheutz P. Dental health in a group of drug addicts attending an addiction clinic. Commun Dent Oral Epidemiol 1984;12:23.

Winkler JR, Murray PA. Periodontal disease: A potential intraoral expression of AIDS may be rapidly progressive periodontitis. Calif Dent Assoc J 1987;15:20.

Patient with DRUG ADDICTION AND A PERIODONTAL PROBLEM

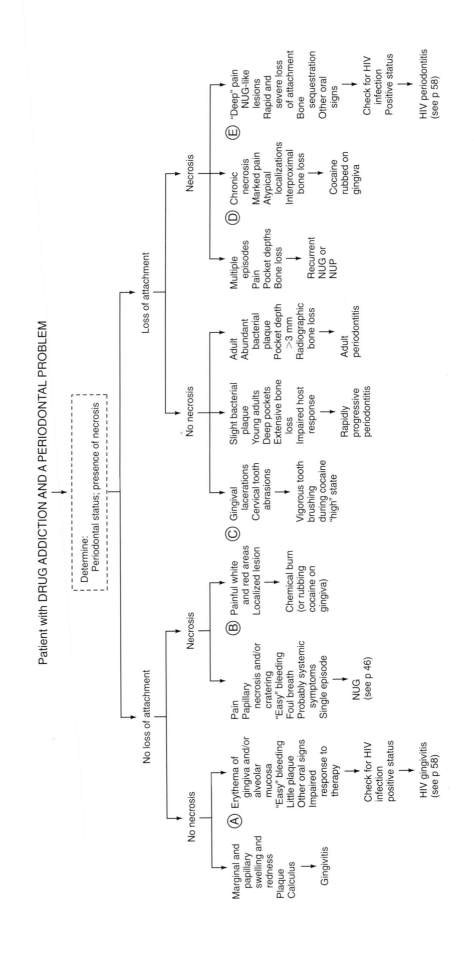

Determine:
Periodontal status; presence of necrosis

No loss of attachment

No necrosis

Ⓐ Marginal and papillary swelling and redness
Plaque
Calculus

→ Gingivitis

Erythema of gingiva and/or alveolar mucosa
"Easy" bleeding
Little plaque
Other oral signs
Impaired response to therapy

→ Check for HIV infection positive status

→ HIV gingivitis (see p 58)

Necrosis

Pain
Papillary necrosis and/or cratering
"Easy" bleeding
Foul breath
Probably systemic symptoms
Single episode

→ NUG (see p 46)

Ⓑ Painful white and red areas
Localized lesion

→ Chemical burn (or rubbing cocaine on gingiva)

Loss of attachment

No necrosis

Ⓒ Gingival lacerations
Cervical tooth abrasions

→ Vigorous tooth brushing during cocaine "high" state

Slight bacterial plaque
Young adults
Deep pockets
Extensive bone loss
Impaired host response

→ Rapidly progressive periodontitis

Adult
Abundant bacterial plaque
Pocket depth >3 mm
Radiographic bone loss

→ Adult periodontitis

Necrosis

Multiple episodes
Pain
Pocket depths
Bone loss

→ Recurrent NUG or NUP

Ⓓ Chronic necrosis
Marked pain
Atypical localizations
Interproximal bone loss

→ Cocaine rubbed on gingiva

Ⓔ "Deep" pain
NUG-like lesions
Rapid and severe loss of attachment
Bone sequestration
Other oral signs

→ Check for HIV infection
Positive status

→ HIV periodontitis (see p 58)

DESQUAMATIVE GINGIVITIS

Alan S. Leider

Desquamative gingivitis is not a disease per se but represents a clinical manifestation of a broad spectrum of mucocutaneous disorders. These may range from a relatively innocuous localized condition involving only the gingiva to that of a more severe, systemic, life-threatening disease affecting extensive areas of the skin and oral mucosa. Clinically, desquamative gingivitis is characterized by a generalized diffuse erythema of the free and attached gingiva (Fig. 1) with areas of vesiculation, erosion, or desquamation. It affects women more often than men; a most patients are middle-aged or older. The differential diagnosis would include specific mucocutaneous dermatoses such as benign mucous membrane pemphigoid, erosive (bullous) lichen planus, pemphigus vulgaris, erythema multiforme, and a nonspecific group of hormonal or idiopathic origin. Distinction between these entities would be based on the presence or absence of eye, skin, or other mucosal lesions as well as on the histopathologic and immunopathologic findings. A definitive diagnosis requires biopsy, with or without immunofluorescent studies.

A. A patient exhibiting desquamative gingivitis with vesiculobullous and erosive lesions of other oral–mucosal tissues and conjunctival eye lesions (Fig. 2) would probably have benign mucous membrane (cicatricial) pemphigoid (BMMP). A routine biopsy specimen would display a sub-basal epithelial–connective tissue split (Fig. 3). Immunofluorescent studies will show linear basement membrane deposits of immunoglobulin (IgG) and complement (C3) (Fig. 4). Although oral lesions may be painful and annoying, eye involvement is more serious and may result in blindness. Treatment consists of topical and/or short-term use of systemic steroids.

B. Desquamative gingivitis in a patient with other oral erosions and peripheral zones of white reticulated striae is suggestive of erosive lichen planus. Cutaneous lesions may be present and appear as scaly keratotic and pruritic plaques on an erythematous base. They are usually observed on the extensor surfaces of the

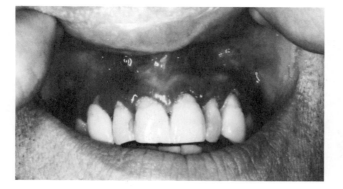

Figure 1. Desquamative gingivitis with generalized diffuse erythema of the free and attached gingiva.

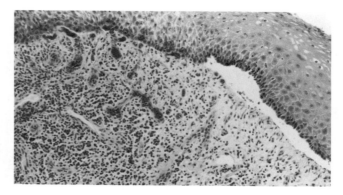

Figure 3. Routine histopathologic section of BMMP showing a subbasal epithelial–connective tissue split.

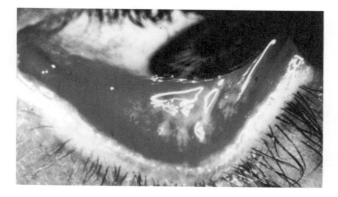

Figure 2. Benign mucous membrane pemphigoid (BMMP) with scarring of the conjuctiva of the eye.

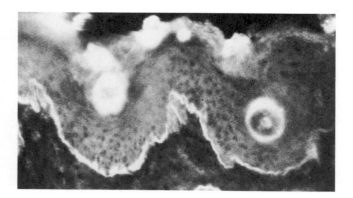

Figure 4. Immunofluorescent sections of BMMP with linear basement membrane deposits of IgG and C_3.

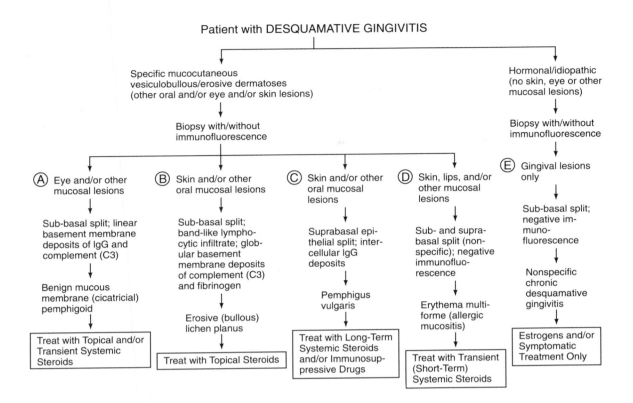

Patient with DESQUAMATIVE GINGIVITIS

Specific mucocutaneous vesiculobullous/erosive dermatoses (other oral and/or eye and/or skin lesions)
→ Biopsy with/without immunofluorescence

(A) Eye and/or other mucosal lesions → Sub-basal split; linear basement membrane deposits of IgG and complement (C3) → Benign mucous membrane (cicatricial) pemphigoid → **Treat with Topical and/or Transient Systemic Steroids**

(B) Skin and/or other oral mucosal lesions → Sub-basal split; band-like lymphocytic infiltrate; globular basement membrane deposits of complement (C3) and fibrinogen → Erosive (bullous) lichen planus → **Treat with Topical Steroids**

(C) Skin and/or oral mucosal lesions → Suprabasal epithelial split; intercellular IgG deposits → Pemphigus vulgaris → **Treat with Long-Term Systemic Steroids and/or Immunosuppressive Drugs**

(D) Skin, lips, and/or other mucosal lesions → Sub- and suprabasal split (nonspecific); negative immunofluorescence → Erythema multiforme (allergic mucositis) → **Treat with Transient (Short-Term) Systemic Steroids**

Hormonal/idiopathic (no skin, eye or other mucosal lesions) → Biopsy with/without immunofluorescence → (E) Gingival lesions only → Sub-basal split; negative immunofluorescence → Nonspecific chronic desquamative gingivitis → **Estrogens and/or Symptomatic Treatment Only**

extremities. A biopsy would exhibit a sub-basal split with a subepithelial, band-like, lymphocytic infiltrate. Globular deposits of complement (C3) and fibrinogen would be seen in the basement membrane with immunofluorescent testing of the submitted tissues. Treatment with topical steroids, such as 0.05% Lidex in Orabase, usually will control the painful erosive and desquamative lesions, but usually will not affect the white components.

C. Desquamative gingivitis in a patient with extensive large bullous and erosive lesions throughout the oral mucosa and skin may suggest pemphigus vulgaris. A bullous lesion may be elicited by rubbing uninvolved oral mucosa or skin. This result is referred to as Nikolsky's sign and is characteristic for pemphigus, but it may also be observed in all the other desquamative lesions under discussion. A suprabasal epithelial split is seen on routine biopsy examination, and immunofluorescence exhibits intercellular IgG deposits. Long-term therapy with systemic steroids and/or immunosuppressive drugs is the treatment of choice. Early diagnosis and initiation of therapy are important in these patients to prevent death from dehydration and septicemia.

D. Extensive hemorrhagic-crusted lesions of the lips, erythematous circular iris, or target lesions on the skin, a wide variety of intraoral, erythematous, and vesiculoerosive lesions, in conjunction with desquamative gingivitis, are highly suggestive of erythema multiforme. When this condition affects the oral mucosa, skin, conjunctiva of the eyes, and external genitalia, it is referred to as Stevens–Johnson syndrome. A biopsy demonstrates a nonspecific suprabasal and sub-basal epithelial split, and immunofluorescent studies are generally negative. Erythema multiforme may represent an allergic mucositis, which is often associated with sulfa drugs, or it may be of idiopathic origin. Treatment consists of short-term (transient) systemic steroids and supportive symptomatic therapy.

E. A patient with desquamative gingivitis without any other lesions or systemic symptomology should be suspected of having nonspecific, chronic desquamative gingivitis of hormonal or idiopathic origin. Although in many cases this represents an early stage of benign mucous membrane pemphigoid, a biopsy will show a sub-basal epithelial–connective tissue split and immunofluorescence is completely negative. The vast majority of these patients are postmenopausal women, and the treatment of choice is estrogens and/or symptomatic therapy only. Patients should avoid spicy or acidic foods, and a palliative mouthwash with elixir of Benadryl and Kaopectate may alleviate the discomfort.

References

Carranza FA Jr. Glickman's clinical periodontology. 6th ed. Philadelphia: WB Saunders, 1984:164.

Daniels TE, Quadra-White C. Direct immunofluorescence in oral mucosal disease. Oral Surg 1981;51:38.

Eversole LR. Clinical outline of oral pathology: Diagnosis and treatment. 2nd ed. Philadelphia: Lea & Febiger, 1984:Chap 5.

Rogers RS III, Sheridan PJ, Nightingale SH. Desquamative gingivitis: Clinical, histopathologic, immunopathologic, and therapeutic observations. J Am Acad Dermatol 1982;7:29.

CRACKED TOOTH SYNDROME

Walter B. Hall

When a patient with a periodontal problem complains of pain localized to one tooth, especially if this is triggered by heavy function, investigate the possibility that the tooth may be cracked (Figs. 1, 2, and 3). If a tooth is cracked superficially, the symptoms may be controlled by crowning that tooth. Selective grinding may be helpful temporarily, but fractures tend to spread within teeth, making crowning the safest long-term solution to controlling these problems. If the crack is symptomatic, it may be extending to involve the pulp. If the crack is deep already, endodontics may be helpful. If the tooth has been treated endodontically and now is symptomatic, the crack may be affecting the periodontal ligament. When a crack is contiguous with a deep pocket, the prognosis for the tooth is guarded at best, and therapy should be planned with this in mind.

A. When a tooth with a periodontal pocket is painful, an endodontic involvement must be ruled out before proceeding with any periodontal surgery. Whether or not the tooth is vital or nonvital to electrical pulp testing or to hot and cold, new periapical radiographs should be obtained and evaluated for evidence of periapical radiolucencies. They should be evaluated visually and with a fiberoptic light source for cracks. The fiberoptic light will stop at the plane of a crack where the light is refracted, and no glow of light will extend to other parts of the tooth if the crack extends to the pulp. The tooth should be tapped and pressed in various directions against each cusp in an attempt to elicit the sharp, brief twinge of pain that is symptomatic of a cracked tooth.

B. If a symptomatic tooth tests vital, a radiograph may still suggest an endodontic problem. If no evidence of a crack (either visual or symptomatic) can be elicited, employ selective grinding to minimize trauma. The tooth should be observed for several months to determine that symptoms have disappeared before any periodontal surgery is undertaken. If evidence of a crack can be elicited, an orthodontic band should be cemented to minimize the likelihood of the crack's spreading. The dentist and patient should decide together either to perform endodontic therapy promptly or to "wait and see" whether symptoms subside before undertaking any periodontal surgery.

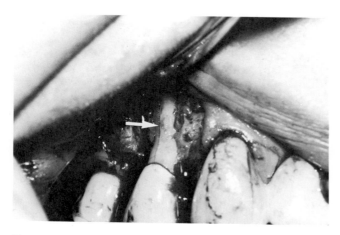

Figure 1. An endodontically treated first premolar with a vertical crack and a resulting deep periodontal defect.

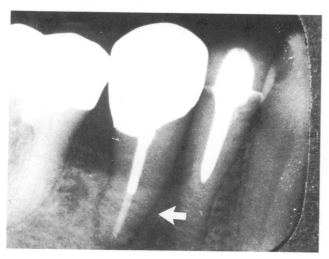

Figure 2. Vertical periodontal defect resulting from a cracked tooth.

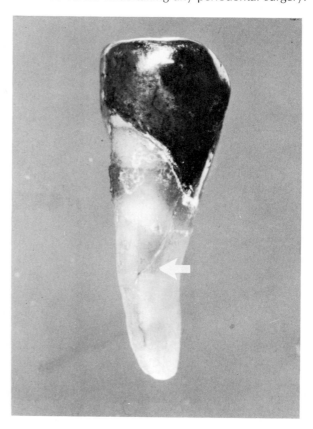

Figure 3. Cracked tooth.

Patient with POCKET DEPTH AND LOCALIZED PAIN OR TWINGES OF PAIN IN A TOOTH

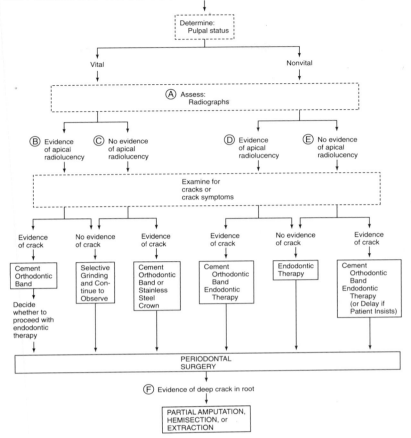

C. If a symptomatic tooth tests vital and has no evidence of periapical radiolucency, examine it for cracks or crack symptoms. If no evidence of a crack is elicited, employ selective grinding and observation for several months before any periodontal procedures are undertaken. If evidence of a crack can be elicited, cement an orthodontic band or a stainless steel crown to minimize fracture spread prior to any periodontal surgery.

D. If a symptomatic tooth tests nonvital, this may be confirmed by a radiographic periapical radiolucency. If so, examine the tooth for cracks. If no evidence of a crack can be elicited, complete endodontic treatment promptly before any periodontal surgery is undertaken. If evidence of a crack is found, cement an orthodontic band to its crown to minimize fracture spreading. A decision by the dentist and patient to initiate endodontic treatment promptly or to "wait and see" should be agreed upon. If symptoms do not subside, endodontics should be undertaken before any periodontal surgery. If symptoms subside, periodontal surgery could be undertaken with full recognition that an endodontic flare up could be precipitated, necessitating prompt treatment.

E. If a symptomatic tooth tests nonvital and radiographic evidence of a periapical radiolucency is not found, evaluate the tooth for evidence of a crack. If no evidence of a crack can be elicited, the tooth should be treated endodontically before any periodontal

surgery is performed. If evidence of a crack can be elicited, cement an orthodontic band to the crown and perform endodontic treatment before any periodontal surgery is undertaken.

F. When periodontal treatment is undertaken in any of these situations, a crack extending down the root where attachment has been lost may become visible. Once the area has been debrided, use the fiberoptic light source to search for cracks. If a deep crack is found, the tooth may have to be extracted or possibly one root of a multirooted tooth may be amputated (in maxillary molars) or the tooth hemisected (in mandibular molars). If a patient elects not to have such a tooth extracted, the dentist should carefully document the patient's choice and his advice that keeping the tooth is risky.

References

Cameron CE. The cracked tooth syndrome: Additional findings. J Am Dent Assoc 1976;93:971.

Eahle WS, Maxwell EH, Braly BV. Fractures of posterior teeth in adults. J Am Dent Assoc 1986;112:215.

Hiatt WH. Incomplete crown-root fracture. J Periodontol 1973;44:369.

Maxwell EH, Braly BV. Incomplete tooth fracture: Prediction and prevention. Cal Dent Assoc J 1977;5:51.

Ritchey B, Mendenhall R, Orban B. Pulpitis resulting from incomplete tooth fracture. Oral Surg Oral Med Oral Pathol 1957;10:665.

PROGNOSIS OF THE DENTITION COMPLICATED BY PERIODONTITIS: INFLUENCING FACTORS

George K. Merijohn

An accurate prognosis should be based upon current established criteria, therapeutic judgment and experience, and the documented successes and failures of the past. The fundamental therapeutic goal for all dental clinicians is the survival of the natural dentition in relative health, comfort, and function, with optimum esthetics, throughout the life of the individual. This goal provides a solid framework for decision making regarding the prognosis of individual teeth.

The decision tree that appears on the opposite page highlights the critical influencing factors that determine the prognosis for the dentition complicated by periodontitis. On the left side are the qualifiers that indicate a worse prognosis. On the right side are the qualifiers that point to a better prognosis. The influencing factors are organized into three major categories: (A) dental factors, (B) medical factors, and (C) psychological factors.

A. Many specific dental conditions can affect the overall prognosis of the dentition. For example, teeth that have moderate-to-advanced furcation bone loss, with close root proximity and difficult access for professional and self-maintenance, will have a worse prognosis than teeth without these afflictions. A comprehensive dental–periodontal examination and recent full-mouth radiographs are prerequisites for decision making. Exacting prognostic treatment planning is essential when a patient needs extensive dental rehabilitation, especially when the overall prognosis hinges on key strategic teeth. Because the prognosis of the dentition can, in certain cases, be enhanced by the strategic placement of endosseous osseointegrated implants, careful evaluation of dentate and edentate alveolar bone quality, quantity, morphology, and location is critical. In order to preserve alveolar bone for future use, consideration must be given to strategic removal of teeth that may have a poor prognosis and whose retention would jeopardize the surrounding alveolar bone.

B. Assessment of the patient's medical status is extremely important because resistance to periodontitis is often diminished when an individual's overall health and/or resistance is compromised. The maintenance of a healthy periodontium requires the responsiveness of a normally functioning host defense system. In addition, hereditary factors and genetic resistance to periodontal diseases have considerable clinical significance.

C. The prognosis of the dentition can be significantly improved when the patient becomes mentally and physically involved with therapy by accepting his individual responsibilities in the treatment process.

References

Hirschfeld L, Wasserman B. A long-term study of tooth loss in 600 treated periodontal patients. J Periodontol 1978; 49:225.

Klavan B, ed. International conference of research in the biology of periodontal disease. Chicago, 1977.

Merijohn GK. Perio Access Periodontal Decision Making, Therapy & Record Keeping System. 2nd ed. San Francisco: Perio Access, 1988:Chap 2.

Nevins M, Becker W, Kornman K, eds. Proceedings of the world workshop in clinical periodontics. Princeton, NJ: American Academy of Periodontology, 1989.

Page RC, Schroeder HE. Periodontitis in man and other animals: A comparative review. Basel: S Karger & Co, 1982.

Ramfjord SP, ed. World workshop in periodontics. Ann Arbor, MI, 1966.

Schluger S, Yuodelis R, Page R, Johnson R. Periodontal diseases. Philadelphia: Lea & Febiger, 1990:341.

Waerhaug J. The furcation problem: Etiology, pathogenesis, diagnosis, therapy, and prognosis. J Clin Periodontol 1980;7:73.

PROGNOSIS OF THE DENTITION COMPLICATED BY PERIODONTITIS: INFLUENCING FACTORS

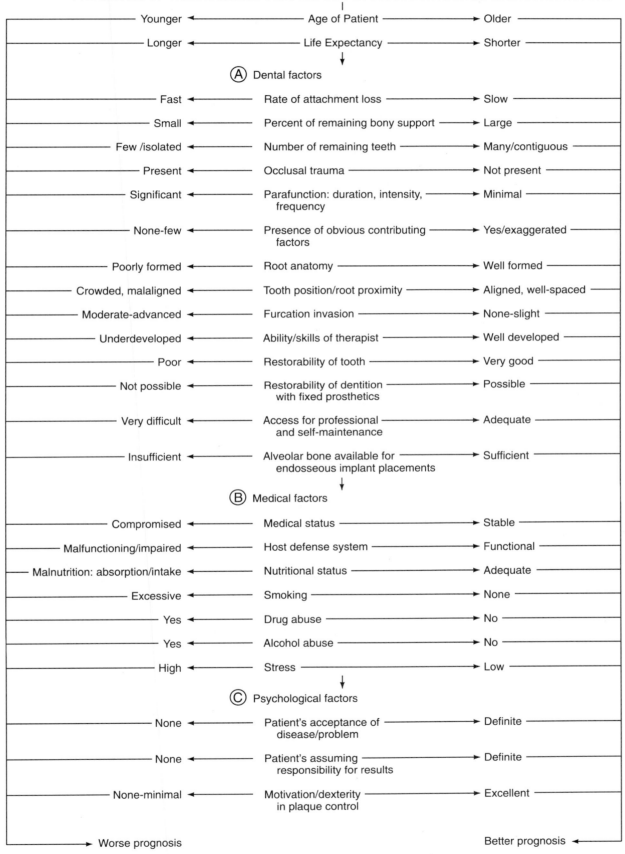

Worse prognosis ←		→ Better prognosis
Younger ←	Age of Patient	→ Older
Longer ←	Life Expectancy	→ Shorter
	A Dental factors	
Fast ←	Rate of attachment loss	→ Slow
Small ←	Percent of remaining bony support	→ Large
Few /isolated ←	Number of remaining teeth	→ Many/contiguous
Present ←	Occlusal trauma	→ Not present
Significant ←	Parafunction: duration, intensity, frequency	→ Minimal
None-few ←	Presence of obvious contributing factors	→ Yes/exaggerated
Poorly formed ←	Root anatomy	→ Well formed
Crowded, malaligned ←	Tooth position/root proximity	→ Aligned, well-spaced
Moderate-advanced ←	Furcation invasion	→ None-slight
Underdeveloped ←	Ability/skills of therapist	→ Well developed
Poor ←	Restorability of tooth	→ Very good
Not possible ←	Restorability of dentition with fixed prosthetics	→ Possible
Very difficult ←	Access for professional and self-maintenance	→ Adequate
Insufficient ←	Alveolar bone available for endosseous implant placements	→ Sufficient
	B Medical factors	
Compromised ←	Medical status	→ Stable
Malfunctioning/impaired ←	Host defense system	→ Functional
Malnutrition: absorption/intake ←	Nutritional status	→ Adequate
Excessive ←	Smoking	→ None
Yes ←	Drug abuse	→ No
Yes ←	Alcohol abuse	→ No
High ←	Stress	→ Low
	C Psychological factors	
None ←	Patient's acceptance of disease/problem	→ Definite
None ←	Patient's assuming responsibility for results	→ Definite
None-minimal ←	Motivation/dexterity in plaque control	→ Excellent

HOPELESS TOOTH

Walter B. Hall

Hopeless teeth are those that cannot be treated with reasonable expectations of eliminating or even controlling their dental problems. Such teeth are not always extracted but in some situations may be maintained, occasionally for years, with full recognition that no means of treating them or stopping their loss of attachment exist. For example, such patients may have lost 50% or more of the attachment on all their remaining teeth. Pocket elimination surgery might be ruled out on the basis of leaving inadequate support to keep the teeth at all with any reasonable degree of comfort or function. A Widman flap might be employed to debride the area once fully, but neither the patient nor the dentist could expect to control the disease process with root planing, even with use of antibiotics. Such teeth might be maintained, if the patient demanded, for some time before abscesses and pain might necessitate their removal. Such patients should proceed with full knowledge that their prognosis is hopeless and be aware of the risks of abscesses and possible danger to general health. The concept of hopelessness, therefore, should be explained fully when such a prognosis is used, so that the patient not only assumes all the attendant risks of keeping such teeth but also is fully informed in the legal sense (see p 224).

In the 1980s, many teeth previously regarded as hopeless became salvageable by means of guided tissue regeneration (GTR), which was pioneered in Sweden. Badly involved Class II furcation involvements, large three-walled infrabony defects, and osseous craters which were nontreatable have become predictably treatable. Significant numbers of formerly hopeless teeth can be saved by this means today. Further advances with this approach, such as GTR for Class III furcations, are imminent, which will further decrease the number of problems that should be regarded as hopeless.

A. Loss of attachment is the most common contributor to a prognosis of "hopeless" for a tooth. When a tooth has lost more than 50% of its attachment, its potential usefulness and ability to be maintained often are related to the status of other teeth in the mouth; thus, if other teeth with adequate support remain, it may be splinted and escape a hopeless prognosis. If not, its long-term prognosis usually should be viewed as hopeless. If a tooth lost less than 50% of its attachment but has a pocket that approaches its apex (or apices), its prognosis will be greatly affected by the character of the adjacent osseous lesion. If the deep pocket is within a narrow, three-walled defect, it may be treatable with a bone regeneration procedure that could greatly improve its prognosis (see p 152). If there is no three-walled defect but the tooth is endodontically involved as well, endodontic treatment could improve its prognosis greatly. If no endodontic lesion is present, the prognosis when neither bone regeneration nor endodontics is to be performed would be hopeless.

Some teeth will continue to be regarded as hopeless because they are not restorable, because they are malposed to an extent not correctable orthodontically, or because of vertical or spiral cracks that extend apically down their roots.

B. If the tooth is a molar with a Class III furcation involvement (see p 146), determine its endodontic status. If endodontic therapy is needed and can be performed, the prognosis for the tooth would be greatly improved. If not, the possibilities of improving the molar's prognosis would be dependent upon the possibility of root amputation or hemisection being employed to eliminate the furcation involvement and to create a maintainable situation on the remaining portion of the tooth. If this could not be done (because of root form or fusion), the prognosis would be hopeless.

Next, assess the endodontic health of a severely periodontally involved tooth. If a tooth is endodontically involved and is not endodontically treatable (i.e., calcified canals, roots too crooked to be obturated, severely internally or externally resorbed or perforated), it should be regarded as hopeless.

C. If the tooth is nonrestorable because of the caries or fracture status of its remaining portion, it should be viewed as hopeless even if it is maintained and the periodontal treatment continues.

If the tooth is not endodontically involved or is endodontically treatable, the next step would be to determine whether it is treatable periodontally.

D. If a periodontally involved tooth is badly malposed, it still might be a useful tooth if it can be treated orthodontically. If a tooth can be moved into, or out of, certain types of osseous defects (see p 128), its prognosis may be greatly improved. If not, its prognosis may be hopeless, regardless of the severity of the periodontal problem.

Usually, a tooth with less than 50% loss of attachment (LOA) is treatable by frequent root planing (see p 142) or with mucogingival osseous surgery (see pp 162 to 192). Teeth with more than 50% LOA usually will require more extensive treatment if they are to be saved.

E. Cracked tooth problems can make a tooth's prognosis hopeless. If cracked tooth syndrome exists and the symptoms are bothersome to the patient, the tooth may have to be removed if the crack extends vertically down the root. If the crack is essentially in the crown, placing a restorative crown may control the symptoms and restrict further crack spreading, so that the prognosis for the tooth could be improved. Vertical cracks in the root of the tooth, however, are not treatable, and the prognosis is hopeless.

Some teeth with more than 50% LOA may be salvaged by GTR with highly predictable success. Teeth with Class II or III furcation involvement (see p 148) may be treatable. Most Class II furcation involvements with greater than 3 mm of horizontal loss into

Patient with a SEVERELY INVOLVED TOOTH

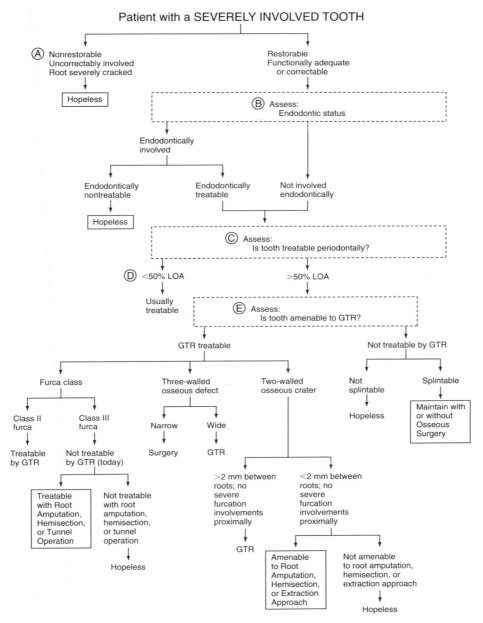

the furca but not "through-and-through" problems are good candidates for GTR. Teeth with Class III furcation involvements may be treatable by GTR in the future, but root amputation, hemisection, or a tunnel operation is more predictable today. If the roots are fused too far apically or are apically fused, such approaches cannot be used, and the tooth should be regarded as hopeless. Teeth with three-walled defects, even of severe depth, will routinely regenerate if the defect is narrow, no more than 1 mm horizontally from tooth to crest of bone. If the three-walled defects are wider, GTR can be expected to be routinely successful. Teeth with a two-walled infrabony crater can be successfully treated by GTR unless their roots are less than 2 mm apart or the proximal furcas are too severely involved to be instrumented owing to restricted access, in which case they should be regarded as hopeless unless root amputation, hemisection, or extraction of one of the involved teeth makes the defect on the remaining

tooth treatable. A tooth with more than 50% LOA that is not amenable to GTR today may still be maintained if it can be splinted to other less involved teeth. If such splinting is not possible, the tooth should be regarded as hopeless.

References

Corn H, Marks MA. Strategic extractions in periodontal therapy. Dent Clin North Am 1969;13:817.

Eakle WJ, Maxwell EH, Braly BV. Fractures of posterior teeth in adults. J Am Dent Assoc 1986;112:215.

Everett FG, Stern IB. When is tooth mobility an indication for extraction? Dent Clin North Am 1969;13:791.

Maxwell EH, Braly BV. Incomplete root fracture: Predictions and prevention. Cal Dent Assoc J 1977;5:51.

Schluger S, Yuodelis R, Page RC, Johnson RH. Periodontal diseases. 2nd ed. Philadelphia: Lea & Febiger, 1990:341.

SEQUENCE OF TREATMENT

Walter B. Hall

When a patient presents with a periodontal problem, a typical sequence of examination and diagnosis precedes treatment planning. Medical, dental, and plaque-control histories should be recorded and amplified upon during radiographic and clinical examination. From these data, diagnoses and prognoses can be developed.

A. For purposes of treatment planning, periodontal problems are divided into acute (symptomatic) problems, in which symptoms are present, and asymptomatic ones, in which no acute problems are present. Symptomatic problems require prompt treatment, usually at the diagnostic visit. Only the four most common symptomatic problems are outlined here. The more common periodontal diseases usually are asymptomatic, and treatment can be planned on a more orderly basis that best fits into the patient's and dentist's schedules.

B. Herpetic gingivostomatitis usually is managed with palliative care (mild pain killers, a topical anesthetic mouthwash), prophylaxis, and instruction about the infectious nature of the problem (see p 48).

C. Necrotizing ulcerative gingivitis and necrotizing ulcerative periodontitis are handled by instrumentation alone or in conjunction with an oral antibiotic, usually penicillin (see p 136).

D. Periodontal abscesses usually are handled by incision and drainage along with antibiotic therapy.

E. Therapy for human immunodeficiency virus (HIV) periodontitis requires close collaboration with the patient's physician in developing a palliative treatment plan (see p 58). Acute or severe episodes of HIV periodontitis in which tissue necrosis is rapid and painful should be treated initially with Betadine, applied several times per day, if bone is exposed; after a week, use chlorhexidine rinses morning and night until necrosis is controlled. Extremely severe episodes may be treated with metronidazole (Flagyl) as the physician directs.

F. Gingivitis of the typical type probably is the most prevalent disease affecting man, and most people experience at least localized inflammations of this type in any given year. Its subgroupings are related to host factors (see p 66). It usually responds favorably to prophylaxis (or root planing, if roots are exposed) and to thorough plaque-removal practices by the patient. In the absence of daily, thorough plaque removal, it will return. Desquamative gingivitis is far less com-mon and usually is the gingival expression of dermatologic diseases (see p 62). Prophylaxis (or root planing), regular plaque removal (often difficult), and topical steroid applications are common treatments.

G. Adult periodontitis is the current name for typical, slowly progressive periodontitis. Its treatment (see p 142) usually consists of initial therapy (root planing, oral hygiene training, occasionally occlusal adjustment, and occasionally temporary splinting or minor tooth movement). After several weeks or months of patient effort, the response is evaluated and decisions are made regarding the comparative value of surgery or continued maintenance.

H. Prepubertal juvenile periodontitis (mixed dentition periodontitis) and rapidly progressive periodontitis are discussed (see pp 44 and 84). Although different bacteria appear to predominate as etiologic agents with these diseases, they are treated in a similar manner. A regimen of tetracycline (250 mg four times daily) or metronidazole (Flagyl) is employed for 3 weeks, during which all root planing is accomplished. This regimen is repeated several times during the first year to contact the virulent bacteria. Often, only regular maintenance or localized surgery is required once this control is established. Such cases are best referred to dental schools or to periodontists (see p 72).

I. Gingival enlargements (often referred to as *hyperplasias*) may result from drug therapy (diphenyl hydantoin, cyclosporine, or nifedipine treatment) (see p 132) or from poor oral hygiene during orthodontic treatment in the pubertal years. They are treated with initial therapy, surgery if the deformities interfere with adequate plaque removal, occlusion, or regular maintenance. Stopping use of the medication or removing the orthodontic bands is necessary in few cases.

References

Barsh LI. Dental treatment planning for the adult patient. Philadelphia: WB Saunders, 1981:152.

Carranza FA Jr. Glickman's clinical periodontology. 7th ed. Philadelphia: WB Saunders, 1990:552.

Genco RJ, Goldman HM, Cohen DW. Contemporary periodontics. St. Louis: CV Mosby, 1990:359.

Grant DA, Stern IB, Listgarten MA. Periodontics. St. Louis: CV Mosby, 1988:592.

Schluger S, Yuodelis R, Page RC, Johnson RH. Periodontal diseases. 2nd ed. Philadelphia: Lea & Febiger, 1990:331.

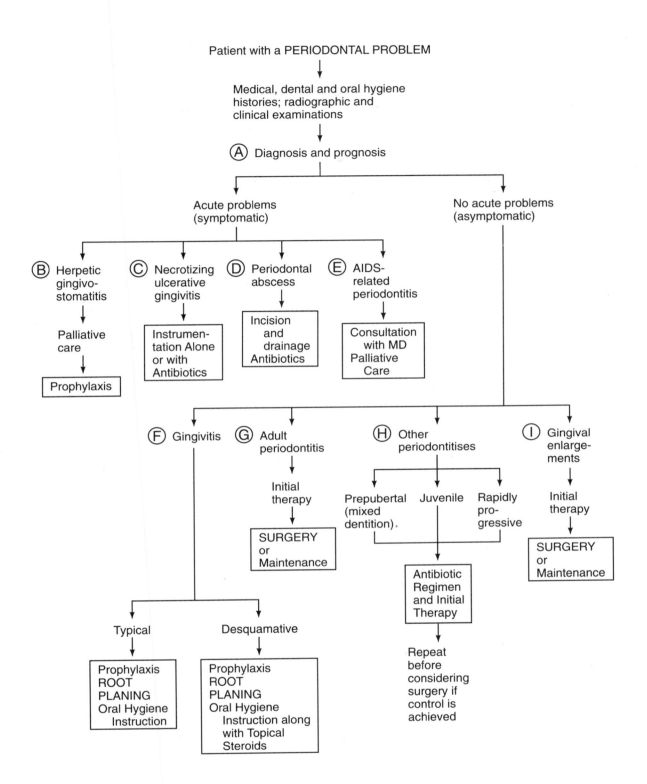

Patient with a PERIODONTAL PROBLEM

Medical, dental and oral hygiene histories; radiographic and clinical examinations

(A) Diagnosis and prognosis

Acute problems (symptomatic)   No acute problems (asymptomatic)

(B) Herpetic gingivo-stomatitis

Palliative care

Prophylaxis

(C) Necrotizing ulcerative gingivitis

Instrumen-tation Alone or with Antibiotics

(D) Periodontal abscess

Incision and drainage Antibiotics

(E) AIDS-related periodontitis

Consultation with MD Palliative Care

(F) Gingivitis

(G) Adult periodontitis

Initial therapy

SURGERY or Maintenance

(H) Other periodontitises

Prepubertal (mixed dentition)   Juvenile   Rapidly pro-gressive

Antibiotic Regimen and Initial Therapy

Repeat before considering surgery if control is achieved

(I) Gingival enlarge-ments

Initial therapy

SURGERY or Maintenance

Typical

Prophylaxis ROOT PLANING Oral Hygiene Instruction

Desquamative

Prophylaxis ROOT PLANING Oral Hygiene Instruction along with Topical Steroids

PROVIDING TREATMENT OR REFERRING TO THE PERIODONTIST

George K. Merijohn

The criteria for deciding whether to treat or refer a patient to the periodontist should be based upon the severity of the diagnosed periodontal problem, the assessment of whether the problem is beyond the skill or management level of the individual dentist or hygienist, and the extent to which treating the patient's problems will require a multidisciplinary approach.

A. A distinction must be made between patients who have previously undergone periodontal surgery and those who have not. For the former, the measurable attachment loss is a result of the disease process and, in many cases, the surgical procedure; therefore, evaluation of disease activity (bleeding or exudate upon probing) and measurement of further attachment loss (periodic comprehensive examinations) become the most important factors in making the diagnosis.

Patients who have had periodontal surgery, perform effective daily plaque control, are on a regular 3-month maintenance therapy cycle, and demonstrate subgingival inflammation and further attachment loss are of extreme concern. Refer these individuals to the periodontist for co-diagnosis and further therapy.

B. Children and adolescents are subject to a wide variety of periodontal infections that can progress rapidly. Because early diagnosis is critical for successful treatment, it is imperative that children and adolescents routinely receive comprehensive periodontal examinations.

C. Nonspecific gingivitis (Case Type I) should be treated by the general dentist and hygienist unless unusual medical, physical, psychological, or other dental factors would make this unfeasible. Under these circumstances, referral to a periodontist would be appropriate. Refer to "Prognosis of the Dentition Complicated by Periodontitis: Influencing Factors."

D. For early (Case Type II) or moderate (Case Type III) periodontitis, decisions on whether or not to refer to a periodontist should be based upon the following: (1) the dentist's and hygienist's ability, skill, interest, and experience in treating more advanced cases; and (2) the extent to which pocket depth, furcation invasion, difficult access, occlusal trauma, anatomic defects, orthodontic, restorative, medical, or psychological parameters affect the patient's prognosis (refer to "Prognosis of the Dentition Complicated by Periodontitis: Influencing Factors"). With advanced (Case Type IV) or refractory (Case Type V) periodontitis, an initial referral to a periodontist for specialized care should be made because of the advanced nature of the disease, complications that can arise with therapy, and the need to evaluate healing carefully after meticulous initial therapy.

E. Initial periodontal therapy includes periodontal scaling and root planing, polishing, instruction in effective daily plaque control, necessary occlusal therapy, and adjunctive antimicrobial therapy when indicated. Also, the therapist should manage other contributing dental factors (extensive decay, grossly defective restorations, etc.) during this phase of therapy.

F. After 3 to 6 weeks, evaluate the success of therapy with a comprehensive examination or periodontal screening. If the dentist determines that the patient will be referred to the periodontist after initial therapy, then a reevaluation (comprehensive examination) is unnecessary because the periodontist will examine the patient at the first visit. Although it is an optional step, the therapist may choose to do a screening exam before referral for the sake of complete documentation. This can be performed at the last scaling and root planing appointment or at a separate appointment. If the patient continues treatment in the general dental office without referral to the periodontist, an extremely important point, from a documentation and medicolegal standpoint, is that this patient must have a comprehensive periodontal examination and the dentist must re-establish the diagnosis.

G. Providing patients with advanced periodontal therapy requires a thorough knowledge and understanding of the following: techniques and concepts of advanced scaling and root planing; rationales, objectives, and methodologies of the various corrective surgical procedures and antimicrobial therapeutic regimens; occlusal and restorative therapy as it relates to the periodontal disease process; and implant prosthesis and surgical therapy.

H. If a patient declines referral to the periodontist, the following should always be recorded in the chart: the diagnosis, the reason for referral, the referral, the patient's reason for declining, treatment and nontreatment risks discussed, alternative therapies described, and final action. These facts are important to record for clinical documentation purposes as well as to decrease your exposure and vulnerability to a periodontal negligence lawsuit.

References

Axelsson P, Lindhe J. Effect of controlled oral hygiene procedures on caries and periodontal disease in adults. J Clin Periodontol 1978;5:131.

Current procedural terminology for periodontics and insurance reporting manual. 6th ed. Chicago: American Academy of Periodontology, 1991.

Guidelines for periodontal therapy. Reprint. Chicago: American Academy of Periodontology, April, 1991.

PROVIDING TREATMENT OR REFERRING TO PERIODONTIST

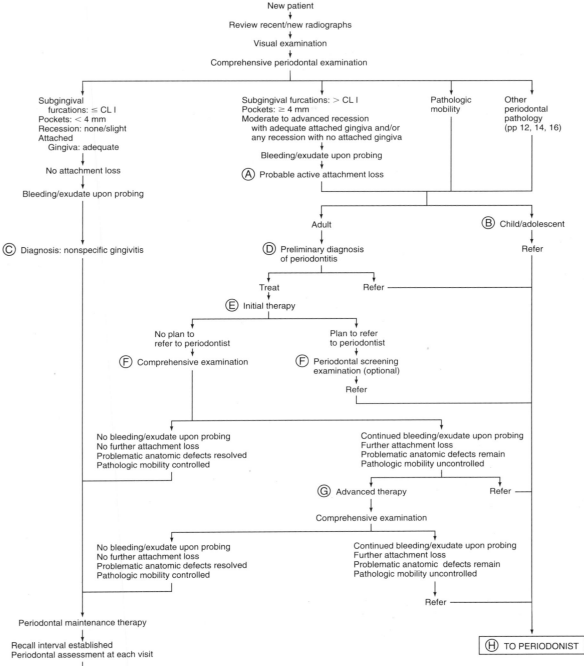

New patient
↓
Review recent/new radiographs
↓
Visual examination
↓
Comprehensive periodontal examination

Subgingival
furcations: ≤ CL I
Pockets: < 4 mm
Recession: none/slight
Attached
  Gingiva: adequate
↓
No attachment loss
↓
Bleeding/exudate upon probing

Ⓒ Diagnosis: nonspecific gingivitis

Subgingival furcations: > CL I
Pockets: ≥ 4 mm
Moderate to advanced recession
  with adequate attached gingiva and/or
  any recession with no attached gingiva
↓
Bleeding/exudate upon probing
↓
Ⓐ Probable active attachment loss

Pathologic
mobility

Other
periodontal
pathology
(pp 12, 14, 16)

Adult

Ⓑ Child/adolescent
Refer

Ⓓ Preliminary diagnosis
of periodontitis

Treat   Refer

Ⓔ Initial therapy

No plan to
refer to periodontist

Ⓕ Comprehensive examination

Plan to refer
to periodontist

Ⓕ Periodontal screening
examination (optional)
↓
Refer

No bleeding/exudate upon probing
No further attachment loss
Problematic anatomic defects resolved
Pathologic mobility controlled

Continued bleeding/exudate upon probing
Further attachment loss
Problematic anatomic defects remain
Pathologic mobility uncontrolled

Ⓖ Advanced therapy   Refer
↓
Comprehensive examination

No bleeding/exudate upon probing
No further attachment loss
Problematic anatomic defects resolved
Pathologic mobility controlled

Continued bleeding/exudate upon probing
Further attachment loss
Problematic anatomic defects remain
Pathologic mobility uncontrolled
↓
Refer

Periodontal maintenance therapy
↓
Recall interval established
Periodontal assessment at each visit
↓
Periodic comprehensive examination

Ⓗ TO PERIODONIST

Knowles JW, Burgett FG, Nissle RR, et al. Results of periodontal treatment related to pocket depth and attachment level, eight years. J Periodontol 1979;50:225.

Merijohn GK. Perio Access Periodontal Decision Making, Therapy and Record Keeping System. 2nd ed. San Francisco: Perio Access, 1988:Chap 3.

Periodontal diseases of children and adolescents. Reprint. Chicago: American Academy of Periodontology, April, 1991.

Periodontal therapy: A summary status report 1987–88. Reprint. Chicago: American Academy of Periodontology, August, 1987.

Ramfjord SP, Knowles JW, Nissle RR, et al. Longitudinal study of periodontal therapy. J Periodontol 1973;44:66.

Schluger S, Yuodelis R, Page R, Johnson R. Periodontal diseases. Philadelphia: Lea & Febiger, 1990:331.

Waerhaug J. The furcation problem: Etiology, pathogenesis, diagnosis, therapy, and prognosis. J Clin Periodontol 1980;7:73.

Waerhaug J. The infrabony pocket and its relationship to trauma from occlusion and subgingival plaque. J Periodontol 1979;50:355.

PROPHYLAXIS VERSUS ROOT PLANING

Walter B. Hall

When examining a patient who has plaque and calculus deposits on several or many teeth, the dentist must decide whether either prophylaxis or root planing or a combination of the two, is the appropriate first step in therapy (Fig. 1). Prophylaxis is defined as the scaling of deposits from the anatomic crown of the tooth, either from enamel or from a restorative material. Root planing is defined as the removal of calculus, most plaque, essentially all cementum, and some dentin from the roots of teeth while planing them to clinic smoothness. The removal of calculus from the crowns (scaling) and the polishing of all exposed tooth surfaces are regarded as part of this process for the sake of ease of documentation and billing. Scaling of the anatomic crowns of teeth is a relatively simple procedure and is of minimal importance. Root planing, however, is one of the most difficult and demanding procedures in dentistry. In planning treatment, the dentist has an obligation to differentiate fairly and correctly between the procedures in order to charge the patient or a third party properly for the work to be done.

A. When only the anatomic crowns (enamel) or restorative materials are exposed and have calculus deposits on them, prophylaxis is the appropriate treatment. The cost of this procedure usually is minimal, as the time, effort, and skill required to perform the procedure usually are minimal. In some cases in which calculus deposits are extensive and of long standing, a higher charge to compensate for the greater time required is justifiable and appropriate.

B. When only a few teeth have roots exposed or many teeth have little root exposure, a charge for prophylaxis and perhaps one quadrant or two of root planing would be appropriate.

C. When most teeth have root exposure of several millimeters or more, a good alternative to root planing is the appropriate treatment plan. The cost of initial root planing might reasonably be set at four or more times the cost of prophylaxis to reflect the greater time, effort, and skill required to perform this procedure.

D. Recall root planing, however, once the roots have been planed by the dentist initially, is a much easier task, because any calculus will be relatively new and will be attached to the previously smoothed dentin much less firmly than the old calculus had been united with cementum. Recall root planing requires a significantly lower fee than the initial planing, perhaps the same as one quadrant initially for the full mouth on recall. Recall instrumentation of exposed roots should not be termed *prophylaxis,* as only scaling calculus deposits from exposed roots would leave a roughened, irregular, or gouged root surface.

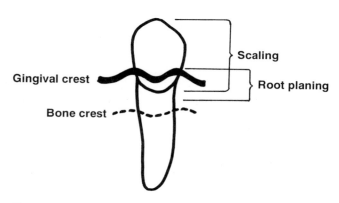

Figure 1. Prophylaxis consists of scaling and polishing natural or restored crowns of teeth, whereas root planing is performed only on natural root structure (cementum or dentin).

References

Hall WB. Clinical practise. In: Steele PF, ed. Dimensions in dental hygiene. 3rd ed. Philadelphia: Lea & Febiger 1982:143.
Hall WB. Procedure code 452: Eliminating the confusion. Cal Dent Assoc J 1983;11:33.

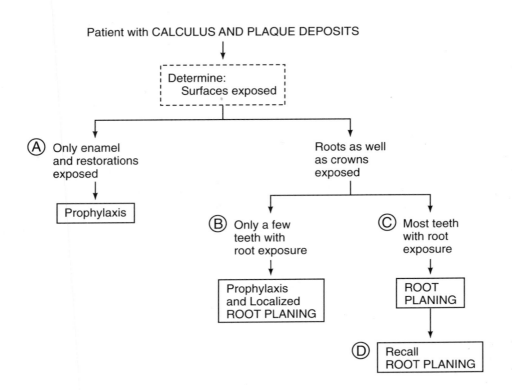

Patient with CALCULUS AND PLAQUE DEPOSITS

Determine:
Surfaces exposed

(A) Only enamel
and restorations
exposed

Prophylaxis

Roots as well
as crowns
exposed

(B) Only a few
teeth with
root exposure

Prophylaxis
and Localized
ROOT PLANING

(C) Most teeth
with root
exposure

ROOT
PLANING

(D) Recall
ROOT PLANING

SURGERY VERSUS REPETITIVE ROOT PLANING

Walter B. Hall

At the time of initial therapy evaluation, the dentist's greatest concern is with what to do next. Broadly speaking, the options are either to do surgery or to maintain the patient with repetitive root planing. The dentist must decide which approach is indicated, but the patient may choose the less desirable option for reasons such as cost or fear. Esthetics becomes a concern when surgery appears to be a reasonable option in maxillary anterior regions. If the probable aesthetic result of surgery, even if therapeutically successful, would be unacceptable to the patient, maintenance would be a reasonable alternative. In cases in which deep and inaccessible pocket areas would remain, the use of a modified Widman flap might be desirable to permit thorough, one-time debridement while minimizing post-surgical exposure. Guided tissue regeneration may permit very significant restitution of periodontal support on teeth with deep osseous defects, making surgery of this type a most desirable option for a patient with localized severe defects.

A. The success of the patient's plaque control efforts is an important factor in deciding whether a patient "merits" surgery. A patient who has been unable to clean the supragingival portions of the teeth before surgery is not a promising candidate to do well with the more tortuous and minimally accessible areas usually exposed following surgery. A patient who has cleaned these areas well is more likely to be able and willing to clean well after surgery.

B. A patient who has removed plaque well usually has a good response to initial therapy. Signs of inflammation are diminished or absent, and both pocket depth and mobility are likely to have decreased. Occasionally, however, a patient's response is not good, despite efforts at plaque control; surgery for such a patient is less likely to be a good alternative.

C. If the patient's response is exceptionally good and there are no requirements that surgery be considered (i.e., pure mucogingival problems, inadequate crown exposure), the patient may do well with only repetitive planing rather than surgery. If there are restorative demands for a surgical approach, however, one should consider surgery unless the esthetic results would be unacceptable. If the patient has localized areas that are inaccessible to root planing, consider surgery. When esthetic concerns exist, a modified Widman flap approach would permit a one-time, thorough debridement, which might be advantageous. A patient whose response has been poor despite good plaque control is not a promising candidate for surgery. If there are no restorative demands for surgery, place the patient on regular, repetitive root planing and evaluation. If there are demanding restorative needs, consider surgery unless the aesthetic results would be unacceptable. If the patient has localized, inaccessible pockets, a modified Widman flap approach or guided tissue regeneration could be employed when esthetics are important, or pocket elimination might be used when esthetics are not a concern or will be minimized restoratively.

D. A patient who has done poorly in plaque control usually shows a poor response to initial therapy; occasionally, however, good responses may occur despite the patient's efforts. For patients with poor oral hygiene who exhibit a good response, surgery may be a practical option if they have restorative needs that would benefit by surgery. If the patient has no esthetic concerns, surgery can be done. If the patient does have aesthetic concerns, maintenance root planing would be a better choice. If the patient with good response but poor oral hygiene has no demanding restorative needs, repeat root planing and evaluate again. If the patient has localized, inaccessible pocket areas, surgery is indicated. If the patient has esthetic concerns, a modified Widman flap approach for one-time, full debridement would be a good choice. If the patient with poor oral hygiene has the expected poor response to initial therapy and no restorative requirements to consider surgery, he should be placed on a repetitive root planing program. If there are restorative requirements, repeat the root planing and evaluate again to see if the patient can improve the oral hygiene to a level at which surgery would be reasonable. If the patient has localized, inaccessible pocket areas, a modified Widman flap approach would permit a one-time, thorough debridement. Guided tissue regeneration could be considered, despite poor oral hygiene, if a very critical tooth could be saved and the patient recognized the risk of continued poor oral hygiene.

References

Carranza FA Jr. Glickman's clinical periodontology. 7th ed. Philadelphia: WB Saunders, 1990:759.

Genco RJ, Goldman HM, Cohen DW. Contemporary periodontics. St. Louis: CV Mosby, 1991:626.

Grant DA, Stern IB, Listgarten MA. Periodontics. St. Louis: CV Mosby, 1988:602.

Lindhe J. Textbook of clinical periodontology. 2nd ed. Copenhagen: Munksgaard, 1989:328.

Schluger S, Yuodelis R, Page RC, Johnson RH. Periodontal diseases. 2nd ed. Philadelphia: Lea & Febiger, 1990:461.

Periodontitis patient for INITIAL THERAPY EVALUATION

Ⓐ Assess:
Oral hygiene

Good oral hygiene

Poor oral hygiene

Ⓑ Assess:
Response to initial therapy

Good response to initial therapy

Poor response to initial therapy

Good response to initial therapy

Poor response to initial therapy

Consider:
Ⓒ Restorative demand for surgery
Esthetic concerns
Ⓓ

Very good response; no restorative demand for surgery

Maintenance

Good response, restorative demand for surgery

Localized, inaccessible areas

Esthetic concern

MODIFIED WIDMAN FLAP PROCEDURE or GUIDED TISSUE REGENERATION

Esthetic concern

Maintenance

No esthetic concern

SURGERY

No esthetic concern

SURGERY

Restorative demand for surgery

Esthetic concern

Maintenance

No esthetic concern

SURGERY

No restorative demand for surgery

Maintenance

Restorative demand for surgery

Esthetic concern

Maintenance

No esthetic concern

SURGERY

No restorative demand for surgery

Repeat PLANING and Reevaluate

Esthetic concern

Maintenance

No esthetic concern

SURGERY

Localized, inaccessible areas

Esthetic concern

MODIFIED WIDMAN FLAP PROCEDURE or GUIDED TISSUE REGENERATION

No esthetic concern

SURGERY

Restorative demand for surgery

Repeat PLANING and Reevaluate

No restorative demand for surgery

Maintenance

SELECTION OF MUCOGINGIVAL–OSSEOUS SURGICAL APPROACHES

Walter B. Hall

Discuss the probability of the need for periodontal surgery with a patient, if indicated, during initial treatment planning. Many patients with complex dental problems will require mucogingival–osseous surgery. Most will have been affected by adult periodontitis and will have a number of teeth with pocket depth, bone loss, and loss of attachment. The character of the bone loss that is present will determine what type of mucogingival–osseous surgery is indicated.

A. First, the dentist must decide whether the problem is one of horizontal bone loss only, one of vertical loss, or a mixed one with some teeth with horizontal and some with vertical bone loss. If the patient has only horizontal bone loss, the severity of loss and the number of severely involved teeth are the factors that would determine the treatment plan. If many teeth are severely affected, mucogingival–osseous surgery would be contraindicated. The teeth should either be extracted or maintained with a hopeless prognosis. The restorative plan would be determined by which, if any, teeth could be utilized. If the horizontal bone loss was not severe or generalized, pocket elimination surgery with osteoplasty to create the most readily maintainable contours would be best.

B. If vertical bone loss is involved, the types of osseous defects that are present will determine which type of

surgery is indicated. One-walled defects that are shallow should be managed with pocket elimination surgery and osseous resection (ostectomy and osteoplasty). If a one-walled defect is moderate to deep, consider the value of the individual tooth to the overall treatment plan. If the tooth is of little value, extraction would be the best approach. If the tooth is critical to the overall treatment plan, employ guided tissue regeneration or guided tissue regeneration with concomitant or second-stage osseous resection.

C. If two-walled defects are present, the surgical approach would depend upon whether the defects are craters (defects between adjacent teeth where facial and lingual cortical plates remain) or the less common type that affects only one tooth in which either a facial or a lingual cortical plate and a wall against the adjacent tooth remain. If a crater is present and it is a shallow defect, pocket elimination surgery with osseous resection would be best. If the crater is a moderate to deep one, use guided tissue regeneration. If the two-walled defect is one that affects only a single tooth, its value to the overall treatment plan would determine whether guided tissue regeneration or extraction would be best.

D. If a three-walled defect is present, its depth and its horizontal width from root to osseous crest determine

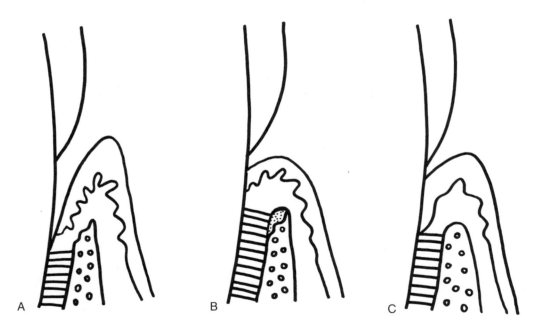

Figure 1. Surgical procedures may result in regeneration of lost bone with new connective tissue attachment of bone to new cementum or in pocket closure by means of a "long" epithelial attachment. **A**, Preoperative defect; **B**, Regeneration; **C**, Pocket closure.

Patient in need of MUCOGINGIVAL–OSSEOUS SURGERY

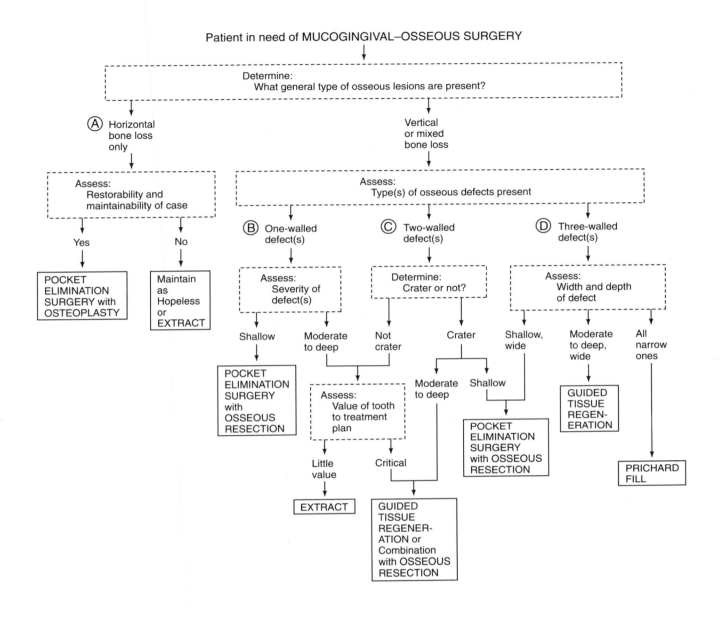

the surgical approach. A narrow defect (less than 1 mm horizontally from root to osseous crest) is amenable to a "Prichard fill" technique, wherein total debridement will be followed by bone fill and new attachment on a predictable basis. If the defect is a wide (more than 1 mm horizontally from root to osseous crest), moderate to deep one, guided tissue regeneration is a predictable means of gaining new attachment. If the defect is a wide, shallow one, pocket elimination with osseous resection is best.

References

Carranza FA Jr. Glickman's clinical periodontology. 7th ed. Philadelphia: WB Saunders, 1990:759.

Genco RJ, Goldman HM, Cohen DW. Contemporary periodontics. St. Louis: CV Mosby, 1990:554.

Pihlstrom BL, Ortiz Campos C, McHugh RB. A randomized four year study of periodontal therapy. J Periodontol 1981;52:227.

Waerhaug J. Healing of the dento-epithelial junction following subgingival plaque control. I. As observed on extracted teeth. J Periodontol 1978;49:119.

Weeks PR. Pros and cons of periodontal pocket elimination procedures. J West Soc Periodontol 1980;28:4.

ADJUNCTIVE PLAQUE CONTROL DEVICES

Walter B. Hall

All patients should use a toothbrush, usually with a sulcular brushing technique. In addition, adjunctive devices can help to clean interproximal areas. Ideally, all patients should also use floss daily; however, some groups of patients are unable to manipulate floss but may be able to use devices that require less dexterity.

A. Patients with a variety of handicaps are unable to use floss, usually because of compromised dexterity. Physical handicaps that restrict arm and hand movement may be of long-term or short-term duration. Arthritis often creates problems with finger movement. Many aged patients lose dexterity. Many mentally handicapped persons, however, can be taught to use floss, although the learning process may be long and tedious. For the handicapped who cannot use hand-held floss, a floss holder may permit its use. Thin, birchwood sticks, shaped to fit interproximal spaces, are easily manipulated and require little dexterity. In Scandinavia, these sticks often are used instead of floss and achieve good removal of interproximal plaque. Stimudents are less satisfactory because of their much larger dimensions. Interproximal brushes, especially those with short handles, are excellent devices for the removal of interproximal plaque.

B. Not all patients who are able to use floss are willing to do so regularly. Some localized situations, also, are better managed with adjunctive devices (Figs. 1 and 2).

C. Where roots are close together, certain devices cannot be inserted into the available space. Where space is adequate, interproximal brushes (especially those with short handles) are most effective and easy to use. The Perio Aide (a round toothpick-holding device) may be quite effective; however, it is much more difficult to use and can cause damage if pressed into pockets or broken off. Super Floss (dental tape with thickened areas at regular intervals) may be effective where plain floss is not; however, it must be used with a "shoe-shine" approach, which can produce "floss cuts" and tooth abrasion. For those situations in which root proximity makes these devices unusable or dangerous, the thin, birchwood sticks may be effective if furcations are not too badly involved.

D. The Interplak brush, a mechanical brush with ten independently moving tufts, has proven especially effective because of its alternating movements; however, it is expensive. The Uni Tuft brush is a single-tufted brush designed to clean such anatomically difficult areas. The Perio Aide also may be useful here.

E. Where roots are close together or irregularly aligned, the thin, birchwood sticks are most effective and easily used.

F. A cut-off toothbrush may be purchased for the distal surfaces of the most posterior teeth, or one can be made easily using an old brush. All of the tufts are cut off close to the handle except for the last few tufts nearest the end of the handle. Once these tufts have been cut off, the remaining tufts can be applied to the distal surface of the most posterior teeth without the missing tufts pushing against the occlusal surface and restricting contact on the distal surface.

G. Many patients have difficulty removing plaque from the lingual surfaces of lingually tilted teeth for much the same reason that the distal surfaces of the most posterior teeth are difficult to clean. The cut-off brush may be used quite effectively in these cases, too.

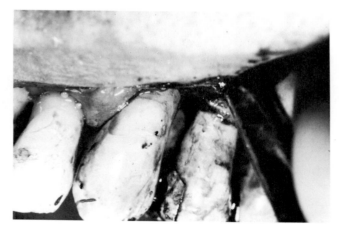

Figure 1. A deep fluting in the root structure of a maxillary first premolar which cannot be cleaned by flossing.

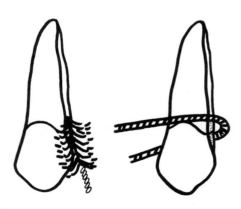

Figure 2. An interproximal brush is more effective than floss for cleaning a deep fluting.

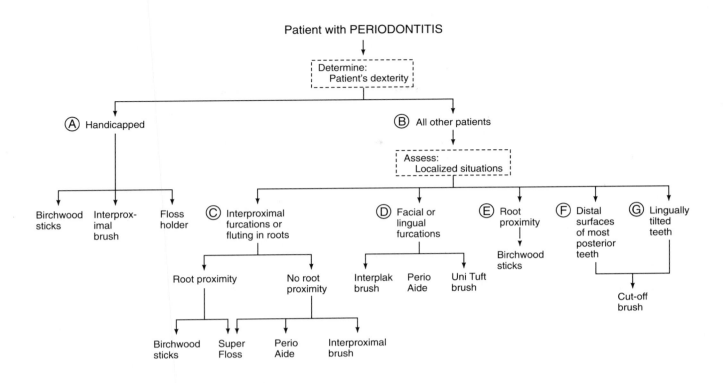

Patient with PERIODONTITIS

Determine:
Patient's dexterity

(A) Handicapped

(B) All other patients

Assess:
Localized situations

Birchwood sticks

Interproximal brush

Floss holder

(C) Interproximal furcations or fluting in roots

Root proximity

No root proximity

Birchwood sticks

Super Floss

Perio Aide

Interproximal brush

(D) Facial or lingual furcations

Interplak brush

Perio Aide

Uni Tuft brush

(E) Root proximity

Birchwood sticks

(F) Distal surfaces of most posterior teeth

(G) Lingually tilted teeth

Cut-off brush

References

Carranza FA, Jr. Glickman's clinical periodontology. 7th ed. Philadelphia: WB Saunders, 1990:699.

Gjermo P, Flotra L. The plaque-removing effect of dental floss and toothpicks: A group comparison study. J Periodont Res 1969;4:170.

Gjermo P, Flotra L. The effect of different methods of interdental cleaning. J Periodont Res 1970;5:230.

Lindhe J. Textbook of clinical periodontology. 2nd ed. Copenhagen: Munksgaard, 1989:346.

Schluger S, Yuodelis R, Page RC, Johnson RH. Periodontal diseases. 2nd ed. Philadelphia: Lea & Febiger, 1990:362.

PERIODONTALLY COMPROMISED POTENTIAL ABUTMENT TEETH

Walter B. Hall

One of the most complex decisions that a dentist must make regularly involves determining the adequacy of periodontally involved teeth to function as abutments in a restorative treatment plan. The dentist must decide by weighing the pros and cons of each of the many factors involved. The patient must be informed of, and able to cope with, various degrees of uncertainty in such complex decisions and must be able to afford the cost of the whole treatment plan before proceeding. If the patient elects not to proceed, the dentist must advise him of the probable consequences of this decision. Such complex situations require careful documentation.

A. The status of the attachment of the potential abutment tooth is very important. A tooth that has lost more than half of its attachment is a poor risk as an abutment; however, if that tooth has a narrow, three-walled osseous defect, it is a candidate for a bone regeneration procedure, and there is a reasonable likelihood of success sufficient to change the prognosis for the tooth. In situations in which guided tissue regeneration has a strong probability of success (i.e., wide three-walled defects, deep Class II furcations, many two-walled infrabony craters), a tooth that would be a poor abutment can be converted to one that may make a good-to-excellent abutment (see pp 152, 154). If this situation does not exist and the tooth has lost more than half of its support, it is unlikely to be a good abutment risk. If the tooth has moderate loss of attachment, it has a reasonable prognosis for successful use as an abutment. If it has little loss of attachment, it is a good candidate.

B. Root form is another important factor to assess. Several radiographs of the tooth can be used to give an important conceptualization of the form for the root (Fig. 1). Exploration of furcations on a multirooted

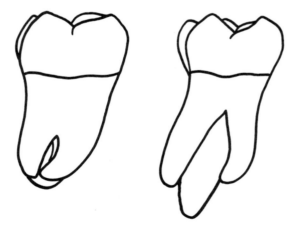

Figure 1. Molar teeth may have fused or spread roots. The spread type usually provides better support as an abutment for a restoration replacing a missing tooth.

tooth can provide useful information on its potential cleansability. Teeth with small or cone-shaped roots are poor abutments as compared with those with large roots (or flared ones on multirooted teeth). If a molar has a Class II furca involvement that is involved 3 mm or more horizontally but is not a Class III ("through-and-through") involvement, it is a good candidate for guided tissue regeneration with eventual use as an abutment (see pp 128 and 134). If a molar has a "through-and-through" involvement, root amputation or hemisection may make its remaining parts useful as an abutment(s) if that approach can be afforded by the patient (see p 138). A molar with minimal furcation involvement and flared roots, however, is a good candidate for abutment.

C. The status of the crown of the potential abutment also is important. If it is badly broken down, it is a poorer candidate than if it can be restored readily. Crown lengthening can improve the potential restorability of some poorer candidates (see pp 234 and 236).

D. The pulpal status affects the potential of a tooth to be used as an abutment. If the tooth has been endodontically treated but either requires further treatment (i.e., apicoectomy) or retreatment or appears to have a cracked root, its usefulness as an abutment depends upon the likelihood of success of the additional treatment. If its root is cracked or it cannot be retreated, it is not a potential abutment. If the earlier endodontic procedure appears satisfactory, the tooth usually is a good potential abutment. If the tooth has an untreated pulpal problem, its potential for use as an abutment depends upon factors affecting the probability for successful endodontic treatment (i.e., accessibility of root canals, presence of pulp stones or internal resorption). If it is treatable, it has good potential as an abutment. A tooth with a healthy pulp, however, is almost always a better abutment candidate than an endodontically treated one, because endodontically treated teeth become more brittle and more susceptible to fractures.

E. The alignment of a tooth affects its usefulness as an abutment. A significant malposed tooth that cannot be orthodontically moved into good alignment is a poor potential abutment. Some periodontally involved teeth are good candidates for orthodontic movement (see p 128) and can become fair-to-good candidates for use as abutments, but only at considerable cost to the patient both in time and in money. A tooth already in normal or usual alignment is always a better candidate for use as an abutment.

F. The number of other abutment teeth and their periodontal statuses affect the potential usability of the tooth in question as an abutment. If few other potential abutments are present and they have much loss of

Patient with PERIODONTALLY COMPROMISED POTENTIAL ABUTMENT TOOTH

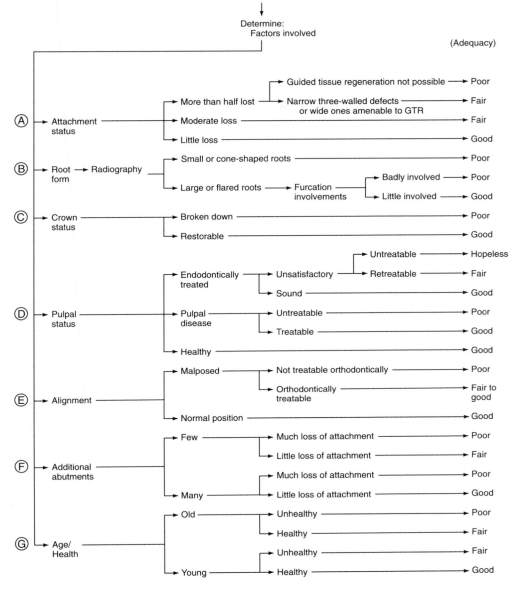

attachment, the tooth in question is a poorer candidate for use as an abutment, because more will be demanded of it. If the other potential abutments, though few in number, have little loss of attachment, the tooth in question is a better candidate. If there are many additional potential abutment teeth, but all or most have significant loss of attachment, the potential use of the tooth in question is less. If the other potential abutments have lost little attachment, the tooth in question has better possibilities for use as an abutment, too.

G. Other factors (such as plaque removal skills of the patient and regularity of dental care) must be weighed by the dentist and patient in deciding upon the potential for a periodontally involved tooth to be used as an abutment. Age and health are two essential factors, however. In one sense, older patients have poorer prognoses than younger ones because their healing capabilities are likely to be lower. In another sense, older patients have better prognoses in that their teeth and dental work will not have to last as long, on the average. A potential abutment tooth that is periodontally compromised in an otherwise healthy patient has a better prognosis, in general, than one in an unhealthy mouth.

References

Grant DA, Stern IB, Listgarten MA. Periodontics. 6th ed. St. Louis: CV Mosby, 1988:982.

Hall WB. Periodontal preparation of the mouth for restoration. Dent Clin North Am 1980;24:195.

Schluger S, Yuodelis R, Page RC, Johnson RH. Periodontal diseases. 2nd ed. Philadelphia: Lea & Febiger, 1990:341.

PERIODONTAL CHEMOTHERAPY

William P. Lundergan

Bacterial plaque is accepted as the primary etiologic agent in the establishment and progression of inflammatory periodontal disease. Recognition of the bacterial etiology stimulated considerable interest in antimicrobial agents as adjuncts to mechanical periodontal therapy. Today, antibiotics and antimicrobial rinses have a role in periodontal therapy, but their use should not be indiscriminate and is not without potential hazards. The clinician should be thoroughly familiar with all potential adverse reactions before prescribing or recommending any chemotherapeutic agent.

A. Patients treated with antibiotic therapy should be closely monitored for therapeutic response and potential side effects. Patients who fail to respond to therapy may require a culture of the subgingival flora with evaluation of antibiotic sensitivity. Pretreatment and post-treatment microbiologic analysis may prove useful in monitoring therapeutic success.

B. The periodontal abscess, pericoronitis, and acute necrotizing ulcerative gingivitis (NUG) are all acute diseases that often present for emergency treatment. Treatment of the acute signs and symptoms is generally best accomplished with local debridement. Antibiotics are usually unnecessary unless the patient is febrile, exhibits lymphadenopathy, is in danger of developing a cellulitis, or does not respond to local debridement within 24 hours. If an antibiotic is indicated, penicillin is the drug of choice. Cephalexin or clindamycin can be used if the infection is not responding in 24 to 48 hours. If the patient is allergic to penicillin, erythromycin is a good alternative. Metronidazole has been used in the treatment of NUG and the acute lesions associated with human immunodeficiency virus (HIV) periodontitis.

C. Antibiotics generally offer no advantage over conventional periodontal therapy (i.e., mechanical plaque control, root planing, elimination of secondary local factors, periodontal surgery, and maintenance) in the treatment of chronic adult periodontitis.

D. Antibiotics can be useful adjuncts to conventional therapy in the treatment of early onset periodontitis (prepubertal periodontitis, juvenile periodontitis, and rapidly progressive periodontitis). The adjunctive use of antibiotics, particularly tetracycline, has been shown to be an effective mode of therapy in treating localized juvenile periodontitis. Optimal dosing regimens, however, have not been determined. Tetracycline hydrochloride, in doses of 250 mg taken every 6 hours for 2 to 6 weeks, has been used. Doxycycline, 100 mg, is generally given daily for 14 days. Metronidazole and amoxicillin of varying amounts have been given in combination three times daily for 7 days. Definitive studies are lacking for prepubertal periodontitis and rapidly progressive periodontitis. Tetracycline should not be used in children under 8 years of age because of the risk for intrinsic staining of permanent teeth. The combination of metronidazole and amoxicillin given three times daily for 7 days should be considered when treating children in this age group. Augmentin (amoxicillin and clavulanic acid) is preferred to amoxicillin because it incorporates the beta-lactanase inhibitor clavulanic acid.

E. Studies suggest that systemic antibiotic therapy can be a useful adjunct to conventional therapy in the treatment of refractory periodontitis. Tetracycline hydrochloride, doxycycline, metronidazole, clindamycin, amoxicillin/clavulanic acid, and metronidazole in combination with amoxicillin and clavulanic acid have all been evaluated. Studies comparing effectiveness of these agents have largely not been done. Tetracycline, 250 mg, is typically given four times daily for 2 to 4 weeks. Doxycycline has a compliance advantage in that it is usually given daily in a single 100-mg dose for 2 to 3 weeks. Metronidazole, 250 mg, is given three times daily for 7 to 10 days. Clindamycin, 150 mg, is given four times daily for 7 days. Clindamycin should be used with caution because of its association with a pseudomembranous colitis that can prove fatal. A 250-mg dose of amoxicillin/clavulanic acid (Augmentin) has been given three times daily for 10 to 14 days. Although no commercial product is currently available, studies have demonstrated that local sustained-release delivery of antibiotics to specific active sites can prove beneficial in the treatment of refractory periodontitis.

F. Human immunodeficiency virus periodontitis often presents with a more acute periodontal lesion characterized by tissue necrosis and sequestration. Treatment of such acute conditions can be augmented with metronidazole, 250 to 500 mg, given three to four times daily for 5 to 7 days. The patient's physician should be consulted before prescribing antibiotic therapy.

G. Chemical plaque control represents an attractive adjunct to mechanical plaque control; thus, several toothpastes and mouthwashes are now being marketed as chemical plaque inhibitors. Current information suggests that some commercial mouthrinses (e.g., Peridex, Viadent, Listerine, and Cepacol) can reduce plaque and decrease gingival inflammation. Supragingival and subgingival irrigation has been evaluated as an alternative mode of delivery for some of those agents. Irrigation has an apparent advantage over rinsing in that it increases the ability of the product to reach the subgingival flora. Compliance and the requirement for some level of patient dexterity are problems commonly associated with irrigation. Although these products can reduce gingival inflammation, little or no information is available regarding the use of these products as a rinse or as an irrigant in

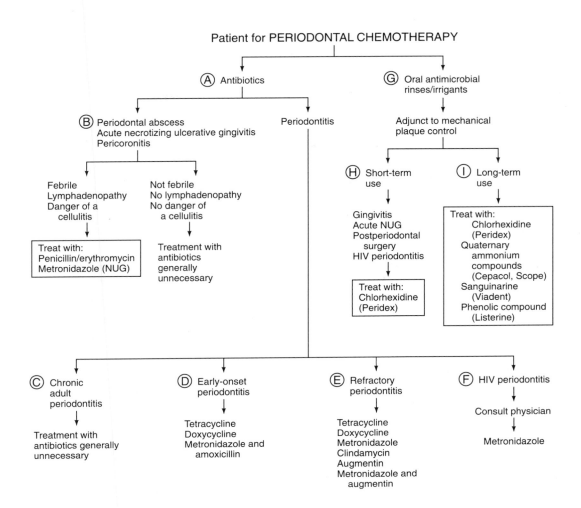

Patient for PERIODONTAL CHEMOTHERAPY

(A) Antibiotics

(G) Oral antimicrobial rinses/irrigants

(B) Periodontal abscess
Acute necrotizing ulcerative gingivitis
Pericoronitis

Periodontitis

Adjunct to mechanical plaque control

Febrile
Lymphadenopathy
Danger of a cellulitis

Not febrile
No lymphadenopathy
No danger of a cellulitis

Treat with:
Penicillin/erythromycin
Metronidazole (NUG)

Treatment with antibiotics generally unnecessary

(H) Short-term use

(I) Long-term use

Gingivitis
Acute NUG
Postperiodontal surgery
HIV periodontitis

Treat with:
Chlorhexidine
(Peridex)

Treat with:
Chlorhexidine
(Peridex)
Quaternary ammonium compounds
(Cepacol, Scope)
Sanguinarine
(Viadent)
Phenolic compound
(Listerine)

(C) Chronic adult periodontitis

Treatment with antibiotics generally unnecessary

(D) Early-onset periodontitis

Tetracycline
Doxycycline
Metronidazole and amoxicillin

(E) Refractory periodontitis

Tetracycline
Doxycycline
Metronidazole
Clindamycin
Augmentin
Metronidazole and augmentin

(F) HIV periodontitis

Consult physician

Metronidazole

preventing and treating periodontitis. Currently, with the exception of Peridex (0.12% chlorhexidine) and Listerine, these antimicrobial products have not been accepted by the American Dental Association's Council on Dental Therapeutics.

H. Numerous studies have demonstrated the safety and effectiveness of chlorhexidine when used in the control of supragingival plaque and gingivitis. Its most appropriate use seems to be as a short-term adjunct to mechanical plaque control. Short-term use of chlorhexidine during the initial healing phase following periodontal surgery may represent one useful application, as gingival and dentinal sensitivity often hamper mechanical plaque control efforts postsurgically. Short-term use of chlorhexidine during the treatment of acute NUG or the acute lesions associated with HIV periodontitis may represent another useful application.

Treatment of NUG requires professional debridement followed by proper home care. Initially, because of gingival discomfort, proper mechanical plaque control is difficult for these patients to achieve. Augmentation with a chemical plaque inhibitor may prove valuable. Antimicrobial agents such as Peridex should be used only under professional supervision, and the therapist should be thoroughly familiar with all potential adverse reactions.

I. The clinician should evaluate carefully the risk-to-benefit ratio before recommending long-term use of Peridex (0.12% chlorhexidine). Stain and increased supragingival calculus can be expected. Stain is especially a problem around silicate composite restorations. Painful gingival and mucosal desquamations have been associated with 0.2% concentrations of chlorhexidine, and some patients experience an alteration in their sense of taste. Bacterial resistance does not seem to develop, but longer evaluation periods are needed. The relationship between the use of chlorhexidine and the rate of formation of subgingival calculus needs to be ascertained. Several other over-the-counter antimicrobial rinses are available, and they have shown some efficacy in reducing plaque and gingivitis. Most of these agents are also associated with varying degrees of tooth discoloration, and some cause a temporary burning sensation.

References

Lindhe J. Textbook of clinical periodontology. Philadelphia: WB Saunders, 1983:335.
Slots J, Rams TE. Antibiotics in periodontal therapy: Advantages and disadvantages. J Clin Periodontal 1990;17:479.

ESTABLISHING THE ADEQUACY OF ATTACHED GINGIVA

Walter B. Hall

When a tooth has a minimal amount of attached gingiva on either its facial or lingual surface, it should be indicated as a potential pure mucogingival problem. The term *inadequate attached gingiva* was coined during the 1960s and has been defined loosely by many investigators. Rather than being a fixed number of millimeters of attached gingiva, it is a clinical estimate by the treating dentist of the adequacy of the attached gingiva on an individual tooth to remain stable and healthy either under conditions imposed by any planned dental treatment or in the absence of any dental treatment involving the tooth (Fig. 1). The "attached gingiva" has been defined by Hall as ". . . that gingiva extending from the free margin of the gingiva to the mucogingival line minus the pocket or sulcus depth measured with a thin probe in the absence of inflammation." That the gingiva is "inadequate" in an individual case is a clinical decision made by the treating dentist based upon a judgment of the tooth's needs within the patient's overall treatment plan. The decision on the need to treat is made with the concurrence of the informed patient (or parent).

A. A simple guideline for determining whether a pure mucogingival problem exists is to record all areas with less than 2 mm of total gingiva as being potential problems because they will have 1 mm or less attached gingiva when crevice depth is subtracted from the total gingiva. This does not mean that all such cases require grafting. Conversely, although a tooth may have more than 2 mm of total gingiva, it may still have 1 mm or less of attached gingiva when crevice depth is subtracted from total gingiva. In such a case, its need for grafting would be treated similarly to any case with 1 mm or less of attached gingiva. It still might require grafting if the tooth were to function as an abutment for a rest-proximal plate-I (RPI) bar-type removable partial denture or an overdenture.

B. For teeth with less than 1 mm of attached gingiva, the patient's age must be considered. Younger patients are more likely to require treatment than are older ones because of the longer period of time in which they could (as a group) expect to keep their teeth.

C. If a young patient has less than 1 mm of attached gingiva on a tooth and is having active recession (i.e., any root exposure at this age), consider using a graft on a periosteal bed which has a high predictability of success. This is preferable to using a graft that is dependent upon new attachment to an exposed root. If the young patient has no recession but restorative procedures (such as Class V restoration) or orthodontic treatment is planned, consider grafting prophylactically. If no such restorative or orthodontic work is planned, observe the area for change at all future visits rather than grafting at this time. If the patient is older, has less than 1 mm of attached gingiva on a tooth, and has active recession, consider grafting at this time. If the situation appears stable (with or without root exposure), the need to treat will depend upon restorative or orthodontic plans. If crowns, bridges, RPI partials, or overdentures are planned involving this tooth or if orthodontic work is planned, consider grafting; if not, observe the area for evidence of change.

D. If the patient has 2 mm or more of attached gingiva on a tooth that will not serve as an abutment for an RPI removable partial or an overdenture, grafting need not be considered. If such a restoration is planned, however, the tooth may require grafting either to create at least 3 mm of attached gingiva over which the RPI clasp would be positioned or to support the movement resulting from an overdenture. If the tooth has 3 mm or more of attached gingiva, grafting is not likely to be needed.

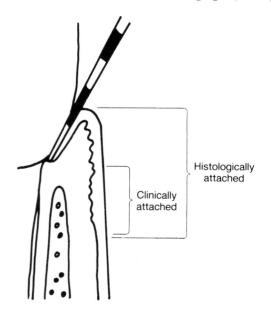

Figure 1. A probe in the sulcus illustrating the difference between clinically and histologically attached gingiva.

References

Hall WB. Present status of soft tissue grafting. J Periodontol 1977;48:587.

Hall WB. Pure mucogingival problems. Berlin: Quintessence Publishing, 1984:61.

Lang NP, Loe H. The relationship between the width of the attached gingiva and gingival health. J Periodontol 1972;43:623.

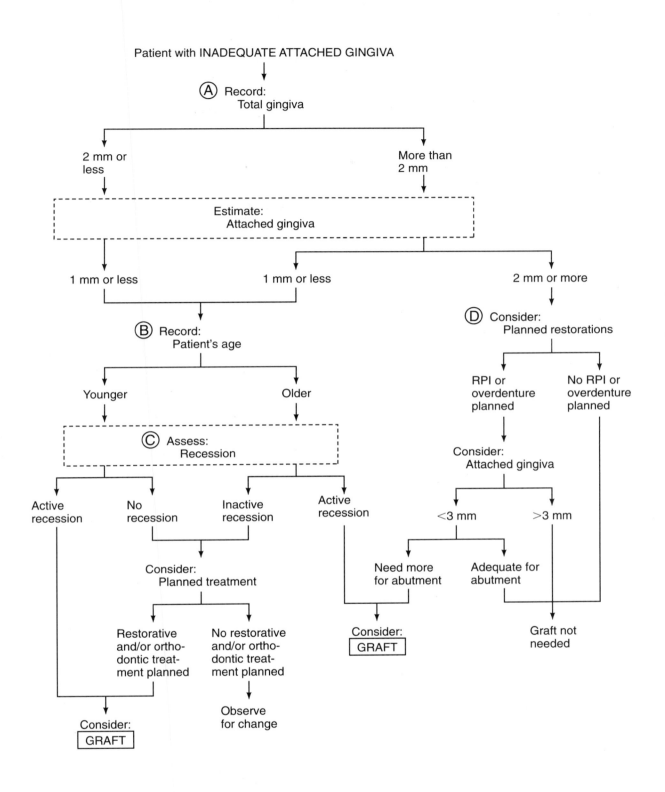

Patient with INADEQUATE ATTACHED GINGIVA

Ⓐ Record:
Total gingiva

2 mm or less   More than 2 mm

Estimate:
Attached gingiva

1 mm or less   1 mm or less   2 mm or more

Ⓑ Record:
Patient's age

Younger   Older

Ⓒ Assess:
Recession

Active recession   No recession   Inactive recession   Active recession

Consider:
Planned treatment

Restorative and/or orthodontic treatment planned   No restorative and/or orthodontic treatment planned

Consider:
GRAFT

Observe for change

Ⓓ Consider:
Planned restorations

RPI or overdenture planned   No RPI or overdenture planned

Consider:
Attached gingiva

<3 mm   >3 mm

Need more for abutment   Adequate for abutment

Consider:
GRAFT

Graft not needed

Lindhe J. Textbook of clinical periodontology. 2nd ed. Copenhagen: Munksgaard, 1989:422.

Maynard JG, Wilson RDK. Physiologic dimensions of the periodontium significant to the restorative dentist. J Periodontol 1979;50:170.

World workshop in clinical periodontics. Chicago: American Academy of Periodontology, 1989:VII-10.

ACTIVE RECESSION VERSUS STABILITY

Walter B. Hall

When a dentist detects a tooth with little or no attached gingiva, it is necessary to determine whether the situation is stable or whether active recession is occurring before one decides to create additional attached gingiva. If a predisposed tooth can be shown to be in a stable state, there is no impetus to graft, whereas there would be if active recession were occurring.

A. When a tooth that is predisposed to recession because of lack of adequate attached gingiva has no root exposure, the situation is stable. If restorative or orthodontic treatment plans indicate that recession could be precipitated on the predisposed tooth by this treatment, consider prophylactic free gingival grafting. If no such treatment is planned, inform the patient about the problem, and either consider prophylactic grafting or evaluate the tooth regularly for indications of change. The dentist and patient together may decide to proceed with restorative work or orthodontics without grafting prophylactically; should recession occur or progress, a connective tissue graft (see p 206) usually would be the treatment of choice in attempting to repair the receded area, but a pedicle graft might be indicated in some cases (i.e., where an adequate connective tissue graft donor site does not exist and an adequate pedicle donor is present) (see p 104).

B. If root exposure is present, earlier records are helpful in determining whether recession is active or the condition is stable. If such records exist and indicate that the situation is stable, continue to observe the area unless restorative or orthodontic plans indicate the need to create more gingiva before proceeding. If comparison with earlier records demonstrates that recession has occurred, gingival grafting is indicated, as it is a more predictable means of covering receded roots than free gingival grafting. When this is not possible, a pedicle graft would be an alternative choice.

C. If no earlier records exist, only the patient's impressions are available to help with the decision whether or not to graft. If the patient believes that recession is occurring actively, a connective tissue graft should be considered. If the patient believes that the root exposure occurred earlier and is stable now, document the problem area and observe it regularly for change unless restorative or orthodontic plans indicate a need to graft now. If there are no earlier records and the patient cannot provide an impression as to the stability of the area of root exposure, document and observe it regularly for change unless other treatment, which is planned, indicates a need to graft now. If treatment is needed now or in the future, a connective tissue graft would be the best approach.

References

Gartrell JR, Mathews DP. Gingival recession: The condition, process and treatment. Dent Clin North Am 1976;20:199.

Hall WB. Pure mucogingival problems. Berlin: Quintessence Publishing, 1984:178.

Rateitschak KH, Egli V, Fingeli G. Recession: A four-year longitudinal study after free gingival grafts. J Clin Periodontol 1979;6:158.

Wilson RD. Marginal tissue recession in general practise: A preliminary study. Int J Periodontol Res Dent 1983;3:41.

World workshop in clinical periodontics. Chicago: American Academy of Periodontology, 1989:VII-10.

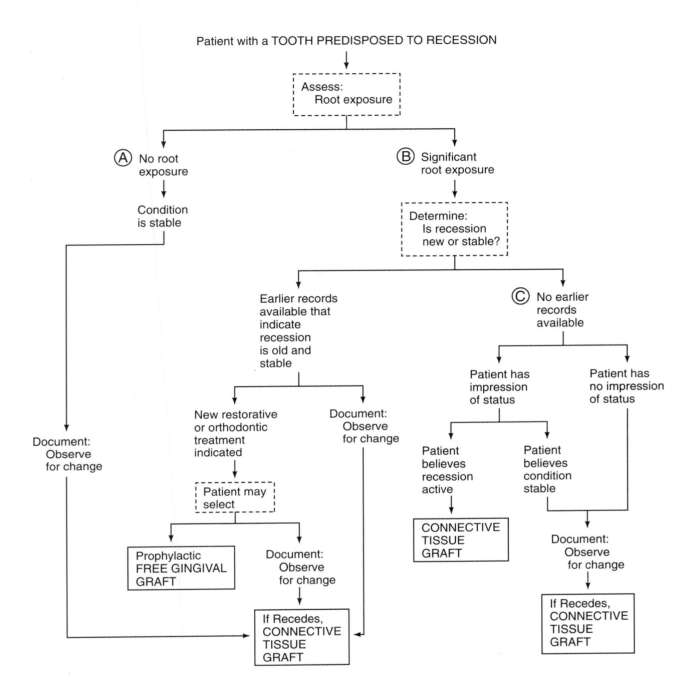

Patient with a TOOTH PREDISPOSED TO RECESSION

Assess:
Root exposure

(A) No root exposure

(B) Significant root exposure

Condition is stable

Determine:
Is recession new or stable?

Document:
Observe for change

Earlier records available that indicate recession is old and stable

(C) No earlier records available

New restorative or orthodontic treatment indicated

Document:
Observe for change

Patient has impression of status

Patient has no impression of status

Patient may select

Patient believes recession active

Patient believes condition stable

Prophylactic FREE GINGIVAL GRAFT

Document:
Observe for change

CONNECTIVE TISSUE GRAFT

Document:
Observe for change

If Recedes, CONNECTIVE TISSUE GRAFT

If Recedes, CONNECTIVE TISSUE GRAFT

PATIENT AGE AND GINGIVAL GRAFTING

Walter B. Hall

When a dentist notes an area of inadequate attached gingiva on a patient's tooth, the age of that patient is an important consideration in deciding when or if gingival grafting should be performed. Generally speaking, the younger the patient, the greater the reason to consider grafting; conversely, the older the patient, the greater the basis for continuing to observe for change. The teeth most likely to have problems of inadequate gingiva are the mandibular incisors, maxillary and mandibular canines, and first premolars. The effects of age on the decision to graft on each of these groups of teeth is different.

A. The mandibular central incisors are the first permanent teeth to erupt. About 12% of these teeth have less than 1 mm of attached gingiva; half of these teeth have some root exposure within 6 months of reaching the plane of occlusion. If active recession is occurring, regardless of the age of the patient, a free gingival graft can be placed to halt further recession and to encourage some "creeping attachment." If little or no recession has occurred, the patient might elect to have the area documented and observed for change. If the recession has been extensive when first detected and significant root exposure has occurred already, a connective tissue graft would be the treatment of choice. If no adequate donor exists (see p 104), a pedicle graft can be employed if an adequate donor site can be found. If an area that has been documented and is being observed begins to recede, a similar decision to employ a connective tissue graft or a pedicle graft should be made. If active recession is not occurring, the decision as to the need for grafting is more complex. For older adults, document the position of the free margin of the gingiva and observe carefully at regular intervals to determine if root exposure is occurring. If a restoration is to be placed close to the gingival margin or subgingivally, assay the need for grafting prior to restoration (see p 92). If the patient is a child or young adult with no root exposure yet, consider prophylactic free gingival grafting to prevent recession. If root exposure already exists but appears to be stable, grafting still should be considered; however, a connective tissue graft or pedicle graft would be the treatment of choice.

B. If a canine or first premolar has an inadequate band of attached gingiva, maxillary teeth often present esthetic concerns or restorative concerns relating to actual or potential root exposure. If active recession is occurring, a connective tissue graft approach is preferable either to cover existing root exposure or to stop further recession, because the color match between adjacent gingiva and the involved area is better than when palatal gingiva is employed in free grafting. When active recession is not occurring and the patient is an older adult, the existing condition need only be documented and observed for change unless restorative plans necessitate grafting beforehand (see p 92). If the patient is a child or younger adult, however, he or his parent may select a prophylactic graft now or wait to observe whether recession is active. If recession does occur, employ a connective tissue graft or, alternatively, a pedicle graft (see p 104). A similar decision should be made if active recession occurs on a maxillary canine or first premolar in the mouth of an older individual.

C. If a mandibular canine or first premolar has an inadequate band of attached gingiva, and active recession is occurring regardless of the age of the patient, a free gingival graft could be employed to stop further recession; however, a connective tissue graft or, alternatively, a pedicle graft would be the treatment of choice to attain root coverage. Also, a broader band of attached gingiva can be placed either to stop further recession or (less predictably) to cover existing exposure. If no active recession is occurring, and no root exposure has occurred earlier, document the position of the free margin of the gingiva and evaluate the area regularly as to whether recession has begun. Restorative needs may indicate grafting even at this time (see p 98). If root exposure already exists or if active recession is documented, a connective tissue graft or, alternatively, a pedicle graft should be placed (see p 104).

References

Hall WB. The current status of mucogingival problems and their therapy. J Periodontol 1981;52:569.

Hall WB. Pure mucogingival problems. Berlin: Quintessence Publishing, 1984:173.

Maynard JG, Ochsenbein C. Mucogingival problems: Prevalence and therapy in children. J Periodontol 1975;46:543.

Wilson RD. Marginal tissue recession in general dental practice: A preliminary study. Int J Periodontol Res Dent 1983;3:41.

World workshop in clinical periodontics. Chicago: American Academy of Periodontology, 1989:VII-1.

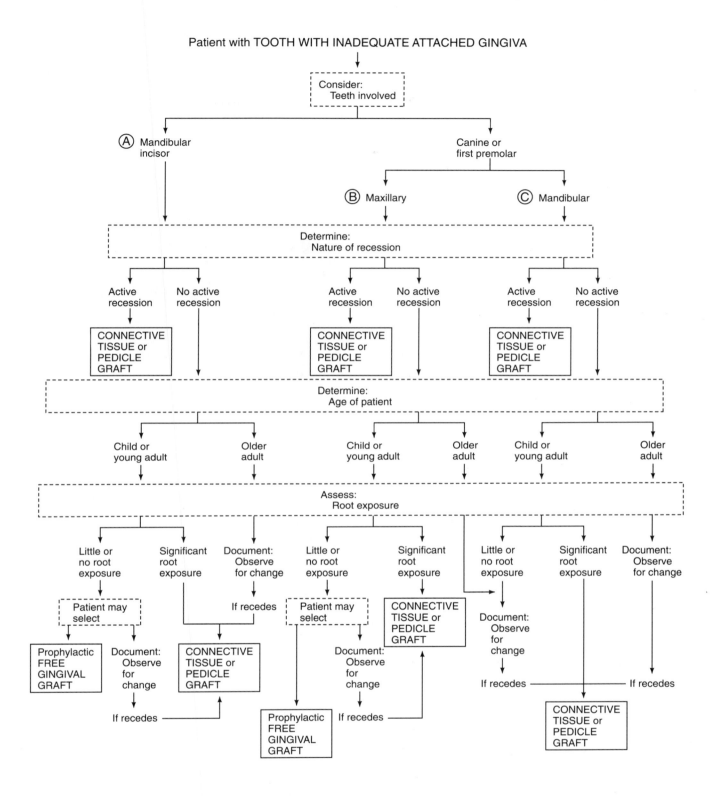

Patient with TOOTH WITH INADEQUATE ATTACHED GINGIVA

Consider:
Teeth involved

(A) Mandibular incisor

Canine or first premolar

(B) Maxillary

(C) Mandibular

Determine:
Nature of recession

Active recession

No active recession

CONNECTIVE TISSUE or PEDICLE GRAFT

Active recession

No active recession

CONNECTIVE TISSUE or PEDICLE GRAFT

Active recession

No active recession

CONNECTIVE TISSUE or PEDICLE GRAFT

Determine:
Age of patient

Child or young adult

Older adult

Child or young adult

Older adult

Child or young adult

Older adult

Assess:
Root exposure

Little or no root exposure

Significant root exposure

Document:
Observe for change

Little or no root exposure

Significant root exposure

Little or no root exposure

Significant root exposure

Document:
Observe for change

Patient may select

If recedes

Patient may select

CONNECTIVE TISSUE or PEDICLE GRAFT

Document:
Observe for change

Prophylactic FREE GINGIVAL GRAFT

Document:
Observe for change

CONNECTIVE TISSUE or PEDICLE GRAFT

Document:
Observe for change

If recedes

If recedes

If recedes

If recedes

Prophylactic FREE GINGIVAL GRAFT

CONNECTIVE TISSUE or PEDICLE GRAFT

CONNECTIVE TISSUE or PEDICLE GRAFT

RESTORATIVE PLANS AND GINGIVAL GRAFTING

Walter B. Hall

Upon determining that a tooth that is predisposed to recession by lack of adequate attached gingiva has restorative needs or is going to be used as an abutment, the dentist must decide whether grafting to increase the band of attached gingiva is indicated. The patient who elects not to proceed with a graft, when indicated, must be informed of the potential problems.

A. If the predisposed tooth requires restoration, the type of restoration and its locale are most important. If the restoration is a Class V but is to be supragingival, there is no need to graft. If the Class V restoration is to be close to the gingiva margin or subgingival, consider a graft. If the restoration is to be of any other class, grafting need not be considered.

B. If the predisposed tooth requires a crown and the crown margins are to be supragingival, there is no need to graft; however, if the crown margin is to be placed at the gingival margin or subgingivally, grafting is indicated, because the diamond bur will cut soft tissue as well as tooth structure when carried subgingivally and will produce recession as a consequence of the soft-tissue curettage. If the entire crown of the tooth is to be visible and recession would expose a chamfer, the patient must be aware that not grafting is likely to result in a visible gold margin apical to the porcelain facing. Grafting beforehand is strongly encouraged, because the successful covering of such an exposed chamfer surgically after crown placement is exceedingly unlikely.

C. If the predisposed tooth is to become an abutment for a fixed bridge, consider grafting whether or not a subgingival margin will be placed in the area of inadequate attached gingiva, because cleaning either under the pontic or between it and the tooth is likely to produce recession. If a three-quarter crown design is to be employed, grafting should be considered but is not as essential as when a full-crown restoration is to be placed.

D. If the predisposed tooth will serve as an abutment for a rest-proximal plate-I (RPI) bar-type removable partial denture, a graft should be placed sufficiently large enough that the entire I-bar will be over the gingiva. If this is not done, the patient who removes the partial denture by placing a fingernail under the apical end of the I-bar is likely to cause wounding and to induce recession (Fig. 1). A graft usually cannot be placed under an existing I-bar, because the space is inadequate for a graft of sufficient thickness to be placed; therefore, a new partial denture would have to be constructed following grafting.

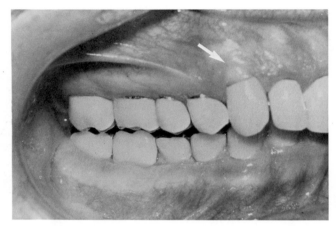

Figure 1. Recession of 3 mm has occurred on the canine (which had inadequate attached gingiva) following crown placement.

E. If the predisposed tooth is to be used as an abutment for an overdenture, much the same situation applies. If recession occurs (which is likely when a full denture is placed in the area), the denture could be relieved and a graft placed, or the denture could be left out while the graft heals. In either case, the graft is likely to be moved about and to fail. Instead, a large flange of acrylic must be cut away, the graft placed, and the overdenture rebased once healing is completed. The more advisable course would be to graft on any predisposed tooth prior to beginning the overdenture treatment. If a graft is to be placed for restorative reasons, the type to be employed would involve considering the options among free gingival grafts, pedicle grafts, or connective tissue grafts (see p 104).

References

Genco EJ, Goldman HM, Cohen DW. Contemporary periodontics. St. Louis: CV Mosby, 1990:621.

Hall, WB. Periodontal preparation of the mouth for restoration. Dent Clin North Am 1980;24:195.

Hall WB. Pure mucogingival problems. Berlin: Quintessence Publishing, 1984:41.

Maynard JG, Wilson RD. Physiologic dimensions of the periodontium significant to the restorative dentist. J Periodontol 1979;50:170.

World workshop in clinical periodontics. Chicago: American Academy of Periodontology, 1989:VII-16.

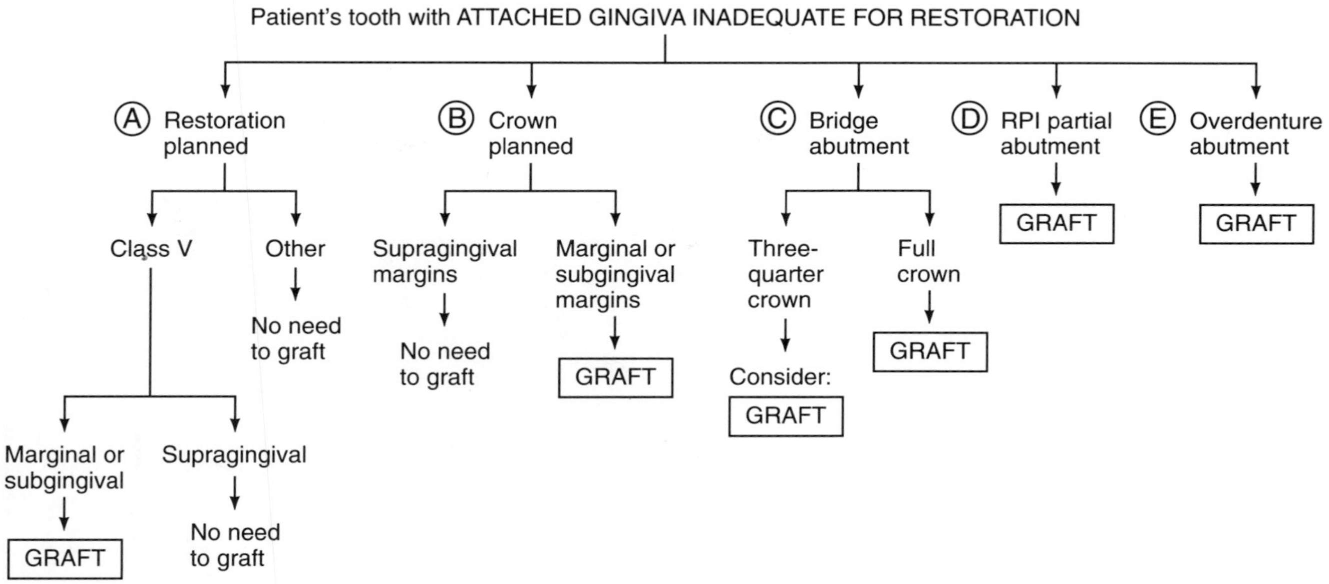

Patient's tooth with ATTACHED GINGIVA INADEQUATE FOR RESTORATION

(A) Restoration planned

Class V

Marginal or subgingival

GRAFT

Supragingival

No need to graft

Other

No need to graft

(B) Crown planned

Supragingival margins

No need to graft

Marginal or subgingival margins

GRAFT

(C) Bridge abutment

Three-quarter crown

Consider:

GRAFT

Full crown

GRAFT

(D) RPI partial abutment

GRAFT

(E) Overdenture abutment

GRAFT

ORTHODONTICS AND GINGIVAL GRAFTING

Walter B. Hall

A patient planning to have orthodontic treatment may have pure mucogingival problems. The dentist must be aware of the relationship of, and the correct sequence of treatment for, orthodontic and pure mucogingival problems when they occur together. Orthodontic and pure mucogingival problems are related, but not in a cause-and-effect manner. A tooth that erupts in a position in which it is in prominent version and, thus, prone to occlusal trauma also is likely to have erupted with minimal attached gingiva. The two problems are related and occur together frequently, but not in a cause-and-effect relationship. Both relate to the prominent eruptive position of the tooth. Understanding this relationship is most important in planning therapy for these cases.

A. The age of the patient is important in deciding how to sequence treatment of combined pure mucogingival and orthodontic problems.

B. If the patient is young and has an overbite—overjet discrepancy that would prohibit free gingival grafting on mandibular incisors prior to some orthodontic movement, proceed with some orthodontic treatment in the maxillary arch prior to grafting so that the graft will not be disturbed directly when the patient closes in centric relation.

C. If the young patient does not have an overbite—overjet problem but has pure mucogingival problems, consider grafting before beginning orthodontic treatment, because the placement of a vestibular arch wire will alter the approach to brushing. Once the arch wire is placed, the brush must be placed apical to it and turned so that the bristle tips contact the teeth and gingiva. The bulkiness of the brush thus positioned causes the lip to press the brush heavily against prominent root surfaces, especially in areas where frena are present. These are the same areas where minimal attached gingiva is present. The patient who struggles to meet the orthodontist's requests for especially good daily plaque removal may wound these predisposed areas, producing recession (Fig. 1). The dentist and patient (and parent when appropriate) should consider gingival grafting of mandibular incisors and all canines that have pure mucogingival problems prior to initiating orthodontic treatment. In the case of predisposed first premolars, another aspect of orthodontic therapy must be considered. In many orthodontic cases, four first premolars or two first premolars are extracted to create space for realigning the remaining teeth. If a first premolar has minimal attached gingiva and is going to be extracted, there is no pure mucogingival concern. If the predisposed tooth is to be retained, however, the need to consider grafting before orthodontic treatment is most important.

D. If the adult patient has no periodontitis, consider grafting of the pure mucogingival problem areas prior

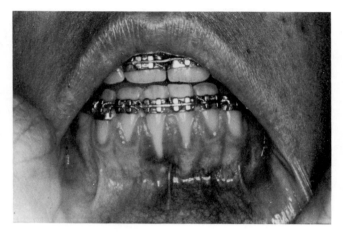

Figure 1. A patient with inadequate attached gingiva who has experienced the illustrated recession since starting orthodontic treatment.

to orthodontic treatment unless the overbite—overjet discrepancy already described exists.

E. If periodontitis is present in the adult patient, the status of potential anchor teeth must be considered first. A molar with a definite furcation involvement or worse (see p 24) is not a good candidate to serve as an anchor tooth. Some teeth with deep pockets may have to be extracted; others may be moved into, or out of, periodontal defects once inflammation is controlled and prognoses have improved (see p 66). If both mucogingival—osseous and pure mucogingival problems exist, their surgical treatment usually is accomplished at the same time. In adult orthodontic cases for which one objective is to move a periodontally involved tooth into, or out of, an osseous defect prior to surgery, the pure mucogingival grafting procedure may be delayed until after the orthodontic goal has been achieved. Then the mucogingival—osseous and pure mucogingival problems can be treated together surgically, if indicated. If there are no periodontitis problems requiring uprighting and no orthodontic movement into defects is being considered, mucogingival—osseous surgery may be employed to correct pocketing and pure mucogingival problems by using an apically positioned flap (see p 164). If problems amenable to guided tissue regeneration exist (see p 148), that approach should be used before orthodontic treatment as a means of regaining lost attachment and creating a greater band of attached gingiva.

References

Boyd RL. Mucogingival considerations and their relationship to orthodontics. J Periodontol 1978;49:67.

Orthodontic patient with PURE MUCOGINGIVAL PROBLEMS

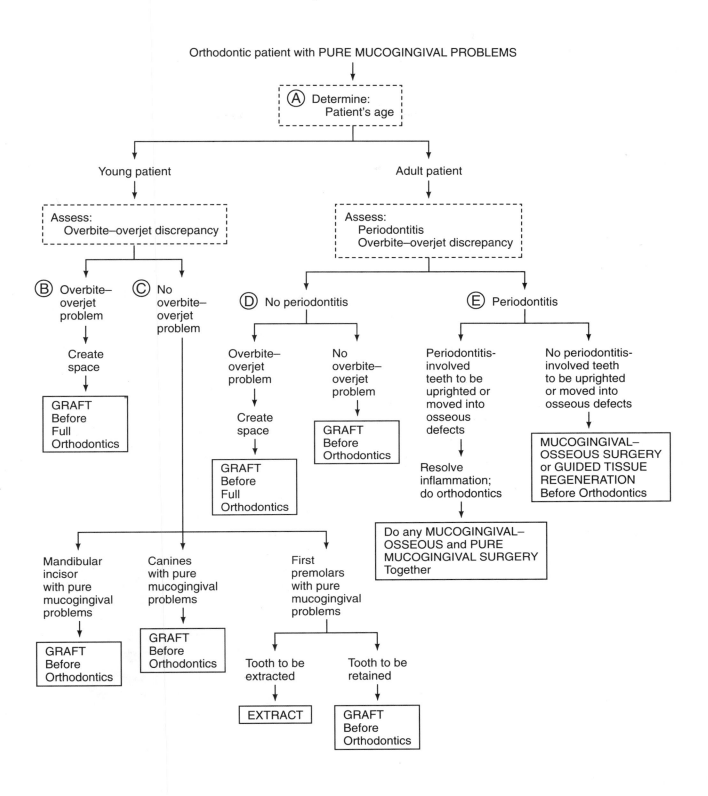

Coatoam GW, Behrents RG, Bissada NF. The width of traumatized gingiva during orthodontic treatment. J Periodontol 1981;52:307.

Dorfman HS. Mucogingival changes resulting from mandibular incisor tooth movement. Am J Orthod 1978;74:286.

Hall WB. Can attached gingiva be increased non-surgically? Quint Int 1982;13:455.

Hall WB. Pure mucogingival problems. Berlin: Quintessence Publishing, 1984:44.

World workshop in clinical periodontics. Chicago: American Academy of Periodontology, 1989:VII-2.

PURE MUCOGINGIVAL CONCERNS OF PATIENTS SCHEDULED FOR ORTHODONTICS: A EUROPEAN VIEW

Giovan Paolo Pini-Prato
Carlo Clauser
Giliana Zuccati

A. Proper plaque control is critical during orthodontic treatment. Orthodontic appliances are a factor in plaque retention; therefore, the patient is required to use a more traumatic method of toothbrushing. Traumatic toothbrushing and plaque accumulation are etiologic factors for recession. Plaque removal may be impaired by anatomic (mucogingival) conditions. Pulling frena or shallow vestibules that affect toothbrushing should be corrected prior to orthodontic treatment.

B. Deep infraosseous impacted teeth (usually upper canines) can be orthodontically guided to erupt in the center of the alveolar crest, where adequate keratinized tissue is physiologically available, thereby preventing any mucogingival problem. To achieve this goal, a full-thickness flap must be raised to bind an attaching device to the tooth. The flap is finally repositioned into its place and the traction chain remains submucosal. In cases of persistent deciduous canine, its empty socket can be used as a path for the traction chain (tunnel traction). (Fig. 1.)

C. Teeth that erupt buccally entrap and destroy the gingiva between the erupting cusp and the deciduous tooth. An adequate amount of uninflamed entrapped gingiva may still be attached to the cementum of the deciduous tooth (Fig. 2, A and B). It can be saved and used as a donor material to create a satisfactory width of gingiva for the permanent tooth.

D. The donor site for interceptive surgery is the area between the erupting cusp and the deciduous tooth. The recipient site is the area immediately apical to the erupting cusp. A flap with two horizontal gingival pedicles is indicated when the tip of a cusp is erupting at the level of the mucogingival junction (MGJ) (see Fig. 2). An apically positioned flap with vertical releasing incisions or a free graft of the entrapped gingiva is indicated when the cusp is erupting apical to the MGJ.

E. An appreciable amount of gingiva is needed to withstand effective toothbrushing and to prevent recession in young orthodontic patients. The risk of recession is higher when the gingiva is thin and narrow and the tooth has to be moved buccally. In case of actual recession, reconstructive surgery is indicated (Fig. 3).

F. The direct mechanical trauma on the gingiva is most often observed in Class II, division 2 malocclusion. It cannot be cured by means of periodontal surgery and requires orthodontic treatment prior to any mucogingival procedure.

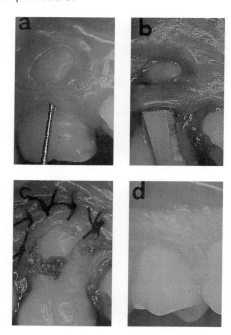

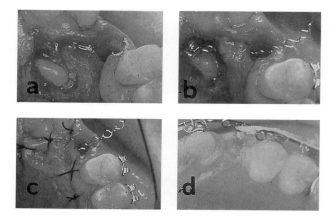

Figure 1. **A,** A full thickness palatal flap has been raised to expose the cusp of an impacted maxillary left canine. **B,** Submucosal traction: a hand-made chain is fixed to the cusp of the canine and passed through the empty socket of the deciduous canine. **C,** The flap is sutured. **D,** The permanent impacted canine is erupting at the center of the alveolar ridge (courtesy Dr. A. Crescini).

Figure 2. **A,** A maxilalry right premolar is erupting buccally. The buccal gingiva remains entrapped between the erupting cusp and the deciduous tooth. **B,** The entrapped gingiva is dissected and displaced apically (bipedicle flap). **C,** Sutures. **D,** Healing after 2 years.

Patient scheduled for ORTHODONTICS

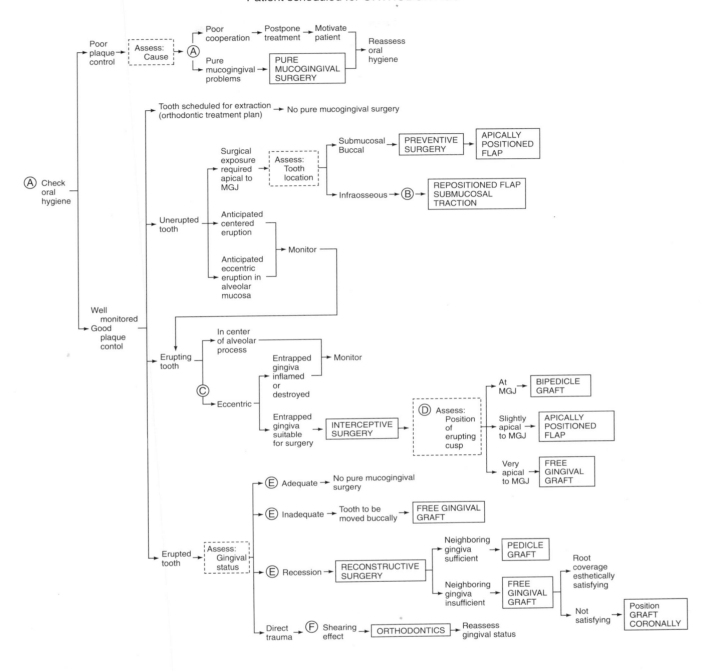

A → Check oral hygiene

- Poor plaque control → Assess: Cause → (A)
  - Poor cooperation → Postpone treatment → Motivate patient → Reassess oral hygiene
  - Pure mucogingival problems → PURE MUCOGINGIVAL SURGERY → Reassess oral hygiene

- Well monitored / Good plaque control

  - Tooth scheduled for extraction (orthodontic treatment plan) → No pure mucogingival surgery

  - Unerupted tooth
    - Surgical exposure required apical to MGJ → Assess: Tooth location
      - Submucosal Buccal → PREVENTIVE SURGERY → APICALLY POSITIONED FLAP
      - Infraosseous → (B) → REPOSITIONED FLAP SUBMUCOSAL TRACTION
    - Anticipated centered eruption → Monitor
    - Anticipated eccentric eruption in alveolar mucosa → Monitor

  - Erupting tooth (C)
    - In center of alveolar process → Monitor
    - Eccentric
      - Entrapped gingiva inflamed or destroyed → Monitor
      - Entrapped gingiva suitable for surgery → INTERCEPTIVE SURGERY → (D) Assess: Position of erupting cusp
        - At MGJ → BIPEDICLE GRAFT
        - Slightly apical to MGJ → APICALLY POSITIONED FLAP
        - Very apical to MGJ → FREE GINGIVAL GRAFT

  - Erupted tooth → Assess: Gingival status
    - (E) Adequate → No pure mucogingival surgery
    - (E) Inadequate → Tooth to be moved buccally → FREE GINGIVAL GRAFT
    - (E) Recession → RECONSTRUCTIVE SURGERY
      - Neighboring gingiva sufficient → PEDICLE GRAFT
      - Neighboring gingiva insufficient → FREE GINGIVAL GRAFT
        - Root coverage esthetically satisfying
        - Not satisfying → Position GRAFT CORONALLY
    - Direct trauma → (F) Shearing effect → ORTHODONTICS → Reassess gingival status

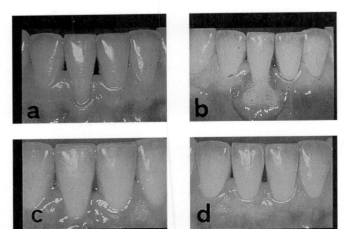

Figure 3. A recession on a mandibular central incisor is treated by free gingival graft before orthodontic treatment.

References

Agudio G, Pini-Prato GP, De Paoli S, Nevins M. Mucogingival interceptive therapy. Int J Periodont Restor Dent 1985;5:49.

Coatoam GW, Beherents RG, Bissada N. The width of keratinized gingiva during orthodontic treatment: Its significance and impact on periodontal status. J Periodontol 1981;52:307.

Crescini A, Pini-Prato GP. Trattamento combinato del canino incluso. Tecnica del doppio arco. Dental Cadmos 1988;56:19.

Hall WB. Gingival augmentation/mucogingival surgery. In: Proceedings of the world workshop in clinical periodontics. Chicago: American Academy of Periodontology, 1989:VII-1.

Maynard G, Ochsenbein C. Mucogingival problems: Prevalence and therapy in children. J Periodontol 1975;46:543.

PREVENTION OF RECESSION

Walter B. Hall

Patients are predisposed to recession when an inadequate band of attached gingiva is present. Gingival augmentation may be performed for prophylactic or therapeutic reasons. Surgical treatment to prevent recession, termed *prophylactic gingival grafting*, has always been a controversial concept. The term was discarded at the World Workshop in Periodontics in 1989. Curiously, that group determined that grafting performed on predisposed individuals to prevent recession during orthodontic therapy was a "therapeutic" rather than a "prophylactic" procedure. The concept of augmenting inadequate gingiva prior to recession, therefore, remains a viable option, but the controversial name has been discarded.

A. When a patient exhibits an inadequate band of attached gingiva (see p 86), determining the nature of any recession is most important. If recession can be documented as being active, the need to consider gingival augmentation is obvious. If the recession is minimal (i.e., less than 1 mm), a free gingival graft to increase the band of attached gingiva is a logical choice unless gingival color in a visible area would interfere (see p 100). If significant recession (i.e., more than 1 mm) already has occurred, a connective tissue graft would be the best choice in order to create an adequate zone of attached gingiva with coverage of some or all exposed roots.

B. If recession cannot be documented as being active, the age of the patient is a significant factor. The approach to treatment decisions is not different whether the patient is young or old; however, the dental needs in the two groups are likely to be different. Younger patients are more likely to consider orthodontics than are older ones. Older patients, however, are more likely to require restorations that involve the marginal gingiva (i.e., crowns, removable prosthetics) than are younger ones.

C. If significant recession (more than 1 mm) has occurred but appears to be stable at the moment, the patient (or parent) may elect to have a connective tissue graft (or, alternatively, a pedicle graft) placed before proceeding either with orthodontics or with a restorative procedure. Alternatively, he may elect to observe the area to determine whether documented recession is occurring before proceeding with gingival augmentation.

D. If no significant recession (less than 1 mm) has occurred in a predisposed youngster or adult, one should consider orthodontic needs. If orthodontic work is planned, the patient or parent may elect to place a free gingival graft apical to the mucogingival junction to increase the band of attached gingiva, which has a high predictability of success, or to document the current status and plan to correct any recession that may occur during therapy, in which case a connective tissue graft (or, alternatively, a pedicle graft) with root coverage as a goal is likely to be preferable. If the tooth involved is going to be extracted (i.e., some first premolars), no augmentation procedure for that area is indicated.

E. If no orthodontic treatment is planned, restorative needs also may influence the need for gingival augmentation. If no Class V restoration or crown is planned in the predisposed area, its current status should be documented; if recession occurs, a connective tissue graft (or alternatively a pedicle graft) would be employed to stop further recession and cover some or all of the exposed root. If a Class V restoration or crown is indicated on a predisposed tooth, where less than 1 mm of recession has occurred already, the patient may elect to have a free gingival graft to augment the inadequate band of attached gingiva or elect to take his chances; if recession does occur, the patient may have the less predictable connective tissue (or pedicle) graft placed to stop further recession and cover the newly exposed root in whole or in part.

References

Ericson I, Lindhe J. Recession in sites with moderate width of paratinized gingiva: An experimental study in the dog. J Clin Periodontol 1984;11:95.

Hall WB. Pure mucogingival problems. Berlin: Quintessence Publishing, 1984:130.

Langer B, Langer L. Subepithelial connective tissue graft technique for root coverage. J Periodontol 1985;56:715.

Maynard JG, Wilson RD. Diagnosis and management of mucogingival problems in children. Dent Clin North Am 1980;24:683.

World workshop in clinical periodontics. Chicago: American Academy of Periodontology, 1989:VII-19.

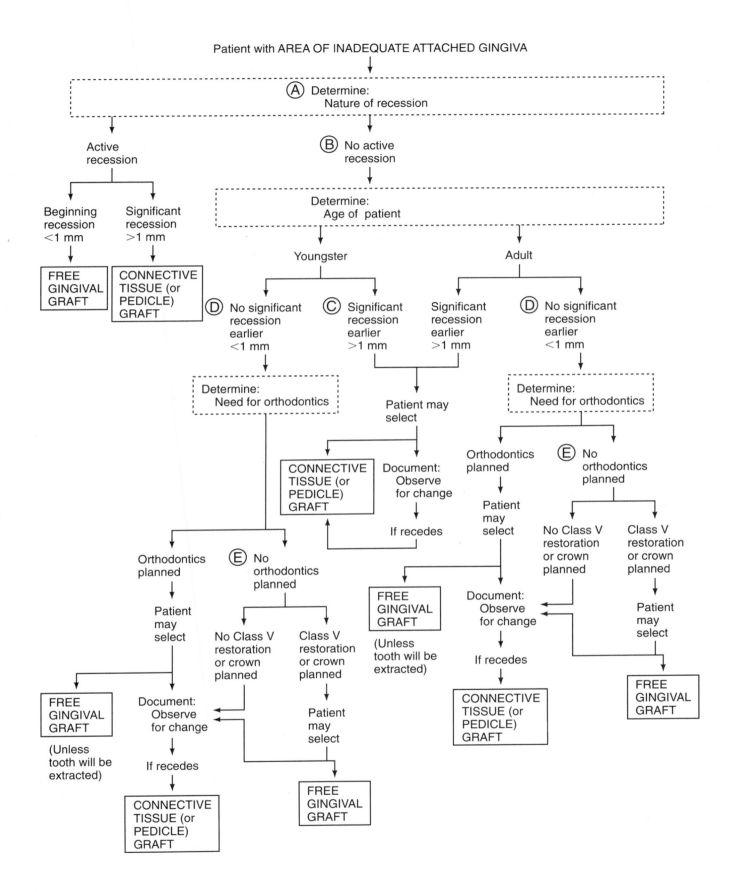

ESTHETICS AND GINGIVAL AUGMENTATION

Edward P. Allen

Treatment of periodontal disease in the maxillary anterior segment may lead to esthetic problems in some patients owing to the destructive nature of the disease process. In order to avoid results that are dissatisfying to the patient, a careful evaluation of esthetic considerations should be part of periodontal treatment planning.

A. First, perform an evaluation of the patient's smile to determine whether there is exposure of papillary and/or marginal gingiva. If the patient has no gingival exposure, then optimal periodontal therapy can be provided without concern for esthetics. If there is a high lip line with gingival exposure, then periodontal therapy may adversely affect esthetics.

B. The potential esthetic impact of periodontal therapy must be discussed with the patient. If the patient is unconcerned with the possible effects, then the appropriate periodontal therapy may be provided. If the patient is concerned with esthetics, a conservative approach is indicated. This may be accomplished by root debridement through a closed approach followed by an evaluation of response to treatment.

C. In moderate-to-severe cases in which disease is controlled by even a conservative approach, esthetics may be compromised to an extent that is unacceptable to the patient. The two options to improve the esthetics at this point would be prosthetic therapy or removal of the teeth with ridge preservation/augmentation therapy, where required, followed by prosthetic therapy.

D. In cases in which the closed debridement has controlled the disease and esthetics are acceptable, the patient may be placed on a systematic maintenance program.

E. When the disease has not been controlled by the initial conservative therapy, a surgical approach including either regenerative therapy, open flap debridement, or pocket elimination therapy is indicated. The surgical therapy would be followed by prosthetic evaluation and therapy as needed for esthetics.

References

Allen EP. Use of mucogingival surgical procedures to enhance esthetics. Dent Clin North Am 1988;32:307.

Hall WB. Periodontal preparation of the mouth for restoration. Dent Clin North Am 1980;24:204.

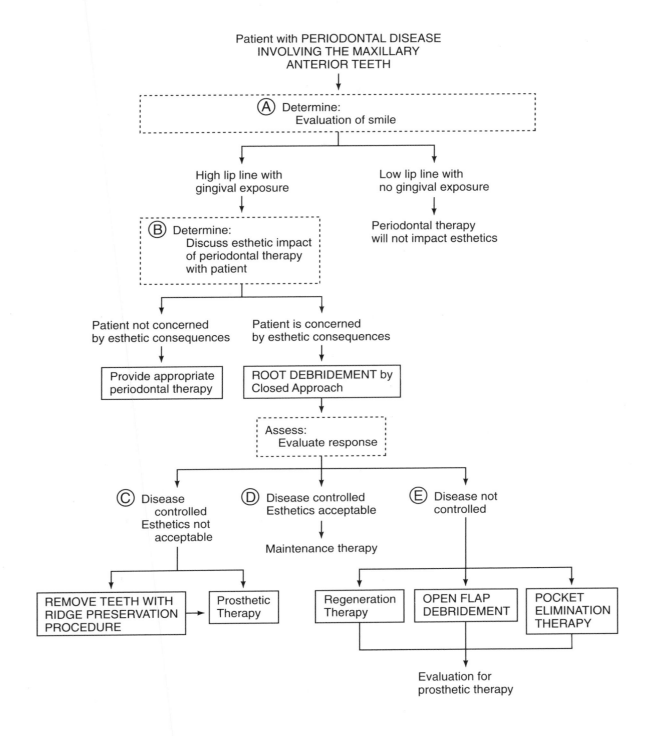

Patient with PERIODONTAL DISEASE
INVOLVING THE MAXILLARY
ANTERIOR TEETH

(A) Determine:
Evaluation of smile

High lip line with
gingival exposure

Low lip line with
no gingival exposure

Periodontal therapy
will not impact esthetics

(B) Determine:
Discuss esthetic impact
of periodontal therapy
with patient

Patient not concerned
by esthetic consequences

Patient is concerned
by esthetic consequences

Provide appropriate
periodontal therapy

ROOT DEBRIDEMENT by
Closed Approach

Assess:
Evaluate response

(C) Disease
controlled
Esthetics not
acceptable

(D) Disease controlled
Esthetics acceptable

Maintenance therapy

(E) Disease not
controlled

REMOVE TEETH WITH
RIDGE PRESERVATION
PROCEDURE

Prosthetic
Therapy

Regeneration
Therapy

OPEN FLAP
DEBRIDEMENT

POCKET
ELIMINATION
THERAPY

Evaluation for
prosthetic therapy

ESTHETIC EVALUATION OF PATIENTS WITH A HIGH LIP LINE

Edward P. Allen

When a patient presents with an esthetic concern due to a high lip line or "gummy" smile, a careful evaluation is indicated. In many cases, this problem can be treated by surgical exposure of more tooth length as the sole treatment or as a finishing procedure following orthognathic therapy. The first step in the esthetic evaluation is a determination of clinical crown length.

A. If the clinical crown length is normal, evaluate the patient for possible vertical maxillary excess (VME). If VME is not present, then the "gummy" smile may be due to excessive muscle activity or a short upper lip, and no treatment is indicated. If VME is present, orthognathic surgery is indicated.

B. If the clinical crown length is less than normal, evaluate the patient for VME; if VME is present, evaluate the patient for orthognathic surgery. Following this evaluation or if there is no VME, determine the length of the anatomic crown by probing for the subgingival location of the cementoenamel junction (CEJ) on the facial aspect of the teeth.

C. Where there is incomplete exposure of the anatomic crown, surgical crown lengthening to the level of the CEJ is indicated. Before surgery, the position and thickness of the marginal bone must be determined by sounding with a periodontal probe. If the bony crest is thick and/or located at the CEJ, flap and osseous surgery will be required to completely expose the anatomic crown. If the margin is thin and approximately 2.0 mm apical to the CEJ, excision of the marginal tissue by internal or external gingivectomy is indicated provided adequate dimensions of gingiva will remain postsurgically. If the gingival dimensions will be inadequate, crown lengthening by flap surgery will be required.

D. In some cases with short clinical crowns, the anatomic crown is also short and may already be completely exposed. Such cases may be treated by flap and osseous surgery for tooth lengthening but must then be treated prosthetically to achieve an esthetic result.

References

Allen EP. Use of mucogingival surgical procedures to enhance esthetics. Dent Clin North Am 1988:307.

Bell WH. Modern practice in orthognathic and reconstructive surgery. Philadelphia: WB Saunders, 1991.

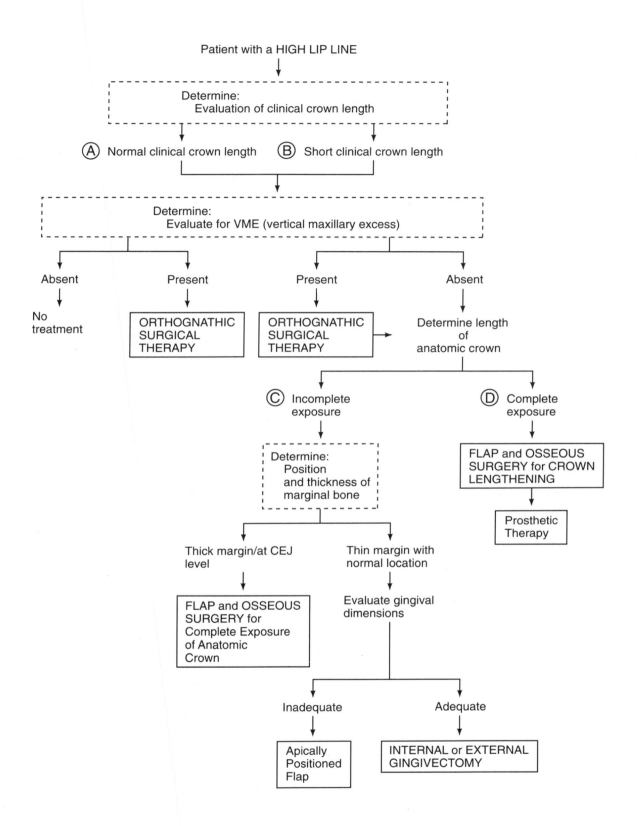

Patient with a HIGH LIP LINE

Determine:
Evaluation of clinical crown length

Ⓐ Normal clinical crown length   Ⓑ Short clinical crown length

Determine:
Evaluate for VME (vertical maxillary excess)

Absent → No treatment

Present → ORTHOGNATHIC SURGICAL THERAPY

Present → ORTHOGNATHIC SURGICAL THERAPY →

Absent → Determine length of anatomic crown

Ⓒ Incomplete exposure

Ⓓ Complete exposure → FLAP and OSSEOUS SURGERY for CROWN LENGTHENING → Prosthetic Therapy

Determine:
Position and thickness of marginal bone

Thick margin/at CEJ level → FLAP and OSSEOUS SURGERY for Complete Exposure of Anatomic Crown

Thin margin with normal location → Evaluate gingival dimensions

Inadequate → Apically Positioned Flap

Adequate → INTERNAL or EXTERNAL GINGIVECTOMY

FREE GINGIVAL GRAFT, CONNECTIVE TISSUE GRAFT, OR PEDICLE GRAFT?

Walter B. Hall

Once the dentist has decided that a pure mucogingival problem requires surgery to create a broader band of attached gingiva, he must select the technique most likely to achieve root coverage or just a broader band of attached gingiva to minimize recession in the future. Esthetics is a prime consideration. Connective tissue grafts and pedicle grafts are more likely than free grafts to be successful in covering roots and in matching the appearance of adjacent gingiva. Connective tissue grafting appears to be more successful than pedicle grafting; therefore, when root coverage is a goal, the connective tissue graft would be preferable to any pedicle graft procedure unless an adequately thick donor site for a connective tissue graft is not available (see p 104).

A. If no esthetic concern exists, as in most mandibular areas and in maxillary molar areas, a free gingival graft is one option. When no existing recession requiring coverage is present, a free gingival graft is an acceptable choice.

B. When no esthetic problem exists but recession requiring root coverage is present, or when an esthetic problem is present, use a connective tissue graft or a pedicle graft for root coverage and for a better esthetic result. Connective tissue grafts have a higher degree of predictability of success than do pedicle grafts.

C. To use the laterally positioned graft, a donor site on adjacent teeth must be wide enough, tall enough, and thick enough to be able to be raised as a flap of approximately 0.5 to 1.0 mm in thickness and laterally positioned to cover the exposed root (or potentially exposed area) and several millimeters of soft tissue on either side of it. The donor site should be about 1.5 times the width of the area to be covered and 2 to 5 mm in height. If such a donor site is not available, consider the next alternative.

D. An obliquely rotated pedicle graft can be used occasionally, when an adequate donor site for a laterally positioned pedicle graft is not present and a papilla adjacent to the receptor area may be of sufficient width and height to be used as a donor site. The pedicle graft will be rotated about 90 degrees to cover the exposed (or potentially exposed) area; therefore, the papilla should be tall enough to cover the receptor site, plus a millimeter more at least mesiodistally. It also should be wide enough to provide sufficient gingiva to cover the exposed root or

to achieve an adequate band of gingiva to minimize recession in the future. The papilla may be taken full thickness, if necessary, as it overlies interproximal bone, which will have a cancellous component subjacent to the cortical plate. It should not have a deep "gingival groove," however, or it may split in two when raised. If no adequate donor site for such a graft exists, consider the next alternative.

E. A double papilla graft is the most difficult of the pedicle grafts to do and is the most likely to fail. The patient should understand these problems before proceeding (see p 202). The donor sites for such a graft are the two adjacent papillae. Together, these papillae must be sufficiently wide when joined to cover the receptor site and a millimeter or more of each on the adjacent papillary donor sites. They should be tall enough to provide a sufficient band of attached gingiva to cover the exposed root or to minimize recession. Thickness, as with obliquely positioned pedicle grafts, is not a problem, but deep "gingival grooves" can make this approach untenable. When the donor sites are not sufficient, a free gingival graft should be considered.

F. Free gingival grafts for covering roots have long been a desired goal of those practicing pure mucogingival surgery. The predictability of success with a free graft is not great, although claims for improved success through root treatment either with citric acid or complicated suturing have been made. The free gingival graft usually is taken from the palate, which may be of a markedly different color than the gingiva adjacent to the area to be grafted. If the donor gingiva is such a poor color match that it would create a greater esthetic problem, if successful, than that created by root exposure, grafting for root coverage should not be attempted.

References

Carranza FA Jr. Glickman's clinical periodontology. 7th ed. Philadelphia: WB Saunders, 1990:883.

Hall WB. Pure mucogingival problems. Berlin: Quintessence Publishing, 1984:129.

Langer B, Langer L. Subepithelial connective tissue graft technique for root coverage. J Periodontol 1983;56:175.

World workshop in clinical periodontics. Chicago: American Academy of Periodontology, 1989:VII-1.

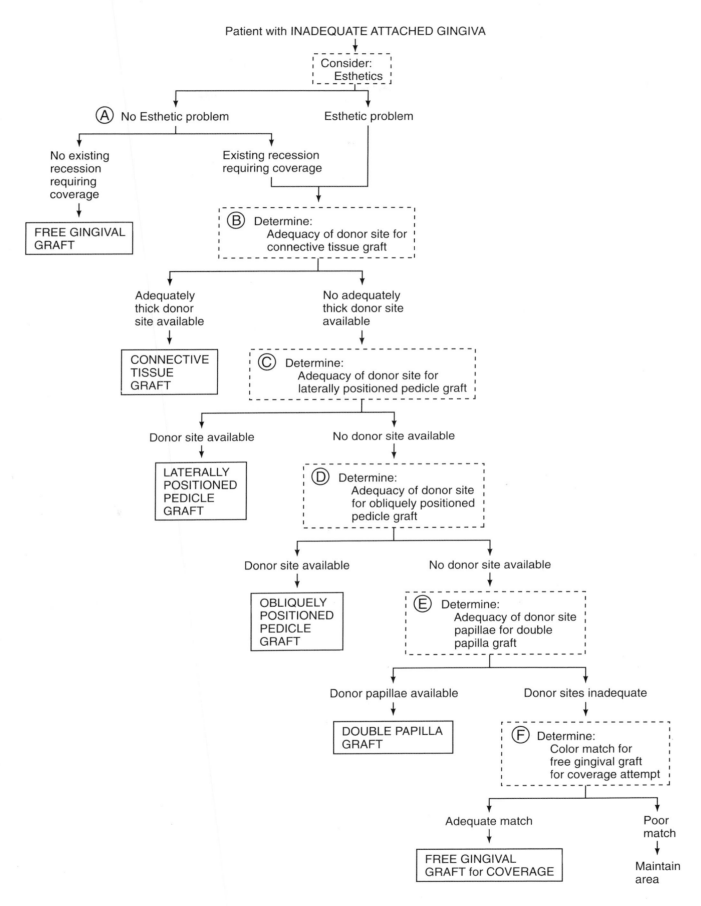

Patient with INADEQUATE ATTACHED GINGIVA

Consider:
Esthetics

Ⓐ No Esthetic problem

Esthetic problem

No existing recession requiring coverage

Existing recession requiring coverage

FREE GINGIVAL GRAFT

Ⓑ Determine:
Adequacy of donor site for connective tissue graft

Adequately thick donor site available

No adequately thick donor site available

CONNECTIVE TISSUE GRAFT

Ⓒ Determine:
Adequacy of donor site for laterally positioned pedicle graft

Donor site available

No donor site available

LATERALLY POSITIONED PEDICLE GRAFT

Ⓓ Determine:
Adequacy of donor site for obliquely positioned pedicle graft

Donor site available

No donor site available

OBLIQUELY POSITIONED PEDICLE GRAFT

Ⓔ Determine:
Adequacy of donor site papillae for double papilla graft

Donor papillae available

Donor sites inadequate

DOUBLE PAPILLA GRAFT

Ⓕ Determine:
Color match for free gingival graft for coverage attempt

Adequate match

Poor match

FREE GINGIVAL GRAFT for COVERAGE

Maintain area

RECESSION TREATMENT: ROOT COVERAGE OR NOT?

Walter B. Hall

When a patient has a root or roots exposed by recession, esthetic needs and restorative needs will influence the need for grafting in an interrelated manner. If the band of attached gingiva is adequate but recession has occurred, surgery may be used to recover exposed roots if an esthetic need exists. If no esthetic need exists, and no restoration affecting the gingival margin is planned, maintenance care alone should suffice. If the band of attached gingiva is "inadequate" in the dentist's opinion, the need to consider gingival augmentation will be greater.

A. First decide upon the "adequacy" of the existing band of attached gingiva. An adequate band of attached gingiva is one that is sufficient to prevent initial or continued recession. The patient's age, other dental needs, oral hygiene status, caries activity, and aesthetic needs are some factors that would influence a decision that treatment is needed if the band of attached gingiva is judged to be "inadequate" to prevent initial or continued recession when resolving his overall dental needs.

B. If the patient has an adequate band of attached gingiva and no cosmetic or esthetic need to attempt root coverage exists, dental health should be maintainable with regular oral hygiene effort, prophylaxis, or root planing. If a Class V restoration or crown is to be placed, the apical margin of the restoration may be placed within the gingival crevice without strong likelihood of inducing recession or placed supragingivally if root sensitivity, caries activity, or other restorative requirements (i.e., crown length) are not involved, then maintenance care should suffice.

C. If root coverage is necessary to meet esthetic or cosmetic goals, and the band of attached gingiva on the tooth or teeth with recession is adequate, a coronally positioned pedicle graft or flap (see p 208) would be the treatment of choice.

D. When an inadequate band of attached gingiva is present and esthetic, cosmetic, or restorative goals indicate the need for root coverage, a coronally positioned pedicle graft (flap) would not likely be successful. In this situation, a connective tissue graft would be most appropriate, particularly if several teeth are involved. If an adequate donor site for such a graft is not available (i.e., the donor site in the rugae area is insufficiently thick), then pedicle grafts should be considered in the sequence described in "Pure Mucogingival Concerns of Patients Scheduled for Orthodontics: A European View" (p 96).

E. If the patient has "inadequate" attached gingiva to meet his dental needs without initiating recession or further recession and no cosmetic or esthetic concern exists, a free gingival graft without root coverage may be performed for stabilization.

References

Allen EP, Miller PD. Coronal positioning of existing gingiva: Short-term results in the treatment of shallow marginal tissue recession. J Periodontol 1989;60:316.

Hall WB. Pure mucogingival problems. Berlin: Quintessence Publishing, 1984:61.

Langer B, Langer L. Subepithelial connective tissue graft technique for root coverage. J Periodontol 1985;56:715.

Matter J. Free gingival grafts for the treatment of gingival recession—a review of some techniques. J Clin Periodontol 1980;9:103.

World workshop in clinical periodontics. Chicago: American Academy of Periodontology, 1989:VII-1

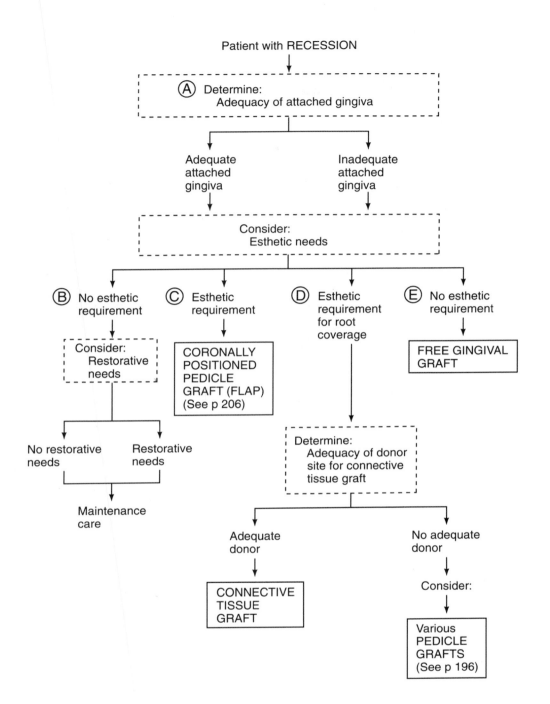

Patient with RECESSION

(A) Determine:
Adequacy of attached gingiva

Adequate attached gingiva → Inadequate attached gingiva

Consider:
Esthetic needs

(B) No esthetic requirement

(C) Esthetic requirement

(D) Esthetic requirement for root coverage

(E) No esthetic requirement

Consider:
Restorative needs

CORONALLY POSITIONED PEDICLE GRAFT (FLAP) (See p 206)

FREE GINGIVAL GRAFT

No restorative needs

Restorative needs

Maintenance care

Determine:
Adequacy of donor site for connective tissue graft

Adequate donor

No adequate donor

CONNECTIVE TISSUE GRAFT

Consider:

Various PEDICLE GRAFTS (See p 196)

DETERMINING THE LEVEL OF ROOT COVERAGE POSSIBLE IN MARGINAL TISSUE RECESSION

Preston D. Miller, Jr.

If root coverage grafting is considered in areas of marginal tissue recession, the recession must be classified so that both the therapist and the patient can visualize the treatment goal. Although many areas of recession can be completely covered with attached tissue, others only lend themselves to partial root coverage; still others, because of anatomic considerations (loss of interdental tissue), are not amenable to root coverage. If complete root coverage cannot be achieved, the patient must then make a value judgment as to whether to proceed with a surgical procedure that will produce partial root coverage or, in some cases, a procedure that only augments gingiva but leaves the recession.

A. To determine the class of recession, first mark the cementoenamel junction with a pencil. If there is interdental loss (loss of papilla height), this marking should be extended to include the cementoenamel junction in the interdental area.

B. Evaluate the level of attached gingiva. If there is no loss of interdental papilla, then generally complete root coverage can be achieved whether or not there is attached gingiva. If there is attached gingiva, this represents Class I recession. If there is no gingiva (alveolar mucosal margin) or if there is unattached gingiva (pocket depth traversing the mucogingival junction), this represents Class II recession.

C. If there is loss of interdental papilla height in conjunction with recession, then the treatment goal is altered, because complete root coverage is not possible. Evaluate the tissue height on the adjacent teeth. A line connecting these points will determine the level of root coverage possible. Mark this level on the root with pencil. If partial root coverage is attainable, this is Class III recession. If no root coverage is possible, this is Class IV recession.

References

Miller PD. Root coverage using a free soft-tissue autograft following citric acid application. Part I: Technique. Int J Periodont Rest Dent 1982;2:65.

Miller PD. A classification of marginal tissue recession. Int J Periodont Rest Dent 1985;2:8.

Miller PD. Root coverage using the free soft-tissue autograft following citric acid application. Part III: A successful and predictable procedure in areas of deep-wide recession. Int J Periodont Rest Dent 1985;2:14.

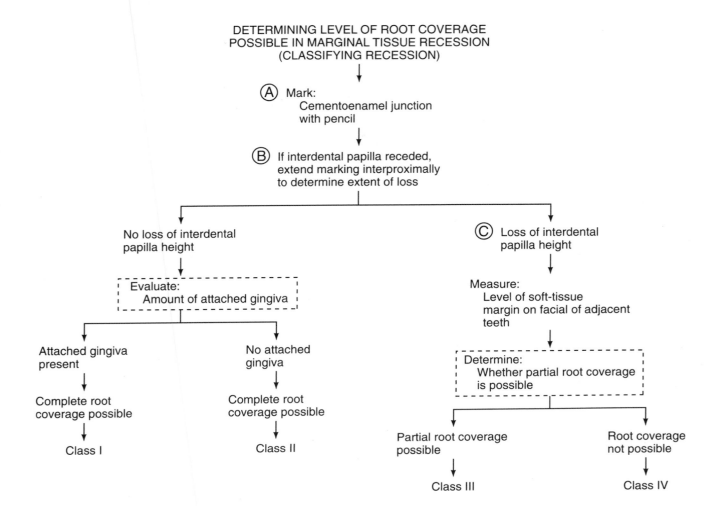

DETERMINING LEVEL OF ROOT COVERAGE
POSSIBLE IN MARGINAL TISSUE RECESSION
(CLASSIFYING RECESSION)

Ⓐ Mark:
Cementoenamel junction
with pencil

Ⓑ If interdental papilla receded,
extend marking interproximally
to determine extent of loss

No loss of interdental
papilla height

Evaluate:
Amount of attached gingiva

Attached gingiva
present

No attached
gingiva

Complete root
coverage possible

Complete root
coverage possible

Class I

Class II

Ⓒ Loss of interdental
papilla height

Measure:
Level of soft-tissue
margin on facial of adjacent
teeth

Determine:
Whether partial root coverage
is possible

Partial root coverage
possible

Root coverage
not possible

Class III

Class IV

CLASS I RECESSION

Preston D. Miller, Jr.

Recession is classified as Class I when the recession does not traverse the mucogingival junction, an adequate amount of attached gingiva is present, and the interdental papilla is at a normal height. Generally, Class I recession is not a clinical problem in and of itself. Problems associated with the root, however, often dictate treatment. On occasion, root sensitivity may be treated with a root coverage procedure. Cervical abrasion or root caries present a special problem (i.e., missing tooth structure) and root coverage surgery may offer the best solution. Ultimately, the patient's desire for improved esthetics may prove to be the overriding factor in electing to proceed with surgery.

A. Evaluate the thickness and height of gingiva. If adequate gingiva is present, both in thickness and height, then a coronally positioned flap becomes the treatment of choice. Arbitrarily, 3 mm of gingival height is considered adequate. At the present time, only clinical judgment can be used to decide on an adequate thickness for gingiva to be coronally positioned (see p 208).

B. Evaluate lost tooth structure. In root caries or cervical abrasion, missing tooth structure may require more than coronally positioning a flap. Although there may be adequate gingival height, generally there is not enough gingival thickness. In this case, consider a graft.

References

Allen EP, Miller PD. Coronal positioning of existing gingiva: Short-term results in the treatment of shallow marginal tissue recession. J Periodontol 1989;66:316.

Miller PD. A classification of marginal tissue recession. Int J Periodont Rest Dent 1985;2:8.

Restrepo OJ. Coronally repositioned flap: Report of four cases. J Periodontol 1973;44:564.

Tarnow DP. Semilunar coronally positioned flap. J Clin Periodontol 1986;13:182.

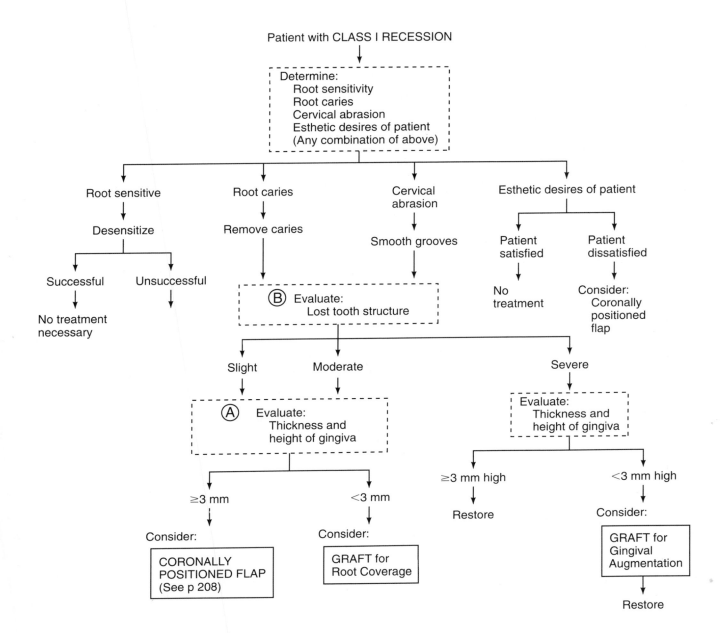

Patient with CLASS I RECESSION

Determine:
Root sensitivity
Root caries
Cervical abrasion
Esthetic desires of patient
(Any combination of above)

Root sensitive → Desensitize
- Successful → No treatment necessary
- Unsuccessful →

Root caries → Remove caries →

Cervical abrasion → Smooth grooves →

Ⓑ Evaluate: Lost tooth structure

- Slight
- Moderate → Ⓐ Evaluate: Thickness and height of gingiva
  - ≥3 mm → Consider: CORONALLY POSITIONED FLAP (See p 208)
  - <3 mm → Consider: GRAFT for Root Coverage

Esthetic desires of patient
- Patient satisfied → No treatment
- Patient dissatisfied → Consider: Coronally positioned flap

Severe → Evaluate: Thickness and height of gingiva
- ≥3 mm high → Restore
- <3 mm high → Consider: GRAFT for Gingival Augmentation → Restore

CLASS II RECESSION

Preston D. Miller, Jr.

Class II recession, unlike Class I recession, does present a clinical problem, because there is no attached gingiva, no loss of interdental papilla height, and complete root coverage is possible. Because there is no gingiva to position coronally, the coronally positioned flap is not a consideration. Root coverage must be accomplished by either the laterally positioned pedicle flap or a free graft.

A. If root caries are present, remove caries. Often this results in a concavity in the root that must be treated by odontoplasty. Odontoplasty can be accomplished with either hand or rotary instruments. If there is cervical abrasion with grooves on cavitation, odontoplasty is required.

B. Evaluate lost tooth structure. If it is slight to moderate, proceed with grafting for root coverage.

C. If the amount of tooth structure loss is severe, then root coverage may not be a viable alternative. In this case, graft for gingival augmentation and then place a restoration.

References

Holbrook T, Ochsenbein C. Complete coverage of the denuded root surface with a one-stage gingival graft. Int J Periodont Rest Dent 1983;3:8.

Langer B, Langer L. Subepithelial connective tissue graft technique for root coverage. J Periodontol 1985;56:715.

Miller PD. A classification of marginal tissue recession. Int J Periodont Rest Dent 1985;2:8.

Miller PD. Root coverage using a free soft-tissue autograft following citric acid application. Part I: Technique. Int J Periodont Rest Dent 1982;2:65.

Miller PD. Root coverage with the free gingival graft: Factors associated with incomplete coverage. J Periodontol 1987;58:674.

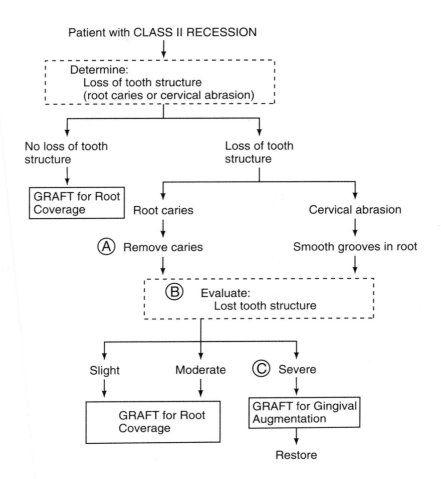

Patient with CLASS II RECESSION

Determine:
Loss of tooth structure
(root caries or cervical abrasion)

No loss of tooth structure

Loss of tooth structure

GRAFT for Root Coverage

Root caries

Cervical abrasion

Ⓐ Remove caries

Smooth grooves in root

Ⓑ Evaluate:
Lost tooth structure

Slight

Moderate

Ⓒ Severe

GRAFT for Root Coverage

GRAFT for Gingival Augmentation

Restore

CLASS III RECESSION AND CLASS IV RECESSION

Preston D. Miller, Jr.

Class III recession is present when a tooth is extruded or there is loss of interdental papilla height. Although complete root coverage is not feasible, partial root coverage may be attempted.

A. The level of root coverage possible is determined by measuring the height of the gingival margin mid-facially on the adjacent teeth. A line connecting these two points will determine the level of root coverage possible.

B. Mark this level with pencil. Place coronal margin of graft at this level to obtain partial root coverage. If partial root coverage is attainable, this is Class III recession.

C. If no root coverage is possible, this is Class IV recession.

References

Holbrook T, Ochsenbein C. Complete coverage of the denuded root surface with a one-stage gingival graft. Int J Periodont Rest Dent 1983;3:8.

Langer B, Langer L. Subepithelial connective tissue graft technique for root coverage. J Periodontol 1985;56:715.

Miller PD. A classification of marginal tissue recession. Int J Periodont Rest Dent 1985;2:8.

Miller PD. Root coverage using a free soft-tissue autograft following citric acid application. Part II: Treatment of the carious root. Int J Periodont Rest Dent 1983;3:8.

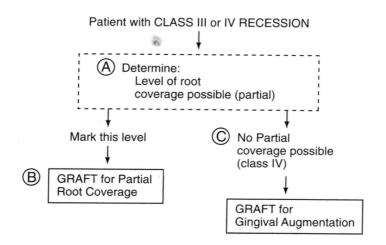

Patient with CLASS III or IV RECESSION

Ⓐ Determine:
Level of root
coverage possible (partial)

Mark this level

Ⓒ No Partial
coverage possible
(class IV)

Ⓑ GRAFT for Partial
Root Coverage

GRAFT for
Gingival Augmentation

DENUDATION VERSUS GINGIVAL GRAFTING

Walter B. Hall

When a dentist has decided that a tooth has inadequate attached gingiva, he must determine what technique to employ in creating a broader band. Among the techniques that could be used are various pedicle grafting techniques (see p 196), free gingival grafting, connective tissue grafting, and denudation. Denudation is a technique that involves leaving bone exposed to granulate and heal over with gingiva; it has the undesirable attributes of slow healing and greater postoperative discomfort. The position of the tooth in the arch, esthetic concerns, pocket depth, and surface (or surfaces) involved must be considered.

A. Mandibular second and third molars are poor candidates for gingival grafting procedures because of the difficulty of access for grafting the thick cortical plate present in the vestibule and the lack of vestibular depth that is common in this site. If the tooth has periodontal pocketing and severe bone loss, it is not a candidate for gingival grafting or denudation but should be either extracted or maintained until lost. If the periodontitis is moderate or less, the apically positioned flap approach to pocket elimination, with the flap positioned so that several millimeters of facial bone is left denuded, would be the technique of choice. If the tooth requiring additional attached gingiva has no periodontitis problem, the apically positioned flap with several millimeters denudation would be the technique of choice. Guided tissue regeneration (see p 148) may be employed to eliminate some pockets and to create a broader band of attached gingiva simultaneously.

B. Any tooth other than the mandibular second or third molar that requires additional attached gingiva has more options for treatment. If the tooth has pocketing and bone loss that is located interproximally, the apically positioned flap for pocket elimination, combined with several millimeters of denudation to gain additional attached gingiva, is a reasonable choice. If

the cratering is deep (i.e., more than 2 mm apical to the facial and lingual cortical plate crests), guided tissue regeneration offers significant advantages for increasing attachment support and the band of attached gingiva (see p 148). If the pocket depth and bone loss are only on the facial or lingual surface and an adequate band of gingiva is present on an adjacent tooth (see p 196), a pedicle graft to cover the exposed root would be one option. Another option would be a connective tissue graft, a technique with greater predictability of success. If no pedicle donor is present, the choice of a connective tissue graft obviously would be the one of choice on the basis of its higher predictability. If no donor for a pedicle graft is available, a free gingival graft could be employed. If no esthetic concerns are present, the graft would be placed apical to existing gingiva; if esthetics are a concern, the graft could be placed so that it covers the root surface as well (see p 106). The gingiva from the donor site must be similar in color to that in areas adjacent to the graft if esthetic demands are to be fulfilled. If the tooth requiring additional attached gingiva is not involved with periodontitis, a gingival grafting procedure appropriate to the area should be selected (see p 104).

References

Hall WB. Pure mucogingival problems. Berlin: Quintessence Publishing, 1984:161.

Karring T, Cumming BR, Oliver RC, Loe H. The origin of granulation tissue and its impact on post-operative results of mucogingival surgery. J Periodontol 1975;45:577.

Robinson PJ, Guernsey LH. Clinical transplantation in dental specialties. St. Louis: CV Mosby, 1980:108.

Schluger S, Yuodelis R, Page RC, Johnson RH. Periodontal diseases. 2nd ed. Philadelphia: Lea & Febiger, 1990:563.

Patient with a TOOTH REQUIRING ADDITIONAL ATTACHED GINGIVA

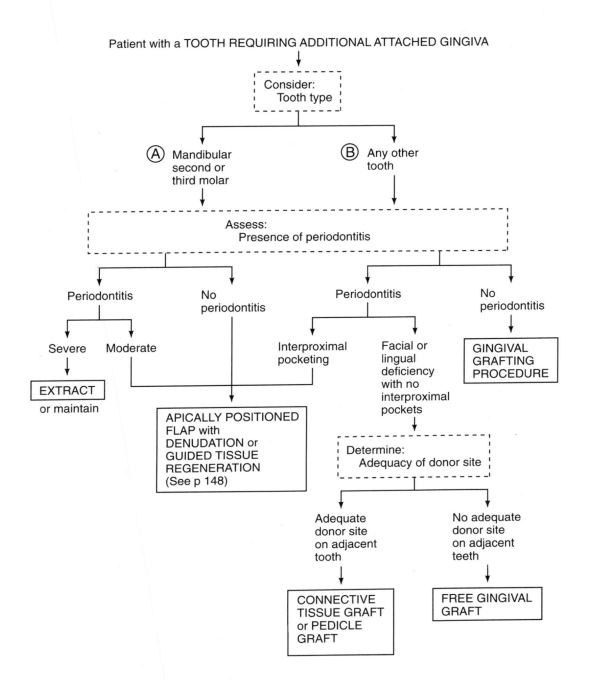

Consider:
Tooth type

Ⓐ Mandibular second or third molar

Ⓑ Any other tooth

Assess:
Presence of periodontitis

Periodontitis

No periodontitis

Periodontitis

No periodontitis

Severe

Moderate

Interproximal pocketing

Facial or lingual deficiency with no interproximal pockets

GINGIVAL GRAFTING PROCEDURE

EXTRACT

or maintain

APICALLY POSITIONED FLAP with DENUDATION or GUIDED TISSUE REGENERATION (See p 148)

Determine:
Adequacy of donor site

Adequate donor site on adjacent tooth

No adequate donor site on adjacent teeth

CONNECTIVE TISSUE GRAFT or PEDICLE GRAFT

FREE GINGIVAL GRAFT

PRIMARY OCCLUSAL TRAUMA

Walter B. Hall

Primary occlusal trauma exists when a tooth with normal support is overloaded and, as a result, is wounded. The problem may be localized, or it may be generalized in several teeth.

A.   Localized, primary occlusal trauma most typically is related to a "high" restoration, a common sequela of the placement of a new restoration in an individual tooth that has been extensively instrumented. An anesthetized patient whose mouth has been opened widely for some time often is unable to detect such an early contact. Selective grinding usually is all that is required to correct the problem; however, severe discrepancies may be resolved best by replacing the restoration.

B.   Malaligned teeth also may be subjected to primary occlusal trauma, especially when they are locked in facial or lingual version. Selective grinding may resolve minor malalignments. Orthodontic movement is often the best choice. In severely crowded situations, however, selective extraction of teeth may be a simple and satisfactory solution.

C.   Generalized, primary occlusal trauma usually is of a different origin. Clenching and grinding habits or bruxism (night grinding) are the most common cause. Occlusal adjustment or, occasionally, selective grinding of a high "trigger" tooth may resolve some problems; however, the psychological component of clenching and grinding habits, especially bruxism, may benefit from psychological counseling in an attempt to control the patient's psychic disturbances. Because such problems are difficult to resolve, a bite guard (night guard) often is used to control the damage done in grinding, especially bruxism. The skill of the dentist in managing such problems, with their complex psychological overtones, often is sorely tried.

D.   Another, less common etiology is "occupational" bruxism, wherein certain occupations may cause patients to grind their teeth. Jobs such as riding a tractor, hauling nets on rocking fishing boats, using a jackhammer, and driving a taxi with bad springs have been implicated. Changing jobs may not be an option open to the patient. If not, a bite guard often can be worn during work hours in such occupations.

E.   *Recreational bruxism* is a term used to describe the extreme gnashing of teeth that accompanies the use of some "recreational" drugs. The best solution to such problems is to discontinue the use of the drugs. Counseling may be helpful in correcting such habits. Occasionally, a bite guard may be helpful when the patient cannot stop using the drug.

F.   Postorthodontic clenching may occur when a major occlusal discrepancy occurs following orthodontic therapy. A so-called "double bite" may have been created in which the patient has a maximal occlusal position a half tooth or more forward of centric relation occlusion. As the patient rocks between these two positions, severe trauma usually occurs. When detected before periodontitis is present, occlusal adjustment may be somewhat helpful; however, the discrepancies often are too great to be ground out. Further orthodontic treatment, even orthognathic surgery, can be undertaken with patient consent. A bite guard may be useful in controlling damage; however, a lifetime of wearing such a device is rarely a palatable alternative. Full-mouth reconstruction to establish a stable, centric relation occlusion is an expensive, but reasonable, alternative.

References

Carranza FA Jr. Glickman's clinical periodontology. 7th ed. Philadelphia: WB Saunders, 1990:722.

Genco RJ, Goldman HM, Cohen DW. Contemporary periodontics. St. Louis: CV Mosby, 1990:493.

Prichard JF. Advanced periodontal disease. 2nd ed. Philadelphia: WB Saunders, 1972:823.

Schluger S, Yuodelis R, Page RC, Johnson RH. Periodontal diseases. 2nd ed. Philadelphia: Lea & Febiger, 1990:388.

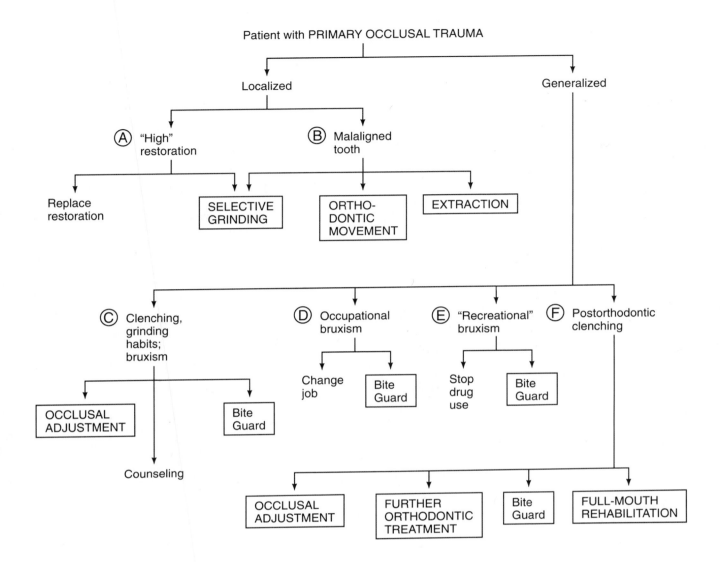

Patient with PRIMARY OCCLUSAL TRAUMA

Localized

Generalized

(A) "High" restoration

(B) Malaligned tooth

Replace restoration

SELECTIVE GRINDING

ORTHO-DONTIC MOVEMENT

EXTRACTION

(C) Clenching, grinding habits; bruxism

(D) Occupational bruxism

(E) "Recreational" bruxism

(F) Postorthodontic clenching

OCCLUSAL ADJUSTMENT

Bite Guard

Counseling

Change job

Bite Guard

Stop drug use

Bite Guard

OCCLUSAL ADJUSTMENT

FURTHER ORTHODONTIC TREATMENT

Bite Guard

FULL-MOUTH REHABILITATION

SECONDARY OCCLUSAL TRAUMA

Walter B. Hall

Secondary occlusal trauma exists when a tooth has lost attachment and bone support to the extent that wounding occurs even with normal occlusal loading. The problem may be localized, or it may be generalized in several teeth.

A. Localized secondary occlusal trauma has a better prognosis than does generalized secondary occlusal trauma. If adjacent teeth have adequate support, selective grinding of the tooth that has lost support can minimize function on that tooth by placing most function on the teeth with good support. If good abutment teeth are available, the tooth that has lost support may be splinted with fixed bridgework to those abutments, minimizing the heavy function on the weakened tooth. The more remaining teeth that have sufficient support to act as abutments or otherwise to assist the compromised tooth, the better the prognosis. If the compromised tooth is amenable to guided tissue regeneration (see p 148), it may be treated, which will obviate the need for splinting; otherwise, it should be extracted and replaced with a bridge.

B. If no good adjacent abutment teeth remain, but the compromised tooth is amenable to guided tissue regeneration, that approach would be the one of choice. If this approach cannot be employed, the tooth should be extracted or may be maintained with full recognition that its prognosis is hopeless (see p 68).

C. When generalized secondary occlusal trauma is present, permanent splinting of all teeth with fixed bridgework may be sufficient to stabilize the problem by tying all compromised teeth together. This approach is a very expensive one and should not be undertaken when all teeth have extensive bone loss. In such badly involved generalized cases, temporary splinting may permit maintaining the teeth for shorter periods of time. Another alternative would be the placement of a bite guard, especially if the patient is a night grinder. If most teeth have lost substantial support, guided tissue regeneration on large numbers of teeth is not practical or predictable as yet; therefore, extraction would be the only reasonable alternative.

References

Carranza FA Jr. Glickman's clinical periodontology. 7th ed. Philadelphia: WB Saunders, 1990:429.

Genco RJ, Goldman HM, Cohen DW. Contemporary periodontics. St. Louis: CV Mosby, 1990:493.

Schluger S, Yuodelis R, Page RC, Johnson RH. Periodontal diseases. 2nd ed. Philadelphia: Lea & Febiger, 1990:405.

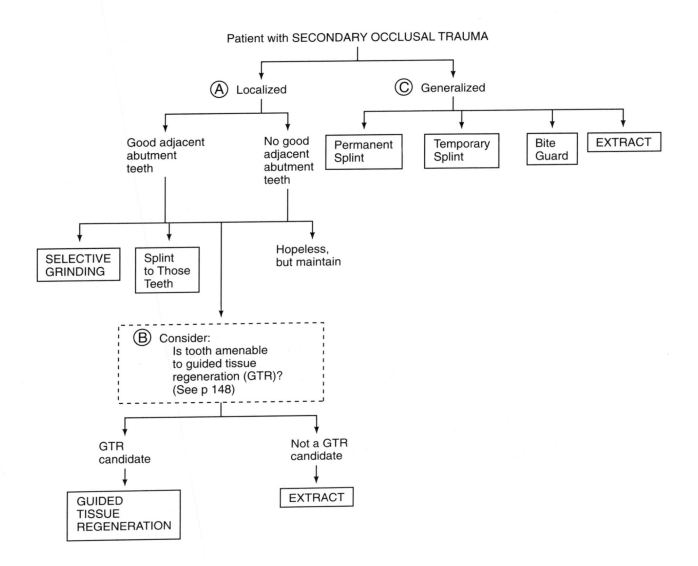

Patient with SECONDARY OCCLUSAL TRAUMA

(A) Localized

(C) Generalized

Good adjacent abutment teeth

No good adjacent abutment teeth

Permanent Splint

Temporary Splint

Bite Guard

EXTRACT

SELECTIVE GRINDING

Splint to Those Teeth

Hopeless, but maintain

(B) Consider: Is tooth amenable to guided tissue regeneration (GTR)? (See p 148)

GTR candidate

Not a GTR candidate

GUIDED TISSUE REGENERATION

EXTRACT

CANINE DISCLUSION (CUSPID RISE) VERSUS GROUP FUNCTION

Walter B. Hall

If, in the opinion of a dentist, a patient would benefit from selective grinding during treatment for periodontitis, the dentist must decide whether establishing canine disclusion (cuspid rise) or group function in lateral movements is best (Fig. 1). Canine disclusion can provide a "cuspid-protected" occlusion in parafunctional lateral movements that may be beneficial when posterior teeth have significant bone loss, considerable occlusal wear, or a number of cracks, and when the patient clenches or grinds the teeth. Canine disclusion is preferable to group function of weakened posterior teeth, but when canine disclusion cannot be employed, group function is used.

A. If both of the canines on one side have little or no bone loss, the first condition indicating the possibility of using canine disclusion is met. The radiographs should show normal-sized maxillary and mandibular canine roots that have little radiographic evidence of bone loss. Probing should confirm that little attachment has been lost. If the canines occlude in lateral movement toward the side on which these teeth are present, canine rise would be a logical objective of selective grinding. If sound maxillary and mandibular canines do not occlude in lateral movement, canine disclusion cannot be attained. If the posterior teeth have little or no bone loss, group function would be the objective. If the posterior teeth have moderate-to-severe bone loss and canines are essentially sound, however, either the canines may be restored to create canine disclusion or orthodontic positioning of the canines can be used to permit it.

B. If one or both canines on one side have moderate-to-severe bone loss, canine disclusion should be discarded as an objective. If the adjacent posterior teeth have little or no bone loss, group function would be the logical objective. If the adjacent posterior teeth have moderate-to-severe bone loss, as do the canines, splinting to distribute the loading more evenly is necessary, especially if the teeth are very mobile. If mobility is minimal, selective grinding to "smooth out" the group function may suffice.

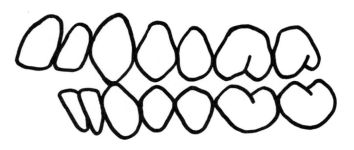

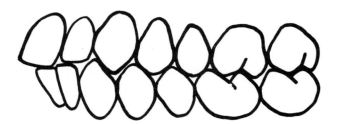

Figure 1. Illustration of working side contacts in canine disclusion or in group function situations.

References

D'Amito A. The canine teeth: Normal functional relation of the natural teeth of man. Cal Dent Assoc J 1958;26:6.

Grant DA, Stern JB, Listgarten MA. Periodontics. 6th ed. St. Louis: CV Mosby, 1988:986.

Ramfjord S, Ash MM. Occlusion. 3rd ed. Philadelphia: WB Saunders, 1983:370.

Schluger S, Yuodelis R, Page RC, Johnson RH. Periodontal diseases. 2nd ed. Philadelphia: Lea & Febiger, 1990:392.

Periodontal patient with NEED FOR SELECTIVE GRINDING

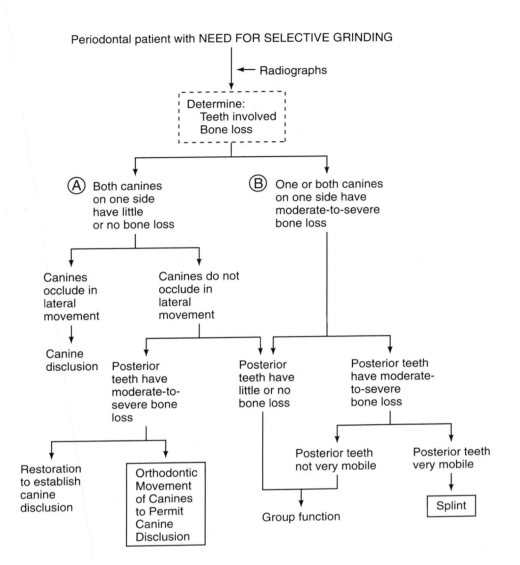

← Radiographs

Determine:
Teeth involved
Bone loss

Ⓐ Both canines on one side have little or no bone loss

Ⓑ One or both canines on one side have moderate-to-severe bone loss

Canines occlude in lateral movement

Canines do not occlude in lateral movement

Canine disclusion

Posterior teeth have moderate-to-severe bone loss

Posterior teeth have little or no bone loss

Posterior teeth have moderate-to-severe bone loss

Restoration to establish canine disclusion

Orthodontic Movement of Canines to Permit Canine Disclusion

Posterior teeth not very mobile

Posterior teeth very mobile

Group function

Splint

SELECTIVE GRINDING VERSUS SPLINTING

Walter B. Hall

If a periodontal patient seeking treatment has loose teeth that would benefit by minimizing further trauma to them, the dentist must decide whether to use selective grinding alone or splinting, or a combination of the two.

A. The loose teeth may be localized or generalized. A localized problem offers more options than does a generalized one. A localized problem may be one of primary or secondary occlusal trauma. A generalized problem may be one mostly of primary, or mostly of secondary, occlusal trauma.

B. Localized loose teeth may have lost little or no bone support but still be mobile. Selective grinding should eliminate such problems of localized primary occlusal trauma.

C. Localized loose teeth, however, could have lost a moderate-to-severe amount of bone. If most other teeth are sound (have little bone loss), selective grinding may reduce the loading to the loose teeth enough that trauma will be minimized. If the adjacent teeth are sound and the loose tooth is moderately involved, splinting may be used to stabilize the loose tooth. If the loose tooth has lost substantial support, guided tissue regeneration (GTR) may be considered. If GTR is a predictable procedure on the severely involved tooth, it should be used (see p 148). If GTR is not possible or acceptable to the patient and the adjacent abutments are adequate, the compromised tooth should be extracted and replaced with a bridge rather than jeopardizing sound abutment teeth to maintain a tooth with a guarded-to-hopeless prognosis.

D. If most teeth are loose but have little or no bone loss, the problem would be one of generalized primary occlusal trauma and can be managed with selective grinding; a night guard along with selective grinding may be required.

E. If most teeth have moderate-to-severe bone loss, generalized secondary occlusal trauma would be the diagnosis. One should assess the possible use of GTR, where predictable, to change individual tooth prognosis. Where practical, GTR should be employed along with temporary or provisional splinting before permanent splinting is employed. In some cases, where the amount of loss of support is less, splinting may be a sufficient treatment along with maintenance or surgery. The age and financial means of the patient would influence the decision to proceed.

References

Carranza FM Jr. Glickman's clinical periodontology. 7th ed. Philadelphia: WB Saunders, 1990:422.

Nyman S, Lindhe J, Lundgren D. The role of occlusion for the stability of fixed bridges in patients with reduced periodontal support. J Clin Periodontol 1975;22:53.

Ramfjord S, Ash MM. Occlusion. 3rd ed. Philadelphia: WB Saunders, 1983:384.

Ringli HH. Splinting of teeth: An objective assessment. Helv Odontol Acta 1971;15:129.

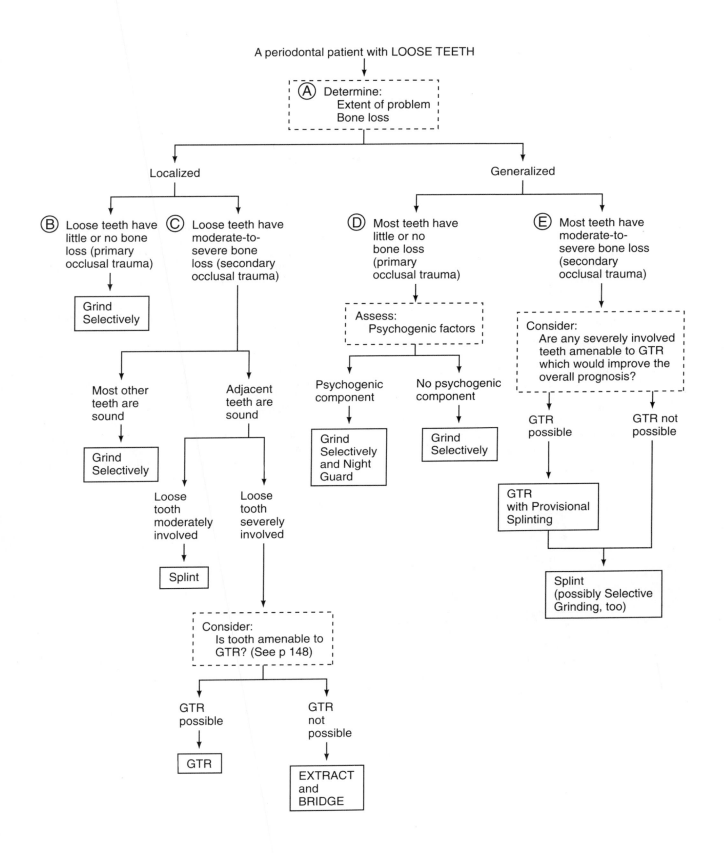

A periodontal patient with LOOSE TEETH

Ⓐ Determine:
Extent of problem
Bone loss

Localized

Generalized

Ⓑ Loose teeth have little or no bone loss (primary occlusal trauma)

Grind Selectively

Ⓒ Loose teeth have moderate-to-severe bone loss (secondary occlusal trauma)

Most other teeth are sound

Grind Selectively

Adjacent teeth are sound

Loose tooth moderately involved

Splint

Loose tooth severely involved

Consider:
Is tooth amenable to GTR? (See p 148)

GTR possible

GTR

GTR not possible

EXTRACT and BRIDGE

Ⓓ Most teeth have little or no bone loss (primary occlusal trauma)

Assess:
Psychogenic factors

Psychogenic component

Grind Selectively and Night Guard

No psychogenic component

Grind Selectively

Ⓔ Most teeth have moderate-to-severe bone loss (secondary occlusal trauma)

Consider:
Are any severely involved teeth amenable to GTR which would improve the overall prognosis?

GTR possible

GTR with Provisional Splinting

GTR not possible

Splint (possibly Selective Grinding, too)

SELECTIVE GRINDING VERSUS NIGHT GUARD

Walter B. Hall

For a periodontal patient with loose or symptomatic teeth who clenches and grinds, the dentist must decide whether selective grinding or night-guard therapy is indicated. Selective grinding either may smooth out the occlusion so that "trigger" discrepancies are eliminated or may only better distribute forces so that less trauma occurs. A night guard (Fig. 1) can be used to control trauma relating to bruxism (parafunctional clenching or grinding at night). Occasionally, a patient may also be able to wear such a guard for periods during the day. If the problems are of psychological origin, selective grinding may be of little help in stopping the clenching and grinding.

A. If the patient has an essentially satisfactory occlusion but still has loose or symptomatic teeth, only a night guard is indicated. The guard will not prevent the patient from clenching and grinding, but it will minimize trauma to the teeth while it is being worn. Such patients usually have a psychogenic need to clench and grind. Not all such patients will wear a night guard. The dentist should explain to the patient the need to wear one in bed and the tendency to salivate more while wearing it, before the patient

decides to have one fabricated. Some patients become so accustomed to a night guard that they cannot sleep if they lose it or forget to bring it with them.

B. Some patients have an inadequate number of teeth or an occlusion that cannot be treated by selective grinding. If a restorative plan that would provide a better, less traumatogenic occlusion cannot be financed by the patient, a night guard may be used to minimize the trauma.

C. In some cases in which the patient has loose or symptomatic teeth and selective grinding is both indicated and feasible, he or she may reject selective grinding. If so, a night guard may be a helpful alternative. If the patient agrees to selective grinding and the dentist can determine a psychogenic component to the etiology of the clenching and grinding, both selective grinding and night guard should be used. Where psychogenic factors are minimal or absent and the dentist can detect "trigger tooth" disharmony, selective grinding alone may be sufficient to control the clenching and grinding, to improve the firmness of teeth, and to minimize the symptoms.

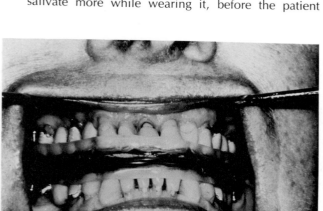

Figure 1. Paired maxillary and mandibular night guards.

References

Glickman I, Ratcliff P, Zander HA, Sugarman M. When and to what extent do you adjust the occlusion during periodontal therapy? J Periodontol 1970;41:536.

Muhlemann HR, Herzog H, Rateitschak KH. Qualitative evaluation of the therapeutic effect of selective grinding. J Periodontol 1957;28:11.

Posselt V, Wolff IB. Treatment of bruxism by bite guards and bite plates. Can Dent Assoc J 1963;29:773.

Ramfjord S, Ash MM. Occlusion. 3rd ed. Philadelphia: WB Saunders, 1983:365.

Schluger S, Yuodelis R, Page RC, Johnson RH. Periodontal diseases. 2nd ed. Philadelphia: Lea & Febiger, 1989: 405.

A periodontal patient with LOOSE OR SYMPTOMATIC TEETH WHO CLENCHES AND GRINDS

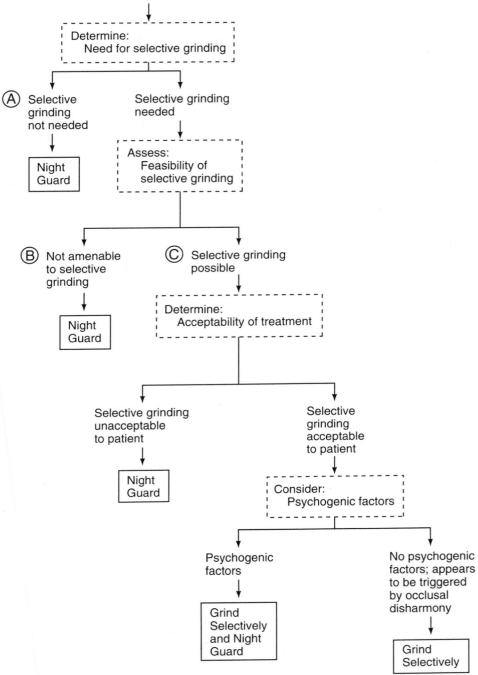

THE ADULT ORTHODONTIC CASE

Timothy F. Geraci

Orthodontic tooth movement in an adult has as its goal the improvement of both the periodontal and restorative environments. The adult orthodontic candidate who presents with preexisting periodontal involvement requires a dentist who has critical diagnostic skills, rigid periodontal therapeutic skills, and a knowledge of the biomechanical movement of teeth. An adult has a static orthodontic environment; the growth period has been completed and cannot be used in diagnostic planning. To make matters more complex, the periodontal status can be either improved or made worse by biomechanical intervention.

A. When the oral hygiene level is not acceptable, the patient should not undergo orthodontic therapy. The inflammatory lesion must be controlled during orthodontic movement. If this is not achieved, the case could be compromised and/or teeth lost as a result of the orthodontics. Thorough root planing and root debridement are basic preorthodontic requirements if pathology is present. Surgical intervention may be required to ensure clean roots or reduction of non-maintainable pocket depth. A periodontal abscess during the active orthodontic phase can be disastrous.

B. Interceptive mucogingival surgery should be performed in areas with potential problems. A compromised solution may result if the problem is not addressed until it is acute. Because of the position of the teeth in the alveolar housing, there may be a partial absence of bone over the facial or lingual root surface and a connective tissue attachment only. Failure to recognize this problem before treatment begins could result in severe root exposure during treatment and/or a tooth that is in a proper position but cannot be restored because of lack of supporting bone.

C. The patient's root form and length are important from the aspect of postorthodontic suitability. Poor root form and length are basic contraindications for orthodontic therapy. At the other end of the spectrum, teeth with long roots may not move easily or move at all.

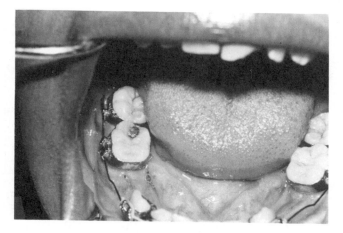

Figure 2. The same teeth with the orthodontic appliance in place to bring the tilted teeth upright.

D. Teeth with preexisting furcation involvements of Class II or more are poor candidates for orthodontic movement. The chances of an abscess or increased bone loss are too great. The involved tooth may be endodontically treated and the root or roots removed if the tooth is critical to the case. A Class I furcation involvement requires the highest priority during orthodontic therapy, and it must be monitored and debrided constantly.

E. Patients who present with preexisting crepitus, muscle tenderness, excessive occlusal wear, restricted mandibular opening, mandibular deviation on opening and closing, or subluxation of the mandible are at high risk for orthodontic tooth movement. These conditions may not improve with orthodontic treatment and, in fact, may worsen. Document these dental findings before beginning tooth movement.

F. If anterior teeth, which have drifted to a facial position, are going to be retracted to a functional position, sufficient overjet and overbite will be required, and an occlusal adjustment may be needed in order to place the mandible in a stable, retruded position. If a suitable overjet/overbite and stable occlusal position cannot be achieved, orthodontic movement cannot be successful. A diagnostic occlusal splint is indicated in preorthodontic therapy in order to determine if the aforementioned objectives can be achieved.

G. Before the dentist initiates minor tooth movement procedures, the patient must be informed of the need to retain teeth in their new position via splinting or fixed bridgework, and the patient should have prior knowledge as to the cost involved in restoring the case. If a tipped tooth is being placed in an upright position for fixed bridgework, occlusal reduction is required during treatment in order to gain space in an occlusal–apical direction in order for the tooth to move. Because of the "increase" in clinical crown

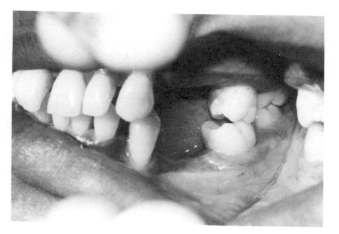

Figure 1. Preoperative view of a tilted molar with a mesial osseous defect prior to uprighting.

CASE PROGNOSIS DEPENDS ON IMPROVING PATIENT'S TOOTH POSITION

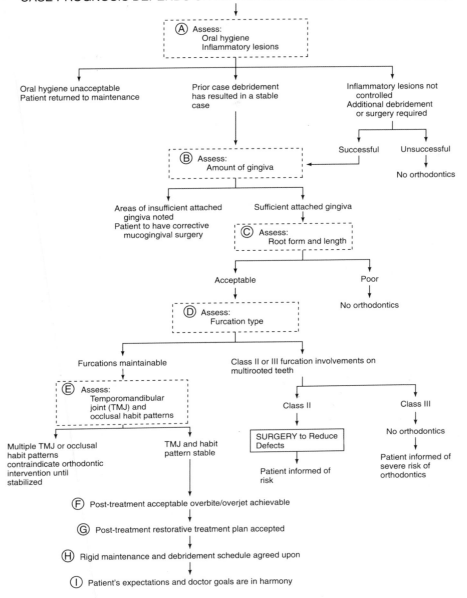

Ⓐ Assess:
Oral hygiene
Inflammatory lesions

Oral hygiene unacceptable
Patient returned to maintenance

Prior case debridement
has resulted in a stable
case

Inflammatory lesions not
controlled
Additional debridement
or surgery required

Successful   Unsuccessful

No orthodontics

Ⓑ Assess:
Amount of gingiva

Areas of insufficient attached
gingiva noted
Patient to have corrective
mucogingival surgery

Sufficient attached gingiva

Ⓒ Assess:
Root form and length

Acceptable   Poor

No orthodontics

Ⓓ Assess:
Furcation type

Furcations maintainable

Class II or III furcation involvements on
multirooted teeth

Ⓔ Assess:
Temporomandibular
joint (TMJ) and
occlusal habit patterns

Class II   Class III

Multiple TMJ or occlusal
habit patterns
contraindicate orthodontic
intervention until
stabilized

TMJ and habit
pattern stable

SURGERY to Reduce
Defects

No orthodontics

Patient informed of
severe risk of
orthodontics

Patient informed of
risk

Ⓕ Post-treatment acceptable overbite/overjet achievable

Ⓖ Post-treatment restorative treatment plan accepted

Ⓗ Rigid maintenance and debridement schedule agreed upon

Ⓘ Patient's expectations and doctor goals are in harmony

---

during the uprighting and the reduction of the occlusal height to gain space, followed by crown preparation, a posterior tooth that has been uprighted may require an endodontic procedure (Figs. 1 and 2).

H. Because orthodontic tooth movement involves a breakdown of bone where pressure is applied and deposition of bone in areas of application of tension, the osseous topography of an area will change as a result of tooth movement. Infrabony defects can be reduced by deposition of bone on the tension side of the root and positioning of the root into an infrabony defect on the pressure side of the root. During the active phase of movement, the roots should be debrided and the soft tissue lining the pockets curetted every 2 weeks. As stated previously, the inflammatory lesion must be controlled during the active phase. Constant debridement of an area will increase the chances for reducing an infrabony defect and the development of a successful case. Patients who do not

present with moderate infrabony lesions should be on a strict 3-month periodontal maintenance program during their orthodontic therapy.

I. Finally, the patient should understand the objectives of minor tooth movement. The expectations of the patient and the goal of the doctor cannot be in conflict, and the dental objectives should be noted and discussed before treatment is initiated.

References

Lindhe J. Clinical periodontology. 2nd ed. Copenhagen: Munksgaard, 1989:564.

Sadowsky C, BeCole E. Long-term effects of orthodontic treatment on periodontal health. Am J Orthod 1981;80:156.

Zachrisson B, Alnaes L. Periodontal condition in orthodontically treated and untreated individuals. Part I. Angle Orthod 1973;43:401; Part II. Angle Orthod 1974;44:43.

PERMANENT SPLINTING

Timothy F. Geraci

A. Patients who have advanced periodontal disease often demonstrate secondary occlusal trauma; thus, the dentist has to treat the additional factors of uncontrolled mobility and occlusal forces that are excessive. Before initiating periodontal therapy, consider how the case is to be restored and if post-treatment mobility will be damaging to the prognosis.

B. At the initial examination, a patient is seen at his worst. A case with poor plaque control, moderate-to-severe subgingival calculus, and chronic inflammation demonstrates measurable mobility patterns. If the case is acutely inflamed, the mobility patterns are significant. The inflammatory lesion does not permit the connective tissue to function as supporting tissue. Establishing good oral hygiene and case debridement by root planing and scaling permit connective tissue fiber groups to reform, which result in decreased mobility patterns.

C. It is not significant that a tooth or teeth demonstrate Class I or Class II mobility patterns. It is significant that a tooth or teeth exhibit fremitus when occlusal forces are introduced or when mobility in lateral and protrusive excursions exists. Adjusting the occlusion to eliminate fremitus and neutralize the excursive forces preempts the need for case stabilization. The need for splinting occurs when the occlusal forces cannot be controlled. Teeth with Class III mobility (depressible) cannot be retained. Teeth commonly become mobile or more mobile after surgery. If the occlusal forces are neutralized, the teeth will return to their presurgical mobility within 18 months after surgery.

D. A splinted case must have the forces of occlusion distributed evenly. If one occlusal area is subject to excessive forces, the traumatic force is transmitted across the splint, and all splinted members are damaged. If this goal cannot be achieved, splinting will be of little value. Splinting will not make a tooth or teeth less mobile. Mobile teeth move in separate planes, and splinting does not permit the individual teeth to move within their planes. If splinted teeth are mobile, nothing has been accomplished. If a case that is in temporary stabilization is mobile, the dentist may elect not to proceed to the permanent prosthetic phase. If the patient has occlusal habit patterns, an occlusal guard will be required in order to compensate for the excessive forces. Permanent splinting permits the dentist greater latitude when restoring a case. If stabilization can be achieved and reciprocal bracing is a reality, the patient has a greater chance to have restored function. The keys to success in a case that exhibits secondary occlusal trauma are control of the occlusal forces and neutralization of the inflammatory process.

References

Glickman I, Stein RS, Smulow JB. The effects of increased periodontal forces upon the periodontium of splinted and non-splinted teeth. J Periodontol 1961;32:290.

Nyman S, Lindhe J, Lundgren P. The role of occlusion for the stability of fixed bridges in patients with reduced periodontal support. J Clin Periodontol 1975;2:53.

Schluger S, Yuodelis R, Page RC, Johnson RH. Periodontal diseases. 2nd ed. Philadelphia: Lea & Febiger, 1990:666.

Patient with SIGNIFICANT MOBILITY PATTERNS PRESENT AT INITIAL EXAMINATION

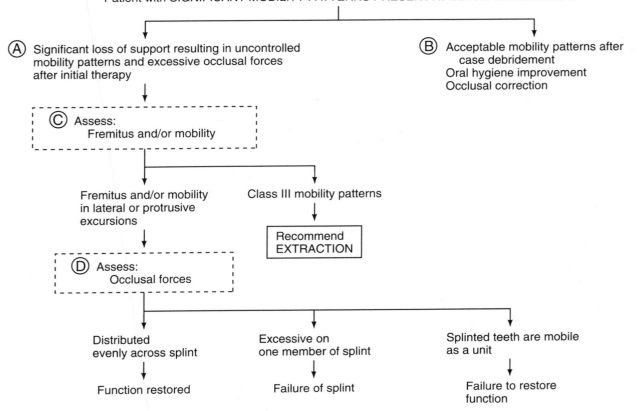

(A) Significant loss of support resulting in uncontrolled mobility patterns and excessive occlusal forces after initial therapy

(B) Acceptable mobility patterns after case debridement
Oral hygiene improvement
Occlusal correction

(C) Assess:
Fremitus and/or mobility

Fremitus and/or mobility in lateral or protrusive excursions

Class III mobility patterns

Recommend EXTRACTION

(D) Assess:
Occlusal forces

Distributed evenly across splint

Excessive on one member of splint

Splinted teeth are mobile as a unit

Function restored

Failure of splint

Failure to restore function

TREATMENT OF GINGIVAL ENLARGEMENTS

William P. Lundergan

Treatment of a gingival enlargement is dependent upon the nature of the enlargement (inflammatory, fibrotic, or neoplastic) and the etiologic factors involved (see p 52). Treatment of inflammatory or fibrotic enlargements generally involves the elimination of local factors followed by surgical treatment of any residual enlargement. Suspected neoplasms require a biopsy to establish or confirm a diagnosis.

A. During the treatment of a gingival abscess or an acute periodontal abscess, the dentist gives a local anesthetic, establishes drainage, and debrides the lesion. In the case of the gingival abscess, blade incision is used to establish drainage. Drainage for the periodontal abscess is achieved with an external incision or by curette via the pocket. Care should be taken not to overinstrument the root surface, as this will decrease the prospects for re-attachment. Once drainage is established, irrigate the lesion with warm saline solution or water. For a periodontal abscess, antibiotics should be prescribed if the patient is experiencing malaise or lymphadenopathy, or is febrile. Analgesics can be prescribed for pain. Following treatment of an acute abscess, the patient should return the next day. The dentist should evaluate the area for further treatment (i.e., surgery) once the acute symptoms have resolved.

B. Treatment of chronic inflammatory gingival enlargements involves a heavy emphasis on proper daily plaque control, elimination of other local irritants (calculus, poor dental restorations, caries, open contacts with food impaction, mouth breathing, orthodontic braces, and poorly fitted removable appliances), and identification of potential systemic factors. Systemic factors may include vitamin deficiency, leukemia, and hormonal changes occurring during pregnancy or puberty or in association with oral contraceptives. Some enlargements may resolve once the etiologic factors are eliminated; however, many are secondarily fibrotic and require surgical treatment to resolve. Evaluate the need for surgery (gingivectomy or flap procedure) once sufficient time has been allowed for response to the initial therapy. Consult the patient's physician if a vitamin C deficiency or leukemia is suspected. Check bleeding and clotting times before treatment for leukemic gingival enlargement.

C. Treatment of a drug-induced gingival enlargement should include a physician consult regarding alternative drug therapy. Drug-induced enlargement may regress or completely resolve once the medication is discontinued. In most cases, however, an alternative drug therapy is not practical. Treatment then involves meticulous plaque control, removal of local irritants, and, once the enlargement interferes with aesthetics or mastication, or presents a significant plaque control problem, gingivectomy or flap surgery. Recurrence is generally a problem, but it can be minimized with proper attention to daily plaque control and to regular professional cleanings. Some clinicians use positive-pressure appliances after surgery to help discourage recurrence.

D. Hereditary gingival fibromatosis is treated surgically (gingivectomy or flap procedure) once it interferes with aesthetics or mastication, or becomes a significant plaque control problem. The condition can recur despite meticulous oral hygiene, and often regresses following tooth extraction.

E. Suspected neoplasms require a biopsy to establish or confirm a diagnosis. Treatment depends on the nature of the neoplasm, and referral to a specialist is often indicated.

References

Carranza FA Jr. Glickman's clinical periodontology. 7th ed. Philadelphia: WB Saunders, 1990:908.

Lundergan WP. Drug-induced gingival enlargements —dilantin hyperplasia and beyond. J Calif Dent Assoc 1989;17:48.

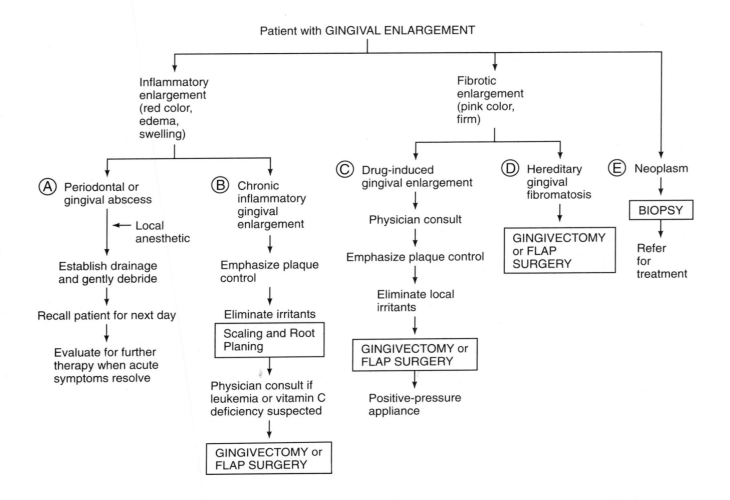

Patient with GINGIVAL ENLARGEMENT

Inflammatory enlargement (red color, edema, swelling)

Fibrotic enlargement (pink color, firm)

(A) Periodontal or gingival abscess

← Local anesthetic

Establish drainage and gently debride

Recall patient for next day

Evaluate for further therapy when acute symptoms resolve

(B) Chronic inflammatory gingival enlargement

Emphasize plaque control

Eliminate irritants

Scaling and Root Planing

Physician consult if leukemia or vitamin C deficiency suspected

GINGIVECTOMY or FLAP SURGERY

(C) Drug-induced gingival enlargement

Physician consult

Emphasize plaque control

Eliminate local irritants

GINGIVECTOMY or FLAP SURGERY

Positive-pressure appliance

(D) Hereditary gingival fibromatosis

GINGIVECTOMY or FLAP SURGERY

(E) Neoplasm

BIOPSY

Refer for treatment

CIRCUMSCRIBED GINGIVAL ENLARGEMENTS

Gonzalo Hernandez Vallejo

Circumscribed gingival enlargements (CGE) include those exophitic lesions that are localized and limited to the gingiva adjacent to a tooth or group of teeth. Circumscribed gingival enlargements may adopt different nonspecific clinical shapes that may aid the clinician in diagnosis. Still, in most instances, biopsy is required to establish the definitive diagnosis. Diagnostic sequence of CGE should include a carefully detailed medical and dental history. Once CGE has been detected, the inflammatory appearance of the lesion has to be assessed.

A. Inflamed lesions are characterized by redness, edema, swelling, and bleeding, and they may appear at the attached or marginal/papillar gingiva (the inflammatory origin of the lesion does not necessarily mean that it appears inflamed). Examination of the morphology of the lesion, accompanied by radiography and probing of the sulcus, is important to assess the diagnosis.

B. Inflamed CGE located at the attached gingiva may adopt a pedunculated/polypoid shape. Dental pain and negative vitality, together with the presence of a polypoid lesion near the border between attached gingiva and alveolar mucosa, suggest a parulis (draining chronic alveolar abscess), which can be easily confirmed by radiograph. If the lesion appears in the socket corresponding to a removed tooth one should suspect an epulis granulomatosum. Presence of partial or complete dentures accompanied by exophitic hyperplastic tissue at the periphery of the prosthesis provides enough information to diagnose an epulis fissuratum.

   Those CGE that display a nodular dome shape, with a smooth, shiny surface, have to be checked for acute infections. Gingival abscess is usually limited to the marginal/interdental gingiva and is clinically characterized by acute pain, redness, and fluctuance with no loss of attachment. Periodontal abscesses, however, show features of periodontal disease and radiographic evidence of bone loss.

C. Inflamed CGE involving marginal/papillar gingiva are common lesions. Radiography is important at the time of evaluating the involvement of the underlying bone. Red polypoid or nodular masses that bleed easily and are accompanied by bone radiolucency may indicate a central giant cell granuloma. When no bone involvement is observed, several conditions must be kept in mind. Chronic inflammatory enlargements sometimes appear as painful, red, localized papillar or marginal masses and are associated with local factors such as bacterial plaque, calculus, and so on. Pyogenic granuloma is an inflammatory hyperplasia that clinically consists of a red/purple, very soft, friable, nodular, or pedunculated mass that frequently shows an eroded or ulcerated surface that bleeds under the slightest trauma. Pregnancy tumor occurs in 3% to 5% of pregnancies; it appears as a spherical or flattened mass located in marginal and interdental papilla. Its surface is dusky red or magenta, and it displays numerous very small red spots. Peripheral giant cell granuloma arises as a nodular or polypoid mass at the gingiva and edentulous alveolar mucosa; its consistency is usually firm, with a smooth or granular surface, and it may become large. Gingival abscess also may appear circumscribed to the marginal/papillar gingiva. Some rarities, such as hemangiomas and Kaposi's sarcoma in cases of acquired immunodeficiency syndrome may resemble the lesions belonging to this group.

D. Noninflamed CGE include those conditions that exhibit clinical characteristics where inflammation is absent. An evaluation of the color of the lesion is extremely important in this group of entities. White color is a typical feature in papillomas and Verruca vulgaris, and they usually show a pedunculated shape with a cauliflower-like appearance. Brown CGE are rare and are associated with hyperparathyroidism; they appear as multiple tumoral lesions accompanied by bone involvement; clinical history, radiography, and biochemical data support the correct diagnosis. Blue lesions include hemangioma, hematoma, eruption cysts, and, less frequently, the blue variety of peripheral giant cell granuloma. Careful examination can give us information about the history of trauma (hematoma) or reveal the presence of unerupted teeth (eruption cyst). Red/pink CGE comprise the majority of gingival tumors and tumor-like conditions. Clinical characteristics are of little help in differentiating those entities; therefore, biopsy is the method of choice to achieve the diagnosis. Clinical diagnosis, however, must be focused on the texture (consistency) of the CGE.

E. Hard lesions with bone-like consistency have to be assessed by radiography. Exostoses are common developmental lesions that can occur in alveolar bone and give a radiopaque image. Radiolucencies accompanied by CGE are associated with central exophitic lesions.

F. Soft-to-firm (not hard) CGE may display normal bone or bone changes under radiographic examination. Radiopaque images can be observed in peripheral fibroma with calcification or in peripheral ossifying fibroma. The presence of radiopaque foci within the tumors, together with the feature of separated teeth in this area, may help in the diagnosis. Radiolucencies appear frequently in cases of central giant cell granuloma, malignant central tumors with peripheral invasion, and cysts. Gingival cysts arising from remnants of odontogenic epithelium may cause erosion of the alveolar bone, giving a circumscript radiolucency.

G. Soft-to-firm masses that concur with normal bone include most of the neoplasias. These conditions have

Patient with CIRCUMSCRIBED GINGIVAL ENLARGEMENT

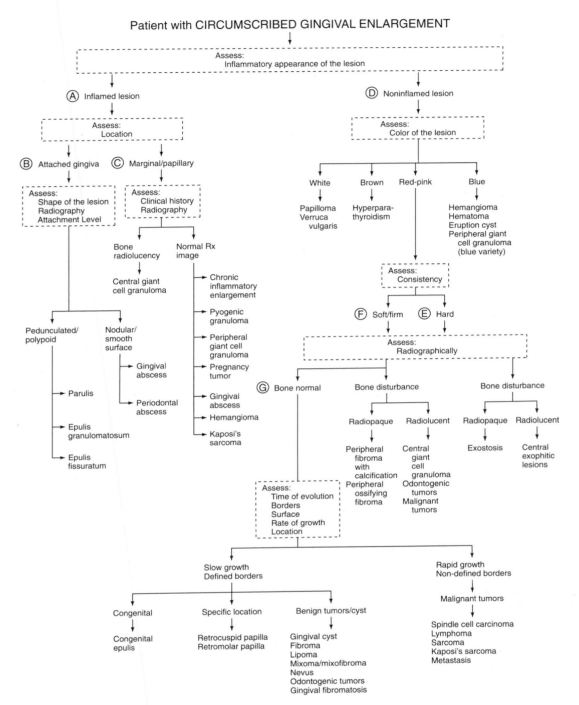

to be evaluated while paying careful attention to the age of the lesion, rate of growth, external aspect of the lesion (surface), and location. Special care has to be taken not to confuse normal anatomic variations such as retromolar papilla and retrocuspid papilla. Congenital epulis appears at birth as a large polypoid swelling and is easily recognizable. Benign tumors and gingival cysts show slow growth and well-defined borders and include a great number of lesions arising from the gingiva; a biopsy is required in all cases. Gingival fibromatosis may appear as a CGE, usually located in the palatal posterior areas.

Those CGE present a rapid rate of growth, and nondefined borders have to be suspected for malig-

nancies, whether growing from gingival tissues, central bone, or metastasis from other locations.

References

Carranza FA Jr. Glickman's clinical periodontology. 7th ed. Philadelphia: WB Saunders, 1990:125.

Eversole LR. Clinical outline of oral pathology. 2nd ed. Philadelphia: Lea & Febiger, 1984:91.

Grant DA, Stern IB, Listgarten MA. Periodontics. 6th ed. St. Louis: CV Mosby, 1988:425.

Wood NK, Goaz PW. Differential diagnosis of oral lesions. 4th ed. St. Louis: CV Mosby, 1991:142.

NECROTIZING ULCERATIVE GINGIVITIS AND PERIODONTITIS: TREATMENT

Gerald J. DeGregori

The successful treatment of necrotizing ulcerative gingivitis and periodontitis demands a definite protocol. The initial goal of treatment is to make the patient more comfortable, which can be accomplished by separating the treatment schedule into two appointments, about 4 days apart. The first appointment is devoted to examination, diagnosis, the prescription of appropriate medications, and a superficial debridement with ultrasonic or hand instruments if heavy calculus deposits interfere with minimal oral hygiene procedures.

A. If the disease is confined to soft tissue only, the dentist should explain the disease process to the patient and give assurance that it is controllable. Direct the patient to rinse the mouth with 50% hydrogen peroxide and 50% warm water for 2 minutes twice a day.

B. Write prescriptions for appropriate antibiotics and analgesics. Explain to the patient the importance of taking the full regimen of antibiotics. The antibiotic of choice is the potassium salt of penicillin V (Pen VK), 500 mg, four times per day for 7 days. Erythromycin, 500 mg, four times per day for 7 days, should be prescribed if the patient is allergic to penicillin. Review possible allergic side effects to the medication.

C. An ideal analgesic is one that not only controls pain but also elevates the patient's mood. A combination of propoxyphene napsylate and acetaminophen (Darvocet N-100) accomplishes such a goal. Explain that the patient will feel better in 24 hours, but stress the necessity of returning for further treatment in 4 days to avoid return of the disease. Explain that the additional treatment consists of a "deep cleaning." The patient should be encouraged to begin minimal oral hygiene procedures with a soft brush made even softer with hot water.

D. When the patient returns in 4 days, perform a full-mouth debridement with lavage, either with an ultrasonic instrument, which is the treatment of choice, or with hand instruments and copious water rinses. Admonish the patient to continue the antibiotics until the 7-day course is completed.

E. If significant soft-tissue damage has occurred, further appointments may be necessary for soft-tissue reconstruction. There is an inherent danger in proceeding too quickly with this step, as the disease may recur after soft-tissue reconstruction and may negate any progress made at this step of treatment.

F. Should the disease proceed into underlying alveolar bone, decide whether conventional periodontal treatment or extraction is necessary. The decision is usually based on the amount of remaining alveolar bone, tooth stability, and root proximity. Recurrence of necrotrizing ulcerative gingivitis is common. For this reason, delay the reconstructive phase of therapy as long as possible to gain assurance of case stability.

G. If the patient is available for only one appointment, the treatment of choice is full-mouth debridement and lavage, preferably using an ultrasonic instrument. Pain control may be a problem because of the degree of inflammation of the gingival tissues. Pain may be overcome by the use of "block" anesthetic procedures plus the use of nitrous oxide and oxygen, conscious sedation. Instrumentation should be followed by at least 4 days of 50% hydrogen peroxide and 50% warm water rinses, for 2 minutes twice a day. Appropriate antibiotic medication should be given for a total of 76 days and analgesics prescribed as necessary for pain control.

References

Carranza FA Jr. Glickman's clinical periodontology. 7th ed. Philadelphia: WB Saunders, 1990:154.

Genco RJ, Goldman HM, Cohen DW. Contemporary periodontics. St. Louis: CV Mosby, 1990:460.

Johnson BD, Engel D. Acute necrotizing gingivitis: A review of diagnosis, etiology and treatment. J Periodontol 1986;57:141.

Schluger S. Necrotizing ulcerative gingivitis in the army: Incidence, communicability and treatment. J Am Dent Assoc 1949;38:174.

Patient with NECROTIZING ULCERATIVE GINGIVITIS/PERIODONTITIS

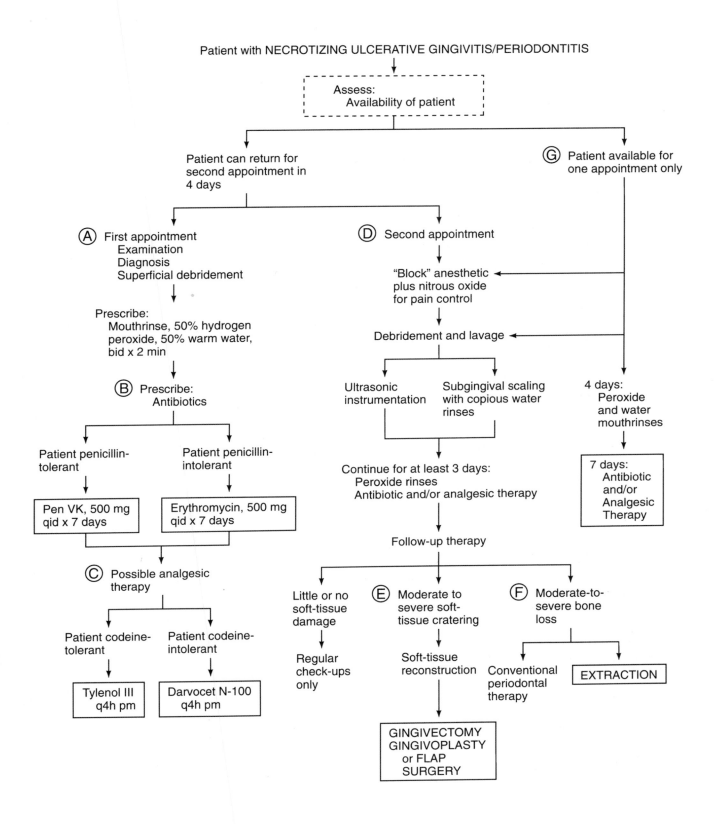

Assess:
Availability of patient

Patient can return for second appointment in 4 days

Ⓖ Patient available for one appointment only

Ⓐ First appointment
Examination
Diagnosis
Superficial debridement

Ⓓ Second appointment

"Block" anesthetic plus nitrous oxide for pain control

Prescribe:
Mouthrinse, 50% hydrogen peroxide, 50% warm water, bid x 2 min

Debridement and lavage

Ⓑ Prescribe:
Antibiotics

Ultrasonic instrumentation

Subgingival scaling with copious water rinses

4 days:
Peroxide and water mouthrinses

Patient penicillin-tolerant

Patient penicillin-intolerant

7 days:
Antibiotic and/or Analgesic Therapy

Pen VK, 500 mg qid x 7 days

Erythromycin, 500 mg qid x 7 days

Continue for at least 3 days:
Peroxide rinses
Antibiotic and/or analgesic therapy

Ⓒ Possible analgesic therapy

Follow-up therapy

Patient codeine-tolerant

Patient codeine-intolerant

Little or no soft-tissue damage

Ⓔ Moderate to severe soft-tissue cratering

Ⓕ Moderate-to-severe bone loss

Tylenol III q4h pm

Darvocet N-100 q4h pm

Regular check-ups only

Soft-tissue reconstruction

Conventional periodontal therapy

EXTRACTION

GINGIVECTOMY
GINGIVOPLASTY
or FLAP
SURGERY

INDICATIONS FOR MOLAR TOOTH RESECTION: HEMISECTION VERSUS ROOT AMPUTATION

Jordi Cambra
Borja Zabelegui

Root resection is a technique for maintaining a portion of a diseased or injured molar by removal of one or more of its roots. Resection may be achieved by hemisection, in which the entire tooth is cut in half and one part is removed, or by root amputation, in which only a root or two are amputated from the remainder of the tooth (Fig. 1). These surgical approaches may be useful in many situations. The indications for selecting hemisection or root amputation are dependent upon the status of the individual molar and its relationships to other teeth. Guided tissue regeneration (GTR) may be a viable option in many cases (see p 148).

A. If a molar has fused roots, neither hemisection nor root amputation is possible. If a Class II furcation is present (see p 144), GTR may be attempted. If a Class III furcation is present (see p 146), extraction or maintenance with a hopeless prognosis is an option.

B. A maxillary molar with advanced involvement of a proximal furcation and separated roots where root proximity is a problem would be treated by root amputation to facilitate access for debridement by the dentist and the patient. Where root proximity is not a complicating factor, a Class II (definite) furcation involvement proximally could be treated by GTR or mucogingival—osseous surgery, or maintained with frequent planing (see p 154). The patient could establish plaque control with an interproximal brush. The same would be true when the facial furcation has a Class II involvement; however, if the furcations join one another (Class III), root amputation is indicated.

C. A mandibular molar with advanced furcation involvement and separated roots that is an existing bridge abutment would be a candidate for root amputation and retention of the existing bridge; however, a similarly involved mandibular molar that is not an existing bridge abutment would be treated by hemisection and crowning. In either case, if a Class II furcation is involved, GTR may be attempted. If a Class III furcation is present, hemisection or root amputation (if it is part of an existing bridge) should be performed.

D. If there is no endodontic involvement, periodontal considerations assume paramount importance. Determine which roots will be amputated. If doubts exist, periodontal surgery with vital resection of the root selected during surgery should be performed before endodontic treatment. If the root to be removed is clearly indicated, endodontics should be done before amputation, but if there is a doubt, surgery and vital root amputation allow for clinical decisions to be made. If the molar is mandibular, and is an abutment for an existing fixed bridge, root amputation may permit retention of that bridge. If it is not an existing abutment, hemisection and then crowning are indicated.

E. When a necrotic pulp condition exists, initiate endodontic treatment before periodontal treatment. The differential diagnosis becomes difficult when the bone loss that is causing a deep pocket formation may be related to failure of the root canal therapy due to technical errors (leaking obturations). Perforations or vertical root fracture with no separation of fragments may cause bone loss defects that mask primary periodontal conditions.

F. If the molar being considered has a cracked or perforated root, part of it may be salvaged by resection. If the tooth is nonsymptomatic, either maintenance with a guarded prognosis or a surgical approach could be considered. If the tooth is symptomatic and not of strategic (long-term) value, it may be extracted; however, if the tooth has strategic value, it should be treated. If the tooth is mandibular and is an abutment for an existing bridge, root amputation should be considered if root canal therapy can be performed on the root that will be retained. If it is not an abutment for an existing bridge, hemisection would be better. If the molar is a maxillary one and a single facial root is cracked or perforated, root amputation would be better if root canal therapy can be performed on remaining roots. If both facial roots are cracked or perforated, hemisection with removal of both facial roots may be a reasonable choice.

References

Amen CR. Hemisection and root amputation. Periodontics 1966;4:197.

Basaraba N. Root amputation and tooth hemisection. Dent Clin North Am 1969;13:121.

Grant DA, Stern IB, Listgarten MA. Periodontics. 6th ed. St. Louis: CV Mosby, 1988:935.

Hiatt WH, Owen CR. Periodontal pocket elimination by combined therapy. Dent Clin North Am 1964;8:133.

Schluger S, Yuodelis RA, Page RC. Periodontal diseases. 2nd ed. Philadelphia: Lea & Febiger, 1990:548.

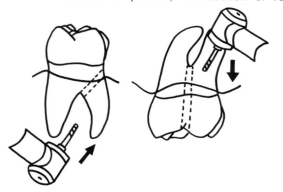

Figure 1. Illustration of hemisection (removal of half a tooth) and root amputation (removal of one root).

HEMISECTION VERSUS ROOT AMPUTATION
Patient with DISEASED or DAMAGED MOLAR

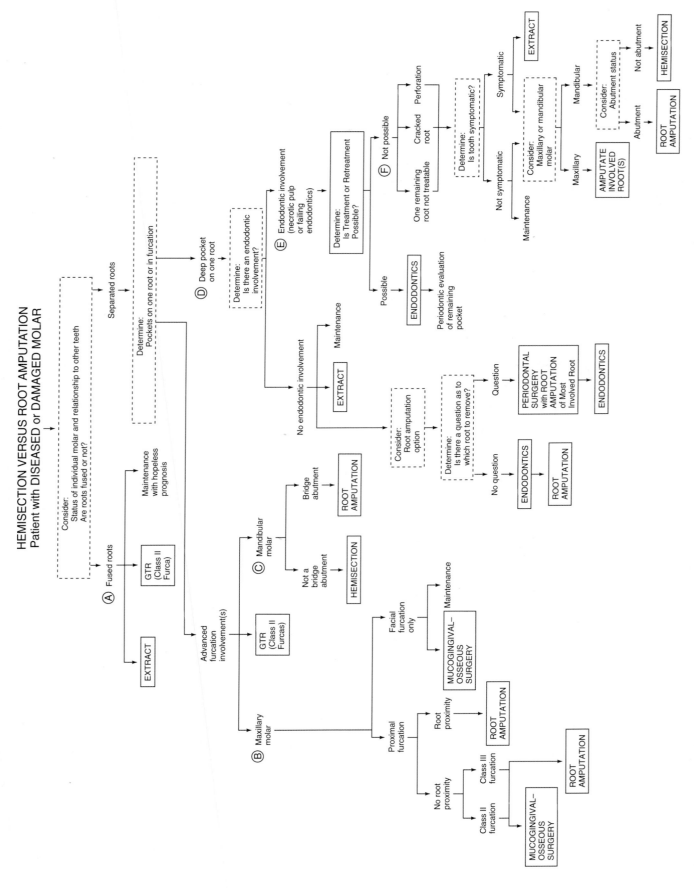

SEQUENCING ENDODONTICS AND ROOT RESECTION

Jordi Cambra
Borja Zabelegui

When a patient has a tooth requiring combined endodontic and periodontal treatment (root resection), the sequencing of the treatment may require considerable thought. Whenever possible, endodontic treatment should be done before root resection so that difficulty in obtaining adequate anesthesia for comfortable root canal therapy will not complicate endodontics following vital root resection. Vital root resection rarely results in complications of serious postoperative pain; however, as necrosis of the exposed pulp proceeds, the ability to obtain adequate anesthesia for comfortable root canal therapy is complicated by increasing acidity, which interferes with the efficacy of the local anesthetic; nevertheless, excellent reasons to accept this problem and to manage it do exist.

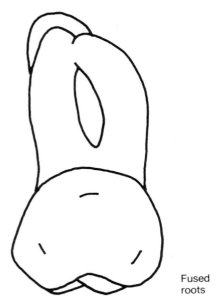

Figure 1. Roots that are fused at their apices are not candidates for root amputation.

Fused
roots

A. If the tooth is nonvital, the problem may be only endodontic, even though probing suggests that deep pockets are present, especially if the problem is severe and acute. If this appears to be the case, endodontics should be done first, because there may be no need for root resection later if pockets no longer can be probed.

B. If root resection will be needed, the first consideration is whether the roots to be resected are fused (Fig. 1). If so, the tooth must be extracted or maintained with a hopeless prognosis.

C. If the roots to be resected are not fused, the dentist must decide whether root canal therapy can be performed on all roots or not. If an untreatable root would be retained, the tooth should be extracted or maintained with a hopeless prognosis if it is symptom-free.

D. If endodontics can be done on all roots, or on all roots that will be retained, the next consideration relates to the certainty regarding which roots will be resected. If doubt exists, periodontal surgery with vital resection of the root selected during surgery should be performed before endodontic treatment. If the roots to be resected are clearly determinable before surgery, endodontic treatment should precede nonvital root resection.

References

Basaraba N. Root amputation and tooth hemisection. Dent Clin North Am 1969;13:121.

Grant DA, Stern IB, Listgarten MA. Periodontics. 6th ed. St. Louis: CV Mosby, 1988:916.

Hiatt WH, Amen CR. Periodontal pocket elimination by combined therapy. Dent Clin North Am 1964;8:133.

Schluger S, Yuodelis RA, Page RC, Johnson RH. Periodontal diseases. 2nd ed. Philadelphia: Lea & Febiger, 1990:549.

Simons HS, Glick DH, Frank AL. The relationship of endodontic–periodontic lesions. J Periodontol 1972;43:202.

Patient with MOLAR REQUIRING ROOT RESECTION

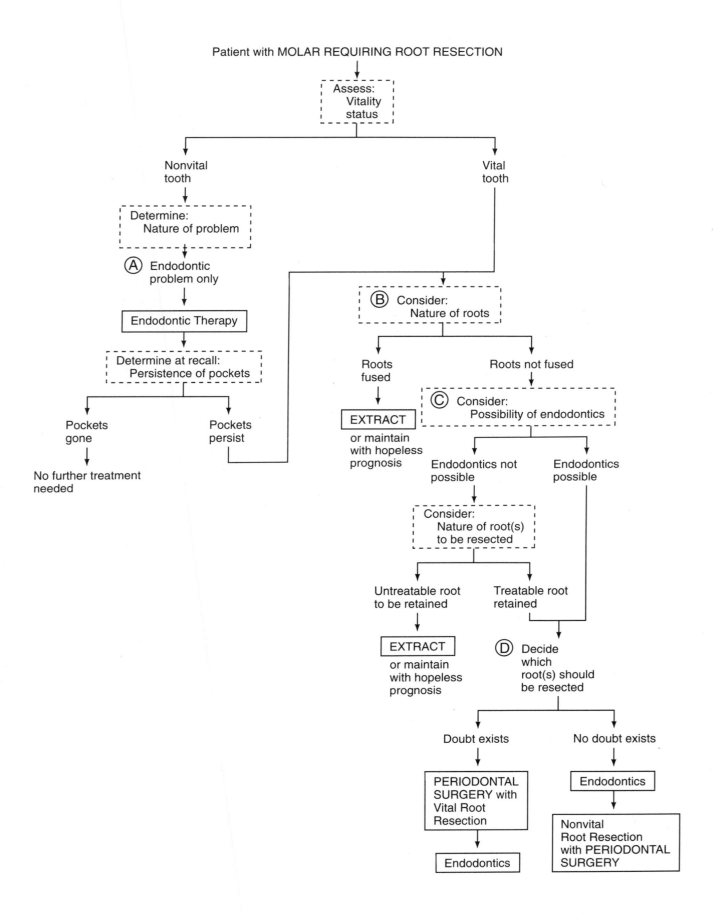

Assess:
Vitality
status

Nonvital
tooth

Vital
tooth

Determine:
Nature of problem

Ⓐ Endodontic
problem only

Ⓑ Consider:
Nature of roots

Endodontic Therapy

Roots
fused

Roots not fused

Determine at recall:
Persistence of pockets

EXTRACT

Ⓒ Consider:
Possibility of endodontics

or maintain
with hopeless
prognosis

Pockets
gone

Pockets
persist

Endodontics not
possible

Endodontics
possible

No further treatment
needed

Consider:
Nature of root(s)
to be resected

Untreatable root
to be retained

Treatable root
retained

EXTRACT

Ⓓ Decide
which
root(s) should
be resected

or maintain
with hopeless
prognosis

Doubt exists

No doubt exists

PERIODONTAL
SURGERY with
Vital Root
Resection

Endodontics

Endodontics

Nonvital
Root Resection
with PERIODONTAL
SURGERY

SURGICAL THERAPY VERSUS MAINTENANCE

Timothy F. Geraci

A. The goal of periodontal therapy is to develop an environment that the patient and the dentist can maintain in a stable status with ease. The possibilities of attaining this goal are a determining factor in evaluating a case for surgery. If initial therapy (i.e., root planing and plaque control) has attained the goal of an easily maintainable case, maintenance planning and monitoring to determine continued stability may be all that is required. If a stable state cannot be attained or maintained with ease, surgical alteration may be useful in achieving this goal. The decision is made at initial therapy evaluation, which should take place several weeks following completion of the initial treatment.

B. If the patient's general health is good, surgery may be considered. If he is seriously compromised (e.g., poorly controlled diabetes, high diastolic blood pressure), surgery may be contraindicated, and the patient should be maintained as well as possible with frequent recall visits for instrumentation and oral hygiene.

C. Plaque control by the patient is a key determining factor in deciding whether surgical therapy has merit or not. If the patient's plaque control on visible, accessible areas of the teeth is not good, mucogingival—osseous surgery would be as likely to compromise the case as to help it. Initial therapy should be repeated. If the patient's plaque control is good (or if there are overriding restorative demands), mucogingival—osseous surgery may be proposed.

D. Bleeding or suppuration on probing is an indication that pocket areas that are inaccessible to plaque control measures at home continue to exhibit active disease. When bleeding or suppuration does not occur on probing, recall maintenance may be an adequate means of stabilizing the case. Restorative needs, however, could be an indication for surgery despite this stability. If plaque control on the visible, accessible parts of teeth is good, but bleeding or suppuration occur on probing, consider surgery.

E. Surgery is indicated if it could make areas more accessible for plaque control and root planing without compromising support of potentially maintainable teeth or creating unacceptable aesthetic situations owing to root exposure. If additional support can be gained by regenerative means, one should vigorously encourage the patient to consider the surgical alternative. If these objectives cannot be obtained surgically, recall maintenance would be the approach of choice. If they can be obtained, propose the surgical alternative to the patient for his acceptance or rejection (see pp 76, 78).

References

Carranza FA Jr. Glickman's clinical periodontology. 7th ed. Philadelphia: WB Saunders, 1990:555.

Lindhe J. Textbook of clinical periodontology. 2nd ed. Copenhagen: Munksgaard, 1989:386.

Lindhe J, Nyman S. The effect of plaque control and surgical pocket elimination on the establishment and maintenance of periodontal health: A longitudinal study of periodontal therapy in cases of advanced periodontal disease. J Clin Periodontol 1985;2:67.

Schluger S, Yuodelis R, Page RC, Johnson RH. Periodontal diseases. 2nd ed. Philadelphia: Lea & Febiger, 1990:461.

Patient with RESIDUAL POCKET DEPTHS AT TIME OF INITIAL THERAPY EVALUATION

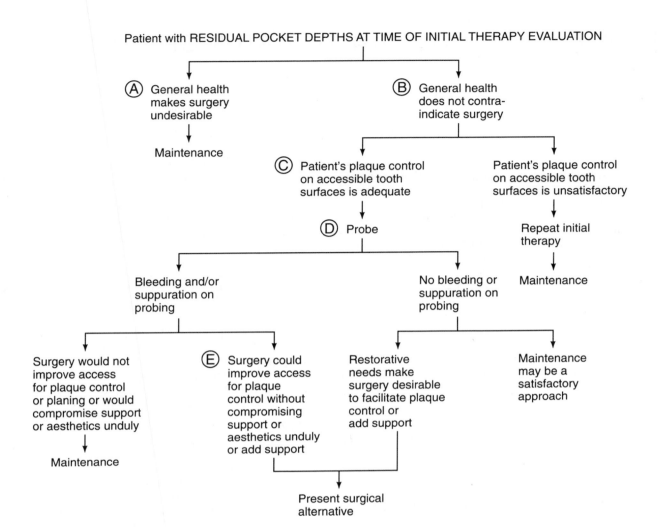

Ⓐ General health makes surgery undesirable
↓
Maintenance

Ⓑ General health does not contra-indicate surgery

Ⓒ Patient's plaque control on accessible tooth surfaces is adequate

Patient's plaque control on accessible tooth surfaces is unsatisfactory
↓
Repeat initial therapy
↓
Maintenance

Ⓓ Probe

Bleeding and/or suppuration on probing

No bleeding or suppuration on probing

Surgery would not improve access for plaque control or planing or would compromise support or aesthetics unduly
↓
Maintenance

Ⓔ Surgery could improve access for plaque control without compromising support or aesthetics unduly or add support

Restorative needs make surgery desirable to facilitate plaque control or add support

Maintenance may be a satisfactory approach

Present surgical alternative

EVALUATION OF FURCATION STATUS OF MOLARS BEFORE SURGERY

Walter B. Hall

When initial therapy evaluation is performed several weeks or more following root planing and any other aspects of initial treatment, the status of furcation involvements of molar teeth becomes an important consideration in deciding whether surgery would be beneficial to the patient. If furcations are readily accessible for plaque removal and root planing, maintenance by regular root planing several times a year is a reasonable option for controlling progress of inflammatory periodontal disease. If the furcations are not accessible for plaque removal and root planing, however, surgery may make them accessible, thus improving the prognosis for the tooth. An individual molar should be treated on the basis of the worst furcation involvement present (Fig. 1).

A. The type of furcation involvement must be assessed in deciding upon treatment options. If the furcations are not involved, maintenance by root planing alone usually is a good option. The status of adjacent teeth and pocket depths on the individual molar may make surgery a desirable option in some cases, even when furcations are not involved. Class I (incipient) and Class II (definite) involvements (see p 24) require considerable decision making. Class III ("through and through") involvements are discussed in the following chapter (see p 146). Mandibular molars have two furcations that must be evaluated in deciding upon further therapy at the time of initial therapy evaluation, whereas maxillary molars have three furcations.

B. If the worst involvement is incipient (Class I), maintenance with regular root planing several times a year usually will suffice. If the roots are fused, a Class I furcation may be all that is present to the apex of the tooth; therefore, pocket depths and type of osseous defect present become critical factors. If pocket depth is slight, the tooth may be maintained; however, if it is extensive, guided tissue regeneration (GTR) may be possible with the expectation of regenerating lost attachment. Most defects associated with fused roots will have three osseous walls, making them good candidates for GTR. Should the roots be tortuous and the defect not accessible to instrumentation surgically, extract the tooth or maintain it with a hopeless prognosis.

C. If the molar has a Class II (definite) involvement, access for plaque removal and root planing is a most important consideration in deciding upon the possible value of surgery. Because maxillary molars have proximal furcations, access is a greater problem in that arch than in the mandibular one. If access is good, maintenance with regular root planing several times a year may be sufficient. The status of adjacent teeth, however, may make including molars with Class II furcations in surgery a desirable option, even though they are accessible for maintenance. If the access is not good, so that adequate plaque removal and root planing are difficult or impossible to accomplish, loss of attachment and type of osseous defect present become the chief factors in deciding upon treatment. If the defect is less than 3 mm straight in, mucogingival–osseous surgery with an apically positioned flap approach will make the area accessible for instrumentation and plaque removal. If the defect is 3 mm or more straight in, a three-walled osseous defect usually will be present on facial or lingual furcas, whereas proximal ones may be two-walled or three-walled. All are good candidates for GTR.

D. Class III "through and through" furcas are not amenable to predictable GTR as yet. The decision-making process for treating them is presented in the next chapter (see p 146).

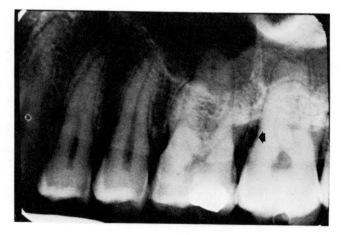

Figure 1. A distal furcation involvement on the first molar with apparent second molar root proximity.

References

Carranza FA Jr. Glickman's clinical periodontology. 7th ed. Philadelphia: WB Saunders, 1990:860.

Genco RJ, Goldman HM, Cohen DW. Contemporary periodontics. St. Louis: CV Mosby, 1990:344.

Hemp SE, Nyman S, Lindhe J. Treatment of multi-rooted teeth: Results after 5 years. J Clin Periodontol 1975;2:126.

Lindhe J. Textbook of clinical periodontology. 2nd ed. Copenhagen: Munksgaard, 1989:515.

Schluger S, Yuodelis R, Page RC, Johnson RH. Periodontal diseases. 2nd ed. Philadelphia: Lea & Febiger, 1990:541.

A MOLAR TOOTH AT INITIAL THERAPY EVALUATION

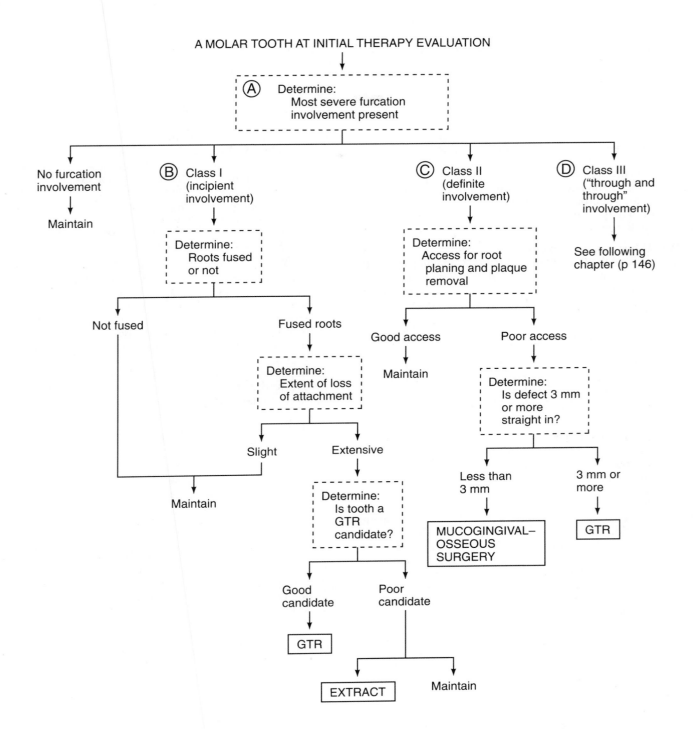

"THROUGH AND THROUGH" FURCATION

Walter B. Hall

Class III or "through and through" furcation involvements are described with other types of furcation involvements (see p 24). Class III involvements require considerable thought in preparing a plan for their treatment. The prognosis for maintaining these teeth is not good; therefore, a definitive approach to therapy is preferred. Extraction of the tooth may be the best approach if adequate abutments for a replacement are available (Fig. 1).

A. When no abutments are available for a fixed bridge to replace the Class III involved tooth, retaining the tooth may be a valid approach. When potential abutments are available, their periodontal status and restorability will determine the options open to the dentist.

B. When no abutments are available, the strategic value of the furcation-involved tooth to the overall treatment plan becomes the most important consideration. If the involved tooth is not important to the treatment plan, it may be either extracted or maintained with a hopeless prognosis. If the involved tooth is essential to the treatment plan, the treatment possibilities discussed in note D apply.

C. If potential abutment teeth to support a replacement for the Class III involved tooth are available, the periodontal status of these teeth becomes the next important concern. If the potential abutment teeth are healthy, extract the badly involved tooth and place a fixed bridge replacement. If the potential abutment teeth have early or moderate periodontal involvement, consider the value of the Class III involved tooth. If keeping the tooth would not appreciably add to the long-term prognosis of the case, extract the tooth, treat the abutment teeth periodontally, and place a replacement fixed bridge. If the Class III involved tooth could add to the long-term prognosis for the case, treatment options discussed in note D apply. If the potential abutment teeth are badly involved periodontally, possible treatment options for the Class III involved teeth would also be those discussed in note D.

D. If the Class III furcation-involved tooth is to be saved or partially saved, the next major decision would concern the possibility of performing endodontics and root resection. If endodontics cannot be performed (because of root canal closure, root tortuosity, etc.) or the roots cannot be resected (because of root fusion, etc.), the tooth would have to be extracted or maintained by root planing with a hopeless prognosis. The treatment options for mandibular and maxillary molars are different.

E. With mandibular molars, if endodontics can be performed on both roots and the roots can be resected, the two separated portions can be retained and crowned. If the roots are close together and orthodontic separation of the hemisected roots is not reasonable or if only one can be treated endodontically, only one root would be fully treated endodontically and the other root would be extracted. If the root to be salvaged can be joined to a satisfactory abutment, a fixed bridge can be used to replace the extracted part of the molar. If the root to be salvaged is adjacent to an abutment and a bridge is not needed, it should be treated endodontically, the tooth hemisected, the other removed, and a crown placed on the salvaged half tooth. If possible, splinting the adjacent tooth to the half tooth and placing a cantilevered bridge could improve the overall case prognosis. This option is a reasonable one.

F. With maxillary molars, if endodontics can be performed on the two roots that are to be retained and a badly involved third root can be resected, perform root amputation following endodontic therapy. The remaining portion of the tooth should be crowned in a manner that would best facilitate plaque removal. If endodontics cannot be performed on the roots to be retained or if the roots are fused to the one to be amputed, extract the tooth or retain it with a hopeless prognosis. If all three furcations are of the Class III type, extraction or maintenance with a hopeless prognosis would also be the options.

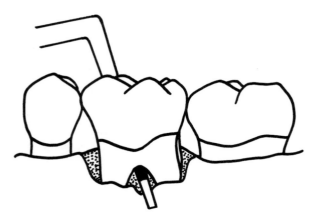

Figure 1. A "through-and-through" (Class III) furcation involvement with good adjacent abutments. The first molar should be considered for extraction.

References

Becker W, Becker B, Berg L, et al. New attachment after treatment with root isolation procedures: Report of treated Class III and Class II furcations and vertical osseous defects. Int J Periodont Restor Dent 1985;5:9.

Carranza FA Jr. Glickman's clinical periodontology. 7th ed. Philadelphia: WB Saunders, 1990:860.

Genco RJ, Goldman HM, Cohen DW. Contemporary periodontics. St. Louis: CV Mosby, 1990:582.

Pontoviero R, Lindhe J, Nyman S, et al. Guided tissue regeneration in the treatment of furcation defects in mandibular molars: A clinical study of degree III involvements. J Clin Periodontol 1989;16:170.

Schluger S, Yuodelis R, Page RC, Johnson RH. Periodontal diseases. 2nd ed. Philadelphia: Lea & Febiger, 1989:549.

Patient's molar with a "THROUGH AND THROUGH" FURCATION INVOLVEMENT

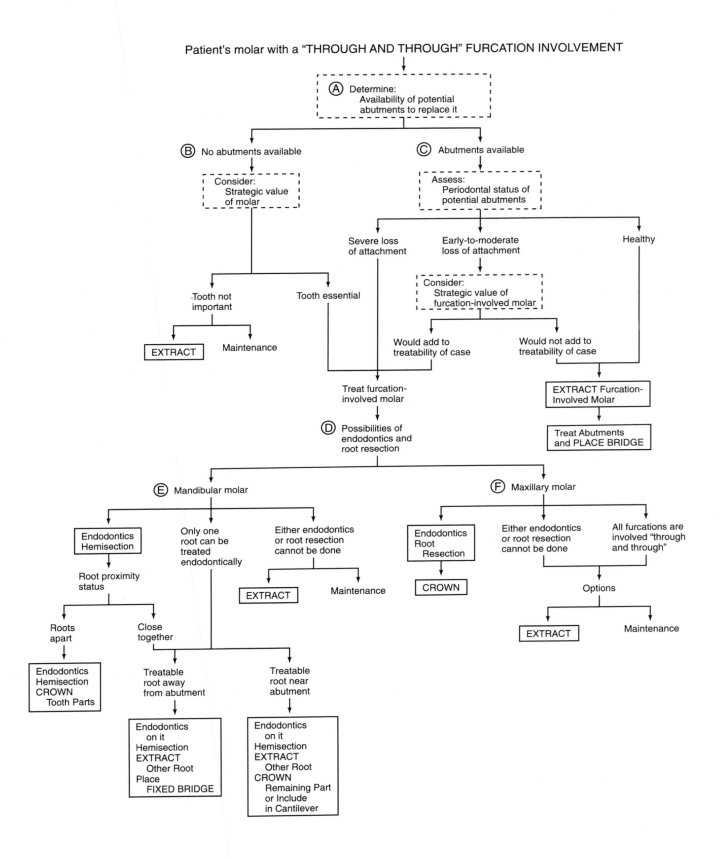

THE EUROPEAN APPROACH TO GUIDED TISSUE REGENERATION: CASE SELECTION

Lavin Flores-de-Jacoby
Axel Zimmerman

Periodontal treatment based on the principles of guided tissue regeneration (GTR) is currently the most advanced of the regenerative methods of periodontal surgery. Guided tissue regeneration does, however, involve a high degree of commitment on the part of both patient and therapist, not least because two surgical interventions are necessary in all events.

To attain optimum clinical results, a number of criteria should be observed when selecting patients, the most important being cooperation by the patient. Only those patients who have been fully informed of the possibilities and limits of GTR should be given this treatment. Competent work by the therapist, then, ensures a good chance of success.

This chapter is designed to help in deciding whether a patient is suitable for GTR. Details such as selection of the appropriate membrane design are dealt with at another level of decision making.

A. Each periodontitis patient is given preliminary treatment consisting of two detailed clinical examinations, a professional supragingival tooth-cleaning session, a subgingival scaling session, and an oral hygiene program.

B. Clinical parameters such as probing attachments (PAL), bleeding on open probing, periodontal recession, tooth mobility, and furcation involvement are determined at the outset of treatment and on re-evaluation after scaling and root planing. The findings are correlated with full-mouth radiographs. Patients with pocket depths of up to 4 mm with no bleeding on probing may require no further treatment except regular recall maintenance. In cases of deeper pocket depths or furcation involvement, consider periodontal surgery. The decision in favor of surgery should be based upon the efficacy of the individual plaque control. For this purpose, a plaque index is recorded during each session. Plaque index values of less than 14% mean that plaque is found at less than 15% of the measuring points in the proximal area. Bleeding on probing is a sign of persistent periodontal inflammation. In conjunction with increased pocket depths, bleeding on probing is an indication for surgical intervention.

C. Vertical osseous defects and furcation involvements are detected by full-mouth radiography or clinically by probing. Use of a Nabers-type probe may be helpful in cases of furcation involvement. Only reflection of a flap provides proof that a defect amenable to GTR is present.

D. Nonvital teeth with a necrotic pulp or irreversible pulpitis require endodontic treatment before surgery. Vitality testing must be performed with the utmost care, as endodontically treated teeth are more susceptible to root resorption.

E. Severely increased tooth mobility (vertical or more than 1 mm horizontal) may cause problems in the healing process of the periodontal ligament and the supporting bone. Perform splinting or occlusal grinding before GTR.

F. Microbiologic investigation is called for in clinically suspicious cases. Only those cases in which the extent or the rate of destruction fails to correlate with the quantity of plaque or the age of the patient are suspect. In these situations testing for periodontopathogens such as *Haemophilus actinomycetemcomitans* or *Porphyromonas* and *Prevotella* may be helpful. Test kits such as latex agglutination test are highly recommended for this purpose. Antibiotics are generally prescribed in accordance with accepted rules. Patients must take an adequately high dose of the appropriate drug for a sufficiently long period (i.e., at least 10 days).

References

Carranza FA Jr. Glickman's clinical periodontology. 7th ed. Philadelphia: WB Saunders, 1990:841.

Flores-de-Jacoby L. New perspectives in periodontal therapy: guided tissue regeneration. Video. Berlin: Quintessenze Verlags-GMBH, 1989.

Gottlow J, Nyman S, Lindhe J, Karring T. New attachment formation as a result of controlled tissue regeneration. J Clin Periodontol 1984;11:494.

Gottlow J, Nyman S, Lindhe J, et al. New attachment formation in human periodontium by guided tissue regeneration. J Clin Periodontol 1986;13:604.

Nyman S, Lindhe J, Karring T, Rylander H. New attachment following surgical treatment of human periodontal disease. J Clin Periodontol 1982;9:290.

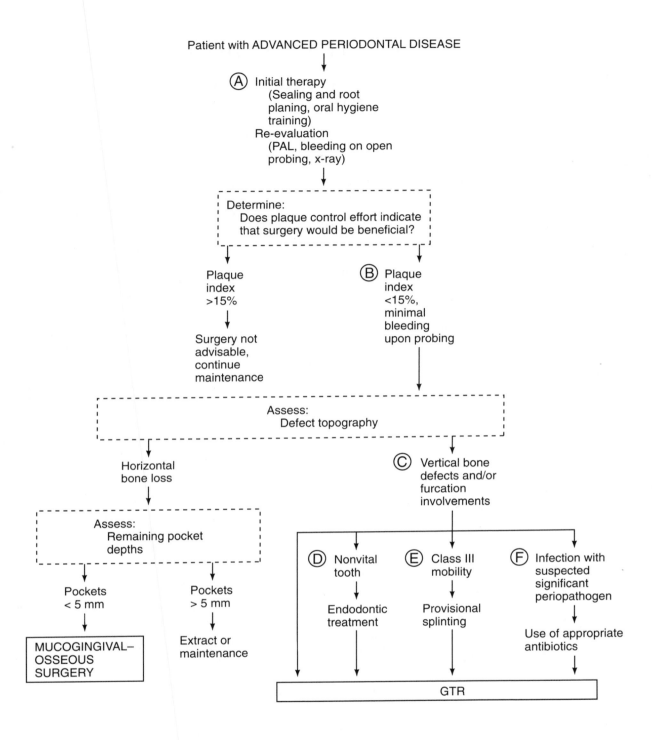

Patient with ADVANCED PERIODONTAL DISEASE

(A) Initial therapy
(Sealing and root
planing, oral hygiene
training)
Re-evaluation
(PAL, bleeding on open
probing, x-ray)

Determine:
Does plaque control effort indicate
that surgery would be beneficial?

Plaque
index
>15%

(B) Plaque
index
<15%,
minimal
bleeding
upon probing

Surgery not
advisable,
continue
maintenance

Assess:
Defect topography

Horizontal
bone loss

(C) Vertical bone
defects and/or
furcation
involvements

Assess:
Remaining pocket
depths

(D) Nonvital
tooth

(E) Class III
mobility

(F) Infection with
suspected
significant
periopathogen

Pockets
< 5 mm

Pockets
> 5 mm

Endodontic
treatment

Provisional
splinting

Use of appropriate
antibiotics

MUCOGINGIVAL–
OSSEOUS
SURGERY

Extract or
maintenance

GTR

THE EUROPEAN APPROACH TO GUIDED TISSUE REGENERATION: MEMBRANE SELECTION

Lavin Flores-de-Jacoby
Axel Zimmerman

The following criteria have been developed as a basis for final case selection and deciding upon the type of membrane to be used.

A. The bone around teeth requiring treatment is exposed using an intrasulcular incision to create mucoperiosteal flaps; vertical relief incisions are made at a distance of at least one premolar's width from the defects to be treated. The mucoperiosteal flap must extend for at least 4 mm beyond the defect margin in an apical direction. When making the incision, it must be designed so that no suture runs across the membrane or across an intra-alveolar defect. An unobstructed view is an essential for optimal cleaning of defects.

B. Use of a membrane (and GTR) can be discontinued in the event that an infraosseous defect is shallow and wide, if bone resorption is found to be mainly horizontal, or if Class I furcation involvement is detected. In these cases, the defect is cleaned thoroughly, any osseous resection is done, and the flaps are closed up again. The usual procedure when teeth are involved in groups is that some of the defects can be treated in the standard way, whereas a few defects will require the use of membranes. More complex cases, in which a number of adjacent defects require the use of membranes, should be embarked upon only if the periodontal surgeon has sufficient experience in the field of GTR. The main problem here is in the management of the covering flaps, which should cover the membrane as much as possible for the full 4-week period in which they remain in situ.

C. Selection of the membrane design is based on the stated intent that the following steps are to be taken in all events. As much as possible, the membrane should be completely covered. Three-walled defects are treated with a single-tooth-narrow or single-tooth-wide membrane depending upon the size of the opening to be covered. If circular or semilunar defects on endstanding teeth, such as distal or second molars, are wide, use a wraparound barrier. Two-walled defects between teeth and some mixed one-walled and two-walled defects require use of interproximal membranes. Class III ("through and through") furcation involvements (although not predictably treatable today) on maxillary molars may be treated with interproximal membranes. Mandibular Class III defects may be treated similarly if there is an adjacent tooth; if a single, isolated tooth is involved, use a wraparound membrane. In some cases with only Class III furcation involvements on lower molars, two single-tooth-wide membranes may be employed. Class II (definite) involvements of facial or lingual furcas only are treated with single-tooth-wide membranes.

The flap is secured with Gore-Tex suturing material. The membrane is left implanted for 4 weeks. In the event that the membrane is exposed for the entire 4 weeks, an application of 0.12 solution of chlorhexidine gluconate twice daily is prescribed.

D. Hopeless teeth are those teeth that are found during surgery to have a functioning remaining periodontium of less than 3 mm. Multirooted molars in which more than half of the roots no longer are supported by bone are also considered hopeless. Grade III mobility does not make a tooth hopeless, as corrective measures can be taken (e.g., presurgical splinting and grinding). Therapeutic efforts may be considered worthwhile even for "hopeless" teeth, provided that the patient has given informed consent.

References

Carranza FA Jr. Glickman's clinical periodontology. 7th ed. Philadelphia: WB Saunders, 1990:841.

Flores-de-Jacoby L. New perspectives in periodontal therapy: guided tissue regeneration. Video. Berlin: Quintessenze Verlags-GMBH, 1989.

Gottlow J, Nyman S, Lindhe J, Karring T. New attachment formation as a result of controlled tissue regeneration. J Clin Periodontol 1984;11:494.

Gottlow J, Nyman S, Lindhe J, et al. New attachment formation in human periodontium by guided tissue regeneration. J Clin Periodontol 1986;13:604.

Nyman S, Lindhe J, Karring T, Rylander H. New attachment following surgical treatment of human periodontal disease. J Clin Periodontol 1982;9:290.

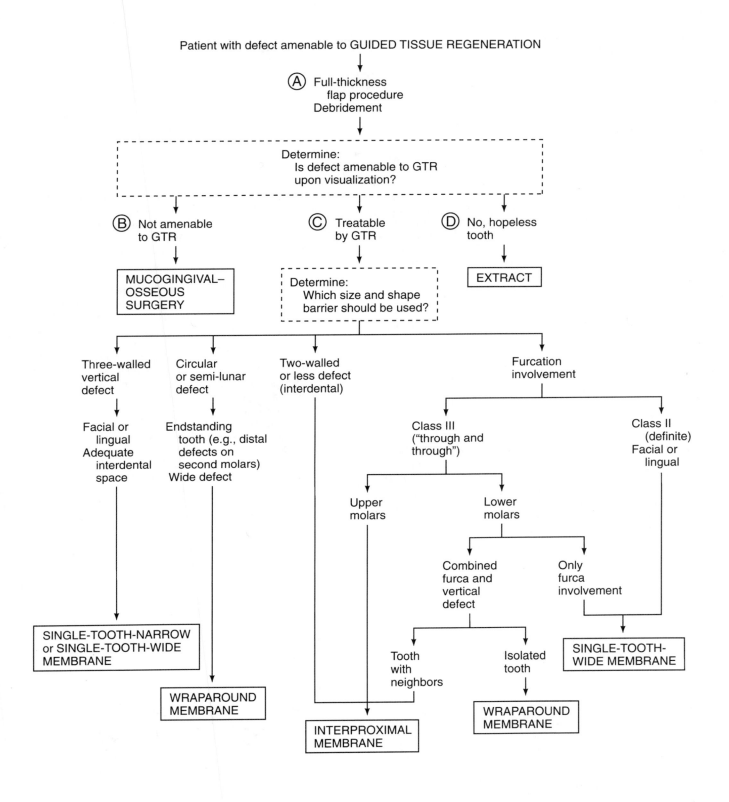

Patient with defect amenable to GUIDED TISSUE REGENERATION

(A) Full-thickness
flap procedure
Debridement

Determine:
Is defect amenable to GTR
upon visualization?

(B) Not amenable
to GTR

(C) Treatable
by GTR

(D) No, hopeless
tooth

MUCOGINGIVAL–
OSSEOUS
SURGERY

Determine:
Which size and shape
barrier should be used?

EXTRACT

Three-walled
vertical
defect

Circular
or semi-lunar
defect

Two-walled
or less defect
(interdental)

Furcation
involvement

Facial or
lingual
Adequate
interdental
space

Endstanding
tooth (e.g., distal
defects on
second molars)
Wide defect

Class III
("through and
through")

Class II
(definite)
Facial or
lingual

Upper
molars

Lower
molars

Combined
furca and
vertical
defect

Only
furca
involvement

SINGLE-TOOTH-NARROW
or SINGLE-TOOTH-WIDE
MEMBRANE

WRAPAROUND
MEMBRANE

Tooth
with
neighbors

Isolated
tooth

SINGLE-TOOTH-
WIDE MEMBRANE

INTERPROXIMAL
MEMBRANE

WRAPAROUND
MEMBRANE

GUIDED TISSUE REGENERATION FOR TREATMENT OF VERTICAL OSSEOUS DEFECTS

Burton E. Becker
William Becker

The biologic principles of GTR are based upon epithelial exclusion and connective tissue exclusion. If the epithelium can be delayed from contacting the root surface long enough for the clot to organize, new cementum, periodontal ligament, and bone may have the potential to regenerate. The use of membranes to exclude the epithelium has been shown to achieve this clinically and histologically.

A. Guided tissue regeneration (GTR) has been shown to be successful treatment for the deep vertical defect. The deep defect is detected accurately by probing depths greater than 5 mm, attachment loss greater than 5 mm, and radiographic evidence of a vertical defect. The Teflon barrier excludes epithelial cells and flap connective tissues. Guided tissue regeneration creates a space for the clot to form in and protects the clot during the early phases of wound healing. Teflon membranes made of e-otfe (Gore-Tex) and resorbable membranes have been used as barriers for GTR.

B. A shallow defect is described as having pocket depths less than 5 mm, attachment loss less than 5 mm, and radiographic evidence of a small vertical defect. This type of defect can be treated with Widman flaps, flap debridement, or apically positioned flaps with or without osseous resection.

C. When osseous defects that are greater than 5 mm in depth are exposed, the number of osseous walls that remain determine treatment options. A deep one-walled defect may require extraction or be amenable to maintenance (even with a poor prognosis) after mucogingival–osseous surgery or a modified Widman flap approach.

D. Two- or three-walled defects that have pocket depths deeper than 5 mm and attachment loss greater than 5 mm can be treated with several modalities of therapy. This type of defect can be treated with flap debridement, GTR, or GTR in combination with either freeze-dried bone or synthetic grafting materials. Guided tissue regeneration has been shown to achieve greater pocket reduction and greater gain of attachment than flap debridement alone, but there is no evidence to suggest that GTR with grafting creates any significant increase in attachment. Synthetic materials act as fillers. Although decreased probing depths have been demonstrated with their use, little or no attachment gain has been shown. Defects that have pocket depths greater than 5 mm, attachment loss greater than 5 mm, and upon entry, two- or three-walled vertical defects deeper than 5 mm in conjunction with a Class II furcation have several options for therapy.

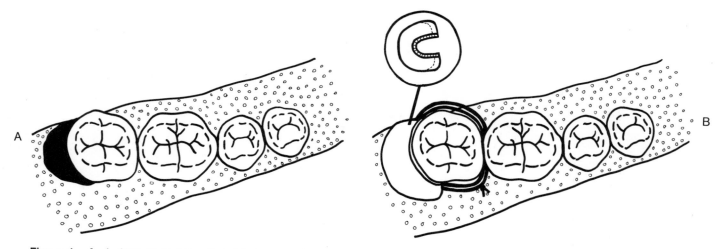

Figure 1. A, A deep vertical 3-walled defect exposed before guided tissue regeneration. **B,** A wrap-around membrane trimmed and sutured in place covering the vertical defect.

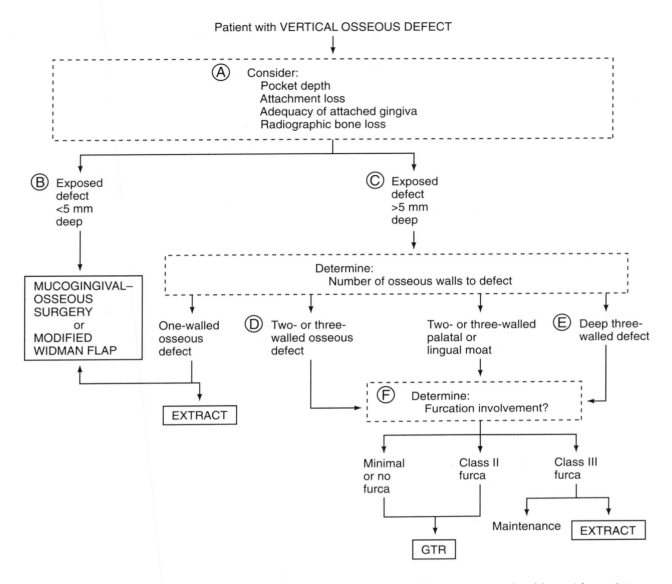

Patient with VERTICAL OSSEOUS DEFECT

(A) Consider:
    Pocket depth
    Attachment loss
    Adequacy of attached gingiva
    Radiographic bone loss

(B) Exposed defect <5 mm deep

(C) Exposed defect >5 mm deep

MUCOGINGIVAL–OSSEOUS SURGERY or MODIFIED WIDMAN FLAP

Determine: Number of osseous walls to defect

One-walled osseous defect

(D) Two- or three-walled osseous defect

Two- or three-walled palatal or lingual moat

(E) Deep three-walled defect

EXTRACT

(F) Determine: Furcation involvement?

Minimal or no furca

Class II furca

Class III furca

Maintenance

EXTRACT

GTR

Flap debridement may be used; however, this type of defect responds well to GTR. Grafting materials may be used with GTR, but there is no evidence that grafting significantly improves the result. The presence of a deep Class II furcation makes this an ideal type of defect to treat with GTR.

E. Most defects that have pocket depths greater than 5 mm and attachment loss greater than 5 mm may be treated with GTR. These defects, which usually are found to wrap around the lingual or palatal aspects of teeth, utilize the barrier to keep the space in the defect open for the clot to form. The deep three-walled intrabony defect is the ideal type of defect for treatment with GTR. This type of defect has been shown to heal with new bone after thorough debridement. Guided tissue regeneration has been shown to provide a predictable reduction in pocket depth and pain and to result in significant new attachment.

F. The presence of a Class II furca will not alter the likelihood of success with GTR. Class III furcas, however, do not yet have a good prognosis for

successful GTR, so one should consider maintenance or extraction.

References

Becker W, Becker B, Berg L, et al. Root isolation for new attachment. J Periodontol 1987;58:819.

Becker W, Becker B, Berg L, et al. New attachment after treatment with root isolation procedures: Report for treated Class III and Class II furcations and vertical defects. Int J Periodont Restor Dent 1988;3(3):9.

Becker W, Becker B, Berg L, et al. Clinical and volumetric analysis of three-walled intrabony defects following open flap debridement. J Periodontol 1986;57:277.

Gottlow J, Nyman S, Karring I, et al. New attachment formation in human periodontium by guided tissue regeneration. J Periodontol. 1986;57:727.

Melcher HH. On the repair potential of periodontal tissues. J Periodontol 1976;47:256.

Schallhorn RG, McClain PR. Combined osseous composite grafting, root conditioning and guided tissue regeneration. Int J Periodont Restor Dent 1988;8(4):9.

GUIDED TISSUE REGENERATION FOR TREATMENT OF FURCATION DEFECTS ON MOLARS

Burton E. Becker
William Becker

The biologic principle of GTR is based on the necessity of epithelial exclusion and flap connective tissue exclusion. If the epithelium can be delayed from contacting the root surface long enough for the clot to organize, new cementum, periodontal ligament, and bone may have the potential to regenerate. The use of membranes to exclude the epithelium and connective tissue has been shown to provide the possibility for new attachment to occur. The principles of guided tissue regeneration (GTR) have been used to treat selected furcation defects in molars.

A. Successful treatment of furcation defects in molars depends on an accurate defect diagnosis. The criteria used for treating furcations with GTR procedures is pocket depth greater than 5 mm, attachment loss greater than 5 mm, presence of an adequate zone of attached gingiva, and radiographic evidence of bone loss. Full-thickness facial and lingual flaps are made, and then further evaluation is required to determine the horizontal depth of the furcation and the presence or absence of a vertical bony defect.

B. Class I furcations require the least amount of therapy. Treatment modalities may vary from oral hygiene, scaling, and root planing to open flap debridement. These defects are often encountered when flaps are done to gain access to interproximal bony defects. They can be managed by various flap-management techniques.

C. Various modalities of therapy can be used to treat Class II furcations with pocket depths of 4 to 6 mm and attachment loss of 3 to 6 mm that are not accompanied by deep horizontal defects into the furcation or deep vertical defects. Widman flaps and flap debridement with and without osseous resection can be used. The flaps can be apically positioned or repositioned. Although GTR could be used, there is no evidence to show that GTR is necessary to either maintain or gain attachment levels in this type of defect. Class II furcation defects that are accompanied by horizontal probing depths greater than 3 mm and vertical defects in the bone of 5 mm or greater can be treated with flaps with or without osseous resection and apically repositioned flaps; however, this type of lesion has been shown to achieve decreased probing depth and attachment level gains predictably with the use of GTR. Class II furcations with vertical bony defects have been treated with bone-grafting materials and synthetic grafts. There is no significant difference in outcome whether one uses membranes with or without grafting materials. Synthetic materials have been shown to decrease pocket depth, but because they act mainly as fillers, no significant accompanying gains in attachment level have been reported.

D. Class III furcation defects are the most difficult defects to treat. They can be treated with maintenance until the tooth is lost in advanced periodontitis. Flap debridement with apically positioned flaps or hemisection has been used. Class III furcations have been treated with GTR, but this has not been found to be predictable, to significantly decrease pocket depth, or to gain attachment level. Maintenance, surgical debridement, root resection, or extraction of the molar with a Class III furcation involvement is an option to be considered.

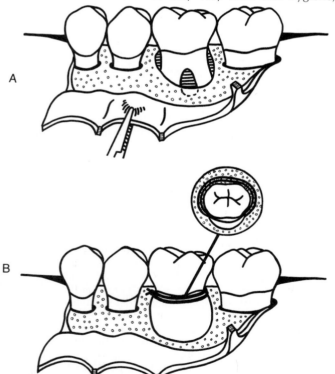

Figure 1. A, A Class II furca exposed before guided tissue regeneration. **B**, A "single tooth wide" membrane trimmed and sutured in place covering the furcation defect.

References

Anderegg OR, Martin SJ, Gray JL, et al. Clinical evaluation of the use of decalcified freeze-dried bone allograft with guided tissue regeneration in the treatment of molar furcation invasions. J Periodontol 1991;62:264.

Becker W, Becker B, Berg L, et al. Root isolation for new attachment. J Periodontol 1987;58:819.

Becker W, Becker B, Berg L, et al. New attachment after treatment with root isolation procedures: Report for

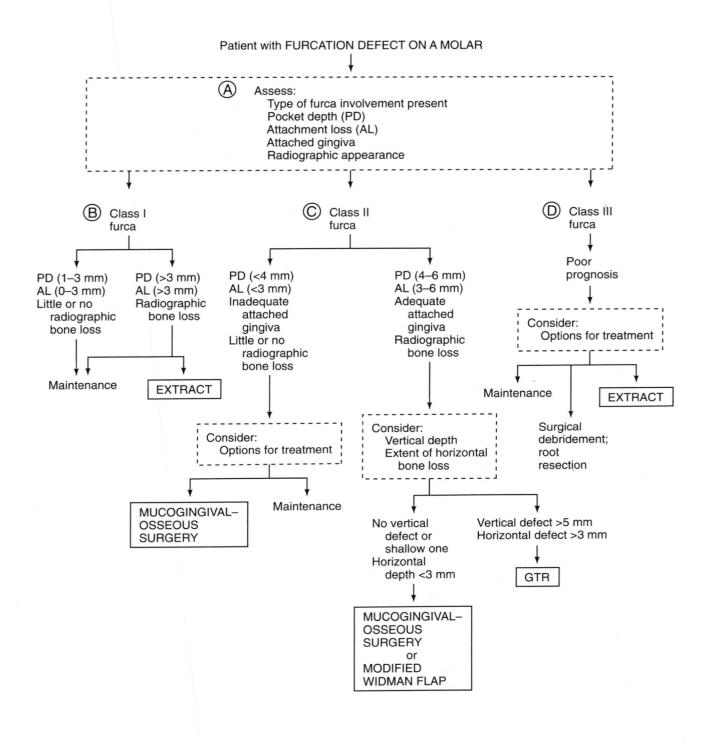

Patient with FURCATION DEFECT ON A MOLAR

Ⓐ Assess:
  Type of furca involvement present
  Pocket depth (PD)
  Attachment loss (AL)
  Attached gingiva
  Radiographic appearance

Ⓑ Class I furca

PD (1–3 mm)
AL (0–3 mm)
Little or no radiographic bone loss

PD (>3 mm)
AL (>3 mm)
Radiographic bone loss

Maintenance

EXTRACT

Ⓒ Class II furca

PD (<4 mm)
AL (<3 mm)
Inadequate attached gingiva
Little or no radiographic bone loss

PD (4–6 mm)
AL (3–6 mm)
Adequate attached gingiva
Radiographic bone loss

Consider:
  Options for treatment

MUCOGINGIVAL–OSSEOUS SURGERY

Maintenance

Consider:
  Vertical depth
  Extent of horizontal bone loss

No vertical defect or shallow one
Horizontal depth <3 mm

Vertical defect >5 mm
Horizontal defect >3 mm

GTR

MUCOGINGIVAL–OSSEOUS SURGERY
or
MODIFIED WIDMAN FLAP

Ⓓ Class III furca

Poor prognosis

Consider:
  Options for treatment

Maintenance

EXTRACT

Surgical debridement; root resection

treated Class III and II furcations and vertical osseous defects. Int J Periodont Restor Dent 1988;3(3):9.

Gottlow J, Nyman S, Karring T, Wennstrom J. New attachment formation in human periodontium by guided tissue regeneration. J Clin Periodontol 1986;57:727.

Melcher AH. On the repair potential of periodontal tissues. J Periodontol 1976;47:256.

Pontoriero R, Lindhe J, Nyman S, et al. Guided tissue regeneration in degree II furcation involved mandibular molars. J Clin Periodontol 1988;15:247.

GUIDED TISSUE REGENERATION IN OSSEOUS DEHISCENCES

Jon Zabelequi
Alberto Sicillia
Jose Maria Tejerina

Very little exists in the current literature about the use of guided tissue regeneration (GTR) in the treatment of osseous dehiscences. The diagnosis of a suspected osseous dehiscence can be made by the "fingertip test," probing, and sounding (see p 194); when present, however, it will be confirmed during the surgery for GTR. The approach should be made through a full-thickness flap.

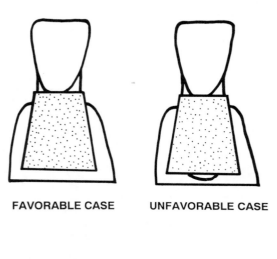

FAVORABLE CASE   **UNFAVORABLE CASE**

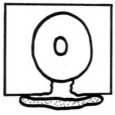   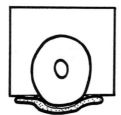

Adequate space is created   Membrane has collapsed
against the tooth

Figure 1. Favorable versus unfavorable cases.

A. In the shallow dehiscences, regeneration is difficult to achieve. Very little regeneration may be obtained, and the cost–benefit relationship, when compared with other kinds of treatment, is unfavorable. Guided tissue regeneration is not recommended.

B. In very deep dehiscences, the prognosis of the affected tooth must be determined. If the prognosis is hopeless (see p 68), the case is unfavorable for GTR.

C. In moderate dehiscences or in deeper ones in which teeth are treatable, this technique must be considered. If the tooth is very prominent in the arch, the case will be unfavorable, and GTR is not recommended.

D. The anatomy of the osseous dehiscence must be such that the membrane can be adapted to the cemento-enamel junction of the teeth in order to cover the defect and the membrane completely and to create a free space under the membrane (Fig. 1, favorable case). If the membrane collapses or doesn't completely close the defect, the case must be considered unfavorable (Fig. 1, unfavorable case). Narrow dehiscences with thick, bony walls make this objective easier. There is a greater quantity of adjacent donor cells, and these are near to the surface where regeneration is desired.

E. An adequate vestibule and the presence of a thick, well-vascularized attached gingiva are fundamental for completely covering the membrane, allowing it to remain stable, and preventing recession, especially if this technique is applied in zones of esthetic importance.

References

Hall WB. Pure mucogingival problems. Berlin: Quintessence Publishing, 1984:36.
World workshop in clinical periodontics. Chicago: American Academy of Periodontology, 1989:Sect VI.

GUIDED TISSUE REGENERATION IN THE TREATMENT OF AN OSSEOUS DEHISCENCE

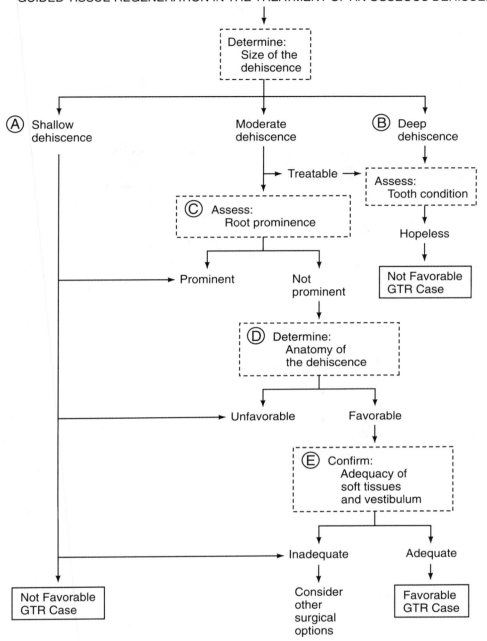

GUIDED TISSUE REGENERATION IN TWO-WALLED OSSEOUS DEFECTS

Jon Zabelequi
Alberto Sicillia
Jose Maria Tejerina

Although a two-walled osseous defect frequently can be diagnosed through a careful clinical and radiographic examination or with sounding, in many cases its presence and morphology up to the moment of the surgical debridement of the defect are not certain. For this reason, the approach must be made through a full-thickness flap to determine whether guided tissue regeneration (GTR) is indicated.

A. In shallow defects, regeneration is difficult to achieve or very little regeneration occurs. When the cost—benefit relationship compared with other kinds of treatment is unfavorable, GTR is not recommended.

B. In very deep defects, the prognosis of the adjacent tooth or teeth must be evaluated. If the prognosis is hopeless (see p 68), the case is unfavorable for GTR.

C. In the moderate defects or in deep ones that are treatable, GTR must be considered. Its application requires an adequate separation of the roots of the adjacent teeth. When less than 2 mm is present, application of the technique is unlikely to be useful.

D. When the separation between adjacent teeth is adequate, the anatomy of the defect and adjacent teeth will determine whether one chooses a GTR technique. Those situations in which it is possible to totally close the entrance of the defect and in which it is possible to create a free space underneath the membrane itself would be favorable for GTR. If the membrane does not totally close the entrance of the defect (a very big entrance defect, or a tooth with marked concavity in its affected surface) or it collapses against the wall of the defect (a defect in which the walls don't adequately support the membrane in the right position), GTR would not be appropriate (Fig. 1). The amount of healthy periodontium close to the defect also is important. Narrow and deep defects are more favorable than those that are wide and shallow.

E. A thick periodontium and an adequate vestibule facilitate the viability and stability of the flap that will cover the membrane, thus reducing the risk of plaque accumulation, which can jeopardize regeneration. The absence of adequate gingiva also can compromise the success of GTR.

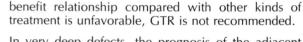

Adequate space is created   **Membrane has collapsed**

FAVORABLE SITUATION   **UNFAVORABLE SITUATION**

Well adapted membrane   **Badly adapted membrane**

Figure 1. Favorable versus unfavorable situations to prevent membrane collapse.

References

Becker W, Becker BE, Berg L, et al. New attachment after treatment with root isolation procedures: Report for treated class II furcations and vertical osseous defects. Int J Periodont Restor Dent 1988;3:2.

Carranza FA Jr. Glickman's clinical periodontology. 7th ed. Philadelphia: WB Saunders, 1990:836.

World workshop in clinical periodontics. Chicago: American Academy of Periodontology, 1989:Sect VI.

GUIDED TISSUE REGENERATION
in TWO-WALLED OSSEOUS DEFECT

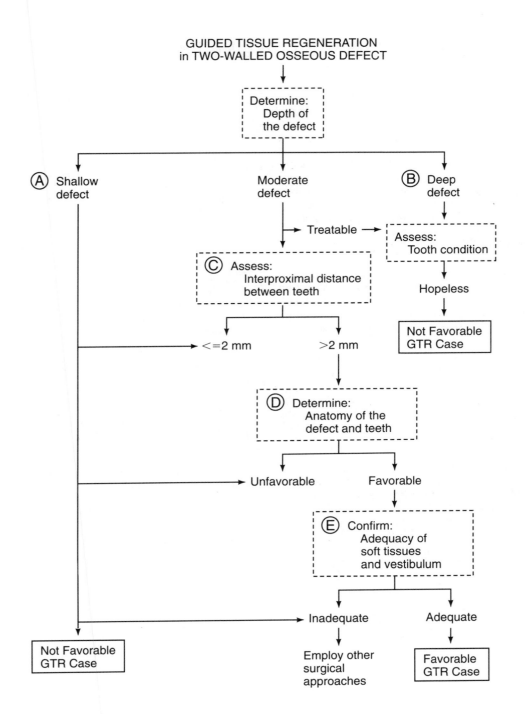

ESTHETIC CONCERNS AND SURGERY

Walter B. Hall

A potential esthetic problem relating to the planning of a periodontal surgical procedure may be evident to a dentist who is considering treatment options. Such problems occur in areas where root exposure can be an unsightly consequence of treatment. This problem is restricted to maxillary anterior, premolar, and, occasionally, first molar teeth. A surgical procedure in this area may be a therapeutic success but an esthetic disaster. To the patient, then, the procedure would not likely be acceptable.

A. A potential esthetic problem, as viewed by the dentist, may not be a problem to the patient. When an informed patient is unconcerned by potential esthetic problems, the dentist should select the best procedure to accomplish therapeutic goals without the restrictions that esthetic concerns might entail (i.e., pocket elimination may be the objective without concern for unsightly root exposure).

B. When the patient perceives esthetics as a prime concern in selecting therapeutic approaches, the dentist must select a treatment approach that will accomplish the most esthetic and therapeutic result.

C. If the roots of the teeth in the surgical segment are round and the pocket depths not so great as to be inaccessible to planing, maintenance with root planing alone (and no surgical exposure) would best meet the esthetic and therapeutic goals of both patient and dentist.

D. If the roots of the teeth in the surgical segment contain flutings or furcation involvements or the pockets are so deep as to be inaccessible for planing, the decision about which type of surgery to employ depends upon the nature of the osseous defects that are present. If only horizontal bone loss is present and it is not severe, the modified Widman flap approach offers an opportunity to thoroughly debride the area, alter root form, and affect esthetics in only a minimally negative way. If vertical defects are present, guided tissue regeneration (GTR) provides a reasonable compromise between the esthetic demands of the patient and the therapeutic goals of the dentist.

References

Allen EP, Gainza CS, Farthing GG, Neubold DA. Improved technique for localized ridge augmentation: A report of 21 cases. J Periodontol 1985;56:195.

Hall WB. Periodontal preparation of the mouth for restoration. Dent Clin North Am 1980;24:204.

Schluger S, Yuodelis R, Page RC, Johnson RH. Periodontal diseases. 2nd ed. Philadelphia: Lea & Febiger, 1989:500.

Seibert J. Reconstruction of deformed partially edentulous ridges using full-thickness grafts: Technique and wound healing. Compend Contin Ed Dent 1983;4:437.

Patient with a POTENTIAL ESTHETIC PROBLEM

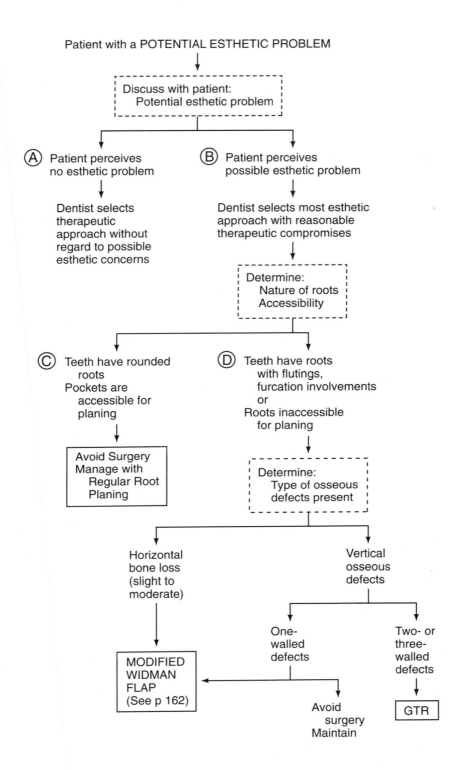

Discuss with patient:
Potential esthetic problem

Ⓐ Patient perceives
no esthetic problem

Ⓑ Patient perceives
possible esthetic problem

Dentist selects
therapeutic
approach without
regard to possible
esthetic concerns

Dentist selects most esthetic
approach with reasonable
therapeutic compromises

Determine:
Nature of roots
Accessibility

Ⓒ Teeth have rounded
roots
Pockets are
accessible for
planing

Ⓓ Teeth have roots
with flutings,
furcation involvements
or
Roots inaccessible
for planing

Avoid Surgery
Manage with
Regular Root
Planing

Determine:
Type of osseous
defects present

Horizontal
bone loss
(slight to
moderate)

Vertical
osseous
defects

One-
walled
defects

Two- or
three-
walled
defects

MODIFIED
WIDMAN
FLAP
(See p 162)

Avoid
surgery
Maintain

GTR

MODIFIED WIDMAN FLAP VERSUS POCKET ELIMINATION

Luther H. Hutchens, Jr.

The decision to perform periodontal surgical procedures in areas of probing pocket depths is delayed until the maximum clinical response has been achieved from the hygienic phase and control of local etiology. After adequate time has elapsed to evaluate the nonsurgical healing response, a decision must then be made to determine if surgical intervention will improve the long-range prognosis of the dentition. Whether to employ a modified Widman flap or pocket elimination procedure depends on the objectives of the therapist and the nature of the pockets (access for instrumentation only or on cleansably deep pockets). Both procedures are acceptable means of treating periodontal pockets. Clinical research trials have shown that pocket elimination therapy reduces pockets initially more effectively; however, studies have failed to correlate pocket elimination to long-term maintenance of probing attachment levels.

A. The presence of probing pocket depths of 4 mm and the radiographic evidence of bone loss (either horizontal or vertical) are usually findings that indicate the need to consider surgical therapy. Also, the presence of bleeding or suppuration on probing in these deeper sites is another clinical finding that may indicate the need for surgery.

B. More localized pockets are found in juvenile periodontitis, areas of foreign-body impactions, endodontic complications, or trauma. Localized pockets often respond favorably to removal of the etiologic factors, such as that achieved with removal of foreign bodies and endodontic therapy. Localized pockets of periodontal origin may require surgical flap procedures.

C. Generalized probing pockets, more usual in the adult periodontitis patient, may be managed by a modified Widman flap or pocket elimination procedure. The decision to perform either procedure will depend upon the treatment philosophy of the therapist. If definitive elimination of the pocket is the treatment goal, then use a flap procedure with ostectomy–osteoplasty. If the goal is root access, pocket reduction, and maximum potential for regeneration, then use the modified Widman flap procedure.

D. In both procedures, an internal bevel incision with a full-thickness mucoperiosteal flap is used to gain access to the diseased root and alveolar bone (Fig. 1). The internal bevel incision is made parallel to the tooth approximately 0.5 to 1.0 mm from the crest of the gingival margin in an attempt to remove the inflamed lining of the periodontal pocket.

E. In situations in which there is minimal attached gingiva, both procedures would require a sulcular-type incision.

F. In the pocket elimination procedure, the flap is

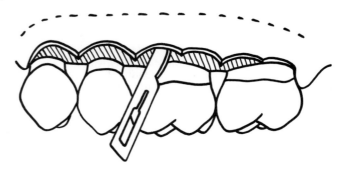

Figure 1. The internal bevel, scalloped incision is utilized for pocket elimination by apically repositioning the flap or for access for debridement with the flap repositioned (modified Widman approach) before closure.

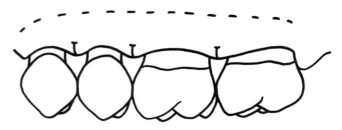

Figure 2. The flap positioned apically for pocket elimination.

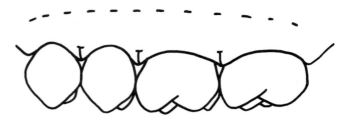

Figure 3. The flap respositioned (modified Widman approach).

elevated far beyond the crest of the bone, allowing good access to the tooth and osseous structures. In the modified Widman flap procedure, the flap is elevated to a lesser degree, exposing only the crestal alveolar bone. In both procedures, the gingival collar of tissue is removed, the defects are thoroughly debrided, and the root surfaces are scaled and planed. In the pocket elimination procedure, the intrabony portions of the bony defects are eliminated by ostectomy–osteo

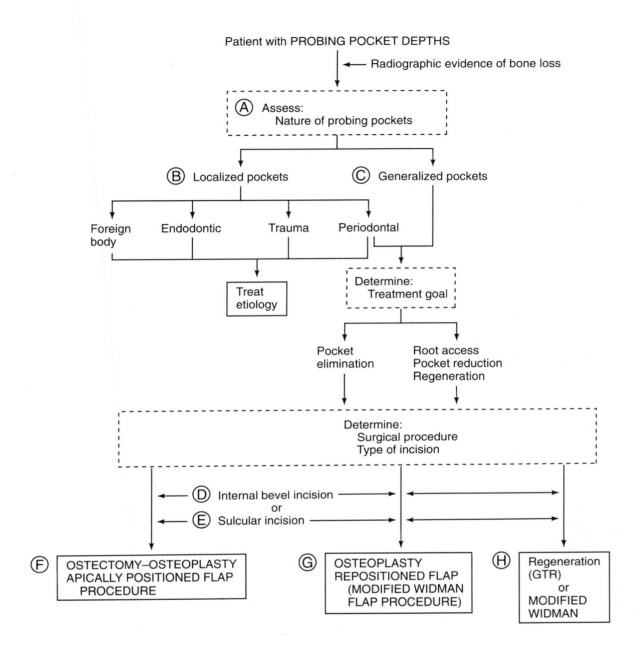

Patient with PROBING POCKET DEPTHS

← Radiographic evidence of bone loss

(A) Assess:
Nature of probing pockets

(B) Localized pockets   (C) Generalized pockets

Foreign body   Endodontic   Trauma   Periodontal

Treat etiology

Determine:
Treatment goal

Pocket elimination   Root access
Pocket reduction
Regeneration

Determine:
Surgical procedure
Type of incision

(D) Internal bevel incision
or
(E) Sulcular incision

(F) OSTECTOMY–OSTEOPLASTY APICALLY POSITIONED FLAP PROCEDURE

(G) OSTEOPLASTY REPOSITIONED FLAP (MODIFIED WIDMAN FLAP PROCEDURE)

(H) Regeneration (GTR) or MODIFIED WIDMAN

plasty in an attempt to create a parabolized positive architecture. Following the removal of the intrabony defects, the flaps are apically positioned at the bony crest and are sutured. (Fig. 2).

G. In contrast, the modified Widman flap procedure does not remove supportive bone by ostectomy but may use osteoplasty to reshape bony contours to allow for better flap adaptation to achieve interproximal primary closure. The modified Widman flap is used to replace the flap at its original position in an attempt to obtain complete flap closure (Fig. 3).

H. The modified Widman flap approach is often utilized with the placement of graft materials (osseous and alloplastic) and synthetic membranes in the treatment of intrabony defects.

References

Becker W, Becker B, Ochsenbein C, et al. A longitudinal study comparing scaling and osseous surgery and modified Widman procedures: Results after 1 year. J Periodont 1988;59:351.

Ochsenbein C. A primary for osseous surgery. Int J Periodont Res Dent 1986;1:9.

Ramfjord SP, Nissle RR. The modified Widman flap. J Periodontol 1974;45:601.

APICALLY POSITIONED FLAP PROCEDURE

Walter B. Hall

The apically positioned flap procedure is the most commonly used surgical approach to pocket elimination and osseous recontouring. Its advantages include its wide spectrum of usefulness, its retention of most existing gingiva, and its ability to solve both mucogingival–osseous and pure mucogingival problems. Because the flaps are fully reflected, the access and vision requirements for doing surgical procedures are achieved. The major disadvantages of the apically positioned flap procedure relate to possible unacceptable aesthetic results in areas where aesthetics may be important and the greater likelihood of root sensitivity because of root exposure.

A. When the flap will extend to a canine tooth or another tooth with a similarly long crown, an envelope flap approach may be used. When access for visibility cannot be obtained adequately with that approach, vertical releasing incisions may be used. Usually they are placed at the proximal line angle of the tooth at the end of a surgical segment.

B. If adequate attached gingiva will remain when the flap is positioned at the crest of the bone, the incision for the flap is made with an internal bevel to the crest of the alveolus on facial and lingual surfaces. It is scalloped interdentally to retain additional gingiva to fit interproximally when the flap is sutured. It should be filleted so that its thickness will be similar over the tooth root and interdentally. If additional attached gingiva is needed, it can be created by leaving several millimeters of coronal bone denuded when the flap is positioned apically. This denuded area will granulate and heal as gingiva, which, when added to the apically positioned old gingiva, will create a band of attached gingiva 2 to 5 mm in height. Such a flap need not be scalloped to fulfill this need.

C. In the apically positioned flap approach, the flap is fully reflected into alveolar mucosa (in contrast to the modified Widman flap approach). Because the palate does not have alveolar mucosa, a gingival flap in that area cannot be apically positioned and is performed differently (see p 166). Next, the remaining interdental and marginal tissue is removed with curettes and chisels, exposing the bone and any osseous defects. These may be treated by osseous recontouring (see p 168) or by bone fill (see p 172). If any defects are amenable to guided tissue regeneration (GTR), this technique should be employed preferentially to pocket elimination, because it provides greater support, better esthetics, and easier cleansability of the area.

D. When the flap is positioned and sutured, if no additional gingiva is to be created by denudation, it may be sutured tightly at the level of the crest of bone and the pack placed. When more attached gingiva is needed, the flap may be positioned so that some bone is exposed, and it may be sutured loosely with suspensory sutures to establish its position before pack placement. Healing is more rapid when the only bone left exposed is between teeth. Ideally performed, the apically positioned flap should result in pocket elimination with improved gingival form, which will facilitate plaque removal by the patient.

References

Ariudo A, Tyrell H. Repositioning and increasing the zone of attached gingiva. J Periodontol 1957;28:106.

Carranza FA Jr. Glickman's clinical periodontology. 7th ed. Philadelphia: WB Saunders, 1990:819.

Genco RJ, Goldman HM, Cohen DW. Contemporary periodontics. St. Louis: CV Mosby, 1990:567.

Lindhe J. Textbook of clinical periodontology. 2nd ed. Copenhagen: Munksgaard, 1989:405.

Nabers CL. Repositioning the attached gingiva. J Periodontol 1954;25:38.

Patient scheduled for POCKET ELIMINATION SURGERY ON THE MANDIBULAR ARCH
OR THE FACIAL ASPECT OF THE MAXILLARY ARCH

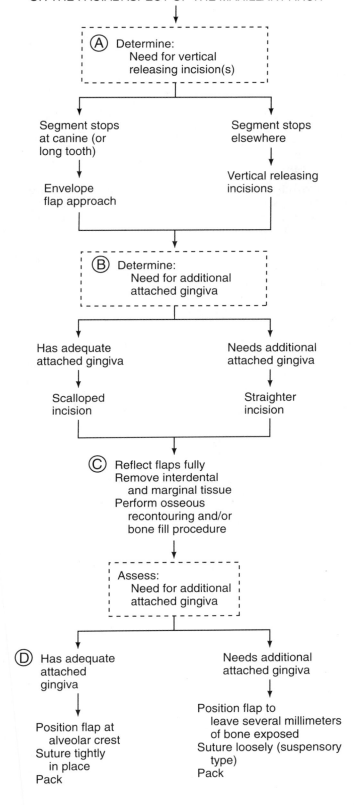

Ⓐ Determine:
   Need for vertical
   releasing incision(s)

Segment stops
at canine (or
long tooth)

Segment stops
elsewhere

Envelope
flap approach

Vertical releasing
incisions

Ⓑ Determine:
   Need for additional
   attached gingiva

Has adequate
attached gingiva

Needs additional
attached gingiva

Scalloped
incision

Straighter
incision

Ⓒ Reflect flaps fully
   Remove interdental
      and marginal tissue
   Perform osseous
      recontouring and/or
      bone fill procedure

Assess:
   Need for additional
   attached gingiva

Ⓓ Has adequate
   attached
   gingiva

Needs additional
attached gingiva

Position flap at
   alveolar crest
Suture tightly
   in place
Pack

Position flap to
   leave several millimeters
   of bone exposed
Suture loosely (suspensory
   type)
Pack

PALATAL FLAP DESIGN

Walter B. Hall

An apically positioned flap approach cannot be employed in mucogingival—osseous surgery involving the palate, because no alveolar mucosa is present on the palate to permit apical positioning. Instead, pocket elimination is achieved by designing a palatal flap that will just cover the contours of the bone created by osseous recontouring to eliminate osseous defects. The conceptualization of the flap design requires skill and experience.

A. When osseous defects are present on the palatal aspects of teeth, the amount of soft tissue that must be eliminated on each tooth is determined by the nature of osseous defects present interproximally and on the palatal aspects of each tooth, an estimate of the amount of osteoplasty needed to facilitate oral hygiene and flap adaptation (see p 170), and/or the amount of soft tissue that will be eliminated by creating a flap of uniform thickness to cover the reshaped bone and to just cover the new osseous crests. Narrow three-walled defects (1 mm or less horizontally from the crest of bone to the tooth) usually will "fill" (see p 180) when fully debrided, whereas other defects (if not treatable by guided tissue regeneration) will require elimination by ostectomy.

B. If defects are sufficiently narrow that bone fill should occur, the margin of the flap will be cut apical to the existing crest of the bone at a distance that is dependent upon the amount of osteoplasty anticipated to create osseous form, which will enhance plaque control possibilities and flap adaptation, and the bulk of connective tissue to be removed in creating a uniformly thick flap. If little osteoplasty or soft-tissue bulk reduction is anticipated, the flap edge will be cut only a little apical to the existing crest of bone. The greater the amount of osteoplasty and or soft-tissue bulk reduction anticipated, the further apically to the existing osseous crest the flap edge should be cut.

C. If the defects are not amenable to osseous fill, ostectomy will be required to eliminate the osseous defects. In deciding how severely to scallop the flap so that it will just cover the new bone margin upon suturing, the dentist must estimate the approximate amount of ostectomy that will be required and correlate those expectations with an estimate of the amount of osteoplasty and/or soft-tissue bulk reduction that will be needed to facilitate plaque control and flap adaptation. If little osteoplasty and/or bulk reduction is anticipated, the scalloping would be less dramatic; the greater the amount of bone or soft-tissue bulk to be removed, the more severely apically the scalloping should be placed.

References

Carranza FA Jr. Glickman's clinical periodontology. 7th ed. Philadelphia: WB Saunders, 1990:814.

Ochsenbein C, Bohannon HM. Palatal approach to osseous surgery. II. Clinical applications J Periodontol 1964; 35:54.

Ochsenbein C, Bohannon HM. Palatal approach to osseous surgery. I. Rationale. J Periodontol 1963;34:60.

Rateitshak KH, Rateitshak EM, Wolf HF, Hassell TM. Color atlas of periodontology. Stuttgart: Georg Thieme Verlag 1985:199.

Schluger S, Yuodelis R, Page RC, Johnson RH. Periodontal diseases. 2nd ed. Philadelphia: CV Mosby, 1990:469.

Patient scheduled for POCKET ELIMINATION SURGERY ON THE PALATE

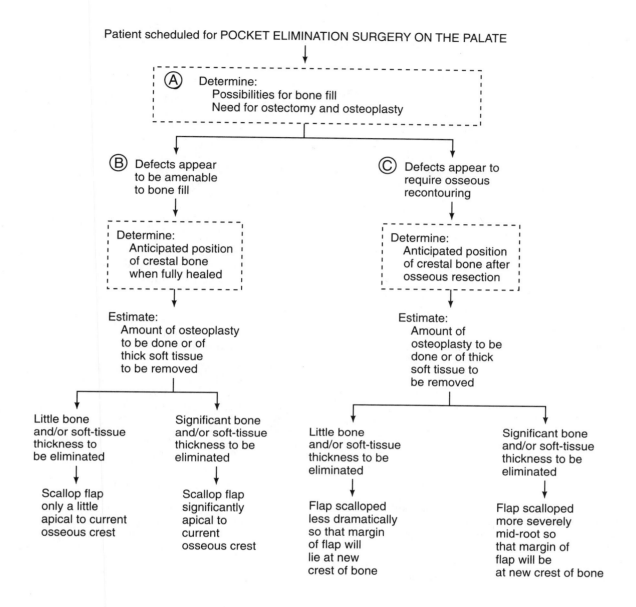

Ⓐ Determine:
   Possibilities for bone fill
   Need for ostectomy and osteoplasty

Ⓑ Defects appear to be amenable to bone fill

Determine:
   Anticipated position of crestal bone when fully healed

Estimate:
   Amount of osteoplasty to be done or of thick soft tissue to be removed

Little bone and/or soft-tissue thickness to be eliminated

Scallop flap only a little apical to current osseous crest

Significant bone and/or soft-tissue thickness to be eliminated

Scallop flap significantly apical to current osseous crest

Ⓒ Defects appear to require osseous recontouring

Determine:
   Anticipated position of crestal bone after osseous resection

Estimate:
   Amount of osteoplasty to be done or of thick soft tissue to be removed

Little bone and/or soft-tissue thickness to be eliminated

Flap scalloped less dramatically so that margin of flap will lie at new crest of bone

Significant bone and/or soft-tissue thickness to be eliminated

Flap scalloped more severely mid-root so that margin of flap will be at new crest of bone

OSSEOUS RECONTOURING

Walter B. Hall

Osseous recontouring includes the full or partial elimination of osseous defects and sculpting of bone to facilitate the closure of flaps and to permit the most ideal access for plaque removal by the patient following healing. It may include both ostectomy (the removal of supporting bone) and osteoplasty (the reshaping of the bony surface). It usually is used following internal bevel, full-thickness, apically positioned flap exposure of the bone surrounding periodontally involved teeth.

A. When pocket elimination surgery employing osseous contouring has been selected as the appropriate method of treating a case, the need for ostectomy relates to the type of osseous defect involved, which is described by numbers of osseous walls remaining (see p 34).

B. When no osseous defects are present, the only ostectomy that might be necessary would be to correct "reversed architecture."

C. When one- and two-walled intrabony defects are present, they are ramped out by eliminating the remaining osseous walls to the level of bone on the adjacent tooth. This procedure usually is done with a round burr and various chisels.

D. When a three-walled intrabony defect is present and guided tissue regeneration cannot be done (see p 180), and if there is a wide gap between crest of bone and tooth (greater than 1 mm from crest to tooth), it would be ramped in the same manner until a narrow (less than 1 mm) gap remained. Narrow three-walled defects routinely "fill" (see p 34) with bone from the walls of the defect, and new attachment (see p 152) usually occurs when the connective tissue regenerates from the periodontal ligament.

E. Interproximal grooving (osteoplasty) is performed to create a festooned form to the fully healed area, to facilitate closure of the flaps interproximally, and to permit greater interproximal penetration of toothbrush bristles while brushing.

F. If exostoses or ledges are present, they are ramped to create an even, flowing surface to facial and lingual bone, which should facilitate flap closure and improve plaque removal possibilities for the patient.

G. When reversed architecture (the more coronal extent of bone facially or lingually than interproximally) is present or occurs following ostectomy, it should be corrected with a chisel to create positive architecture (the more apical positioning of bone facially or lingually than interproximally). Creating positive architecture when reversed architecture is encountered is illustrated below.

H. Upon completion of the osseous recontouring, the roots should be planed to remove any nicks created by the instrumentation, the flaps are sutured in place, a dressing is placed, and postoperative instructions are given to the patient.

References

Grant DA, Stern IB, Listgarten MA. Periodontics. 6th ed. St. Louis: CV Mosby, 1988:838.

Heins PG. Osseous surgery: An evaluation after twenty years. Dent Clin North Am 1969;13:75.

Prichard JF. A technique for treating intrabony pockets based on alveolar process morphology. Dent Clin North Am 1968;85.

Schluger S. Osseous resection—a basic principle in periodontal surgery. Oral Surg 1949;2:316.

Schluger S, Yuodelis R, Page R, Johnson RH. Periodontal diseases. 2nd ed. Philadelphia: Lea & Febiger, 1990:501.

Patient for POCKET ELIMINATION SURGERY WITH FLAPS REFLECTED

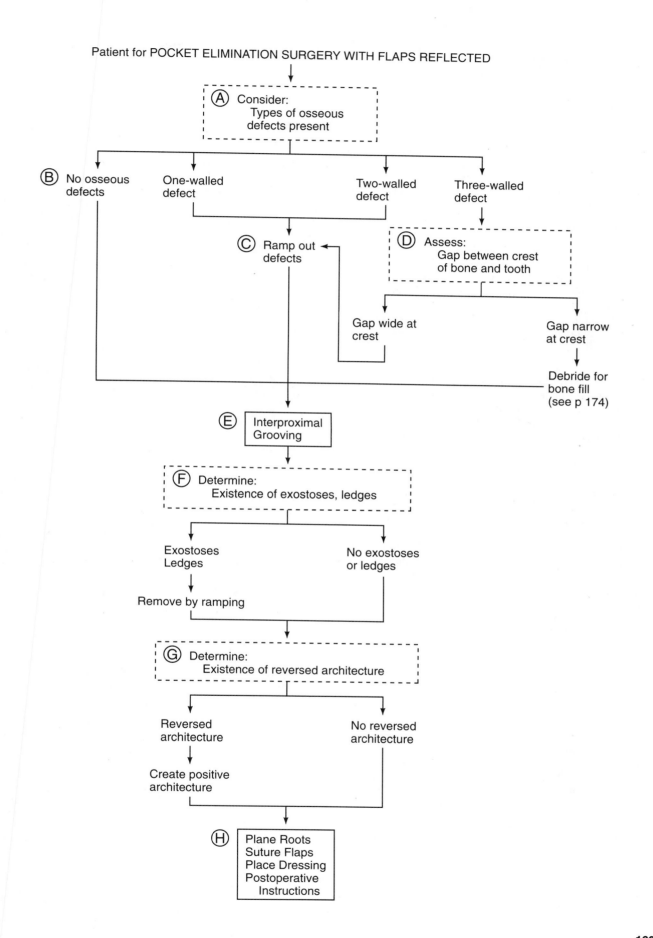

A Consider:
Types of osseous defects present

B No osseous defects

One-walled defect

Two-walled defect

Three-walled defect

C Ramp out defects

D Assess:
Gap between crest of bone and tooth

Gap wide at crest

Gap narrow at crest

Debride for bone fill
(see p 174)

E Interproximal Grooving

F Determine:
Existence of exostoses, ledges

Exostoses Ledges

No exostoses or ledges

Remove by ramping

G Determine:
Existence of reversed architecture

Reversed architecture

No reversed architecture

Create positive architecture

H Plane Roots
Suture Flaps
Place Dressing
Postoperative Instructions

OSTEOPLASTY

Luther H. Hutchens, Jr.

By definition, opsteoplasty is "the reshaping of the alveolar process to achieve a more physiologic form without removal of alveolar (supporting) bone." Osteoplasty is used frequently in periodontal therapy to reshape osseous structures around the teeth.

A. Maxillary and mandibular facial and/or lingual exostoses or tori often are present as a result of a hereditary anatomic bony variation or as a result of heavy occlusal loading or parafunctional habits. The presence of exostoses or tori may necessitate bone reshaping to improve periodontal health and patient comfort. Normal crestal alveolar bone also may require reshaping in some clinical situations in which there are heavy marginal ledges and increased cortical plate thickness in interproximal and interradicular areas.

B. Patient discomfort is often a chief complaint because of the presence of exostoses or tori. These bony prominences are subject both to trauma and to aphthae and/or herpetic ulcerations. Reduction of these bony contours can be achieved with flap access and osteoplasty using rotary surgical burrs and hand instruments.

C. Osteoplasty may be required to facilitate pocket reduction/elimination, flap placement, oral hygiene, or restorative procedures. If the therapist determines that intrabony pockets should be eliminated and the removal of supportive osseous structures is required to create a normal parabolized osseous architecture (ostectomy), then osteoplasty of the crestal bone height and the thickness of the bone is often required prior to the ostectomy procedure. Also, interproximal and interradicular vertical grooving is sometimes necessary to create a physiologic form to which the gingival tissues can adapt (Fig. 1). Reshaping of cortical projections and facial and lingual ledges also

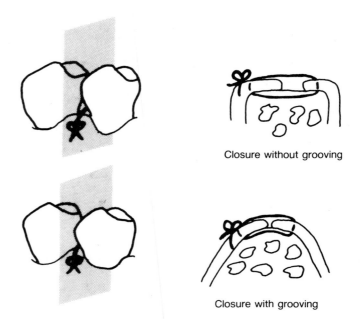

Figure 2. Illustration of closure without and with grooving.

facilitates flap placement when efforts are being made to obtain primary closure in the interproximal space (Fig. 2). Ideal closure of the interdental area will facilitate pocket reduction and allow good flap adaptation. The use of the modified Widman flap often requires some osteoplasty to allow for tight closure in repositioning of the flap. Marginal bone osteoplasty also is used to facilitate procedures as well as the patient's oral hygiene. Patients who are unable to obtain optimal plaque control in marginal areas because of excessive contours of bone or because of deep subgingival restorative margins may benefit from osteoplasty of the crestal bone. This situation is particularly true in Class II furcation areas, where access for oral hygiene is difficult.

D. Edentulous ridge modifications often are required to facilitate the placement of fixed prosthetic pontics and to increase access for patient oral hygiene after the prosthesis is placed. Decreased ridge height and/or excessive ridge thickness may require reshaping of the alveolar ridge before prosthetic placement. Ridge modification in the anterior part of the mouth often improves restorative esthetics. Osteoplasty to flatten the edentulous ridge is often required to facilitate the surgical placement of root-form implants.

E. Extensive subgingival caries, faulty restorations, pin perforations, and root proximity are some of the clinical situations that often require surgical exposure of the tooth to facilitate an adequate restoration. Although both ostectomy and osteoplasty are usually

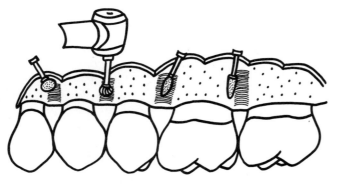

Figure 1. Osseous grooving, performed with various rotating burrs or stones, permits better adaptation of flaps to facilitate plaque removal after healing. Illustration shows diamond stones and a round burr being used for grooving.

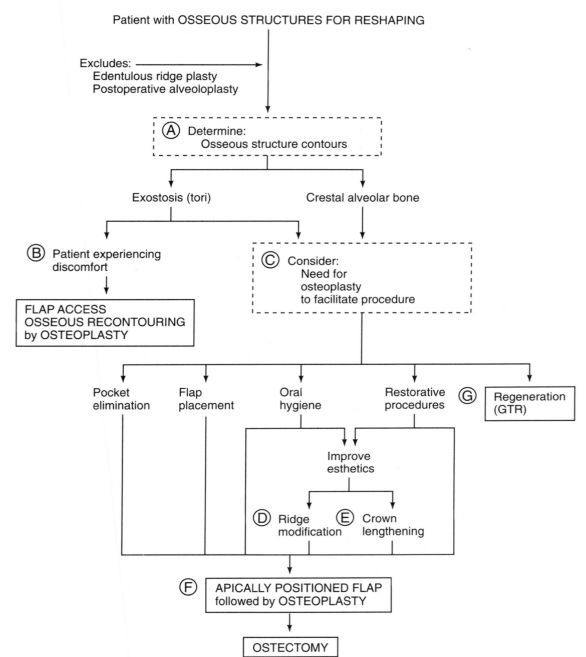

Patient with OSSEOUS STRUCTURES FOR RESHAPING

Excludes:
Edentulous ridge plasty
Postoperative alveoloplasty

(A) Determine:
Osseous structure contours

Exostosis (tori)   Crestal alveolar bone

(B) Patient experiencing discomfort

FLAP ACCESS
OSSEOUS RECONTOURING
by OSTEOPLASTY

(C) Consider:
Need for osteoplasty to facilitate procedure

Pocket elimination   Flap placement   Oral hygiene   Restorative procedures   (G) Regeneration (GTR)

Improve esthetics

(D) Ridge modification   (E) Crown lengthening

(F) APICALLY POSITIONED FLAP followed by OSTEOPLASTY

OSTECTOMY

required in this procedure, many times osteoplasty of the crestal areas facilitates apical flap placement and allows for better access for the restoration. Exposure of short clinical crowns by osseous reshaping and apical flap positioning often can improve anterior esthetics.

F. With the exception of the repositioned flap (see p 162), exostoses or tori removal, and ridge modifications, most osteoplasty procedures are preceded by apically positioning the flap at the osseous margin. Osteoplasty done in conjunction with pocket elimination or crown extension procedures usually will require removal of supportive bone (ostectomy) and apically positioned flaps.

G. Regeneration procedures utilizing implant materials (osseous autografts, allografts, or alloplastic grafts)

may necessitate osteoplasty to improve the coronal positioning of the flap for implant coverage. Guided tissue regeneration (GTR) may also require osteoplasty to improve flap coverage of synthetic membranes.

References

Schluger S, Yuodelis R, Page R, Johnson R. Periodontal diseases. 2nd ed. Philadelphia: Lea & Febiger, 1990: Chap 3.
Yuodelis RA, Smith DH. Corrections of periodontal abnormalities as a preliminary phase of oral rehabilitation. Dent Clin North Am 1976;20:181.

BONE FILL—REGENERATIVE PROCEDURES

E. Barrie Kenney

Bone fill—regenerative procedures are used to treat advanced periodontal disease that has resulted in intrabony defects. Initial therapy should precede these surgical approaches so that inflammation is minimal and there is elimination of any active, purulent lesions.

A. The control of plaque is the most important determinant of success in all surgical procedures directed at periodontal defects. In patients with poor plaque control, surgery should be postponed until an acceptable level of plaque is obtained. The management of patients on completion of bone fill—regenerative surgical procedures must also emphasize control of bacterial plaque in order to maintain the beneficial results of the surgery. Generally, postsurgical patients will be seen every 2 or 3 months for maintenance scaling and polishing.

B. Patients with evidence of pockets without bone loss will require surgery directed at reducing the suprabony pockets, such as flap curettage or gingivectomy. In the anterior portion of the mouth, it may be better to maintain these areas with a nonsurgical approach if postsurgical gingival recession would create an esthetic compromise.

C. Teeth with advanced bone loss will become more mobile after periodontal surgery. In those cases in which the prognosis is very poor, the teeth are generally best treated with a conservative approach of maintenance. If bone fill—regenerative procedures are used, both patient and surgeon should appreciate that the outcome is unpredictable.

D. When a tooth has lost 80% or more of its bone and has three mobility after initial therapy, then bone fill—regenerative procedures have little, if any, chance of success.

E. Horizontal bone loss on the facial or lingual surfaces cannot be expected to regenerate new bone. These regions should be managed with flap procedures without any grafting procedure.

F. Vertical bone loss with a resultant intrabony defect in the facial or lingual surfaces can result in moat-shaped defects. These areas respond well to bone fill procedures.

G. Horizontal defects in the interproximal regions have not responded well to bone fill procedures. Until evidence of regeneration of bone is available, these areas are best treated with conventional flap procedures with or without osseous surgery.

H. In buccal or lingual furcations where there has been bone loss extending apically less than 4 mm from the crotch of the furca, the defect can be well managed with osseous surgery and apically positioned flaps. This will result in a papilla-like projection of gingival tissue in the furcation with pocket depths of 2 to 3 mm.

I. There have been a number of reports of successful treatment of Class II furcations using such bone fill—regenerative procedures as guided tissue regeneration, porous hydroxylapatite, and coronally repositioned flaps. Combinations of bone graft materials with guided tissue regeneration or coronally repositioned flaps also have been beneficial.

J. Crater defects are best managed with nonregenerative surgical procedures. Extremely deep craters that are not suitable for osseous surgery can be treated with bone fill—regenerative procedures, but the outcome is not predictable.

K. Interproximal intrabony defects are best managed with bone fill—regenerative procedures. A wide variety of approaches, including autogenous bone grafts, decalcified freeze-dried bone, porous hydroxylapatite, and guided tissue regeneration, have given favorable results with these lesions.

L. Class III furcations in lower molars generally have a poor prognosis. If the appropriate anatomic conditions are present, such as adequate root separation, a short root trunk, treatable pulp canals, and an adequate residual bone-encased root volume, then hemisection with the use of one or both roots is indicated.

M. Class III furcations have a limited ability to respond to bone fill—regenerative procedures. Any surgical approach to these areas will carry with it a guarded prognosis for the future periodontal health of the affected teeth.

References

Gantes B, Martin M, Garret S, et al. Treatment of periodontal furcation defects. II. Bone regeneration in mandibular class II defects. J Clin Periodontol 1988;15:232.

Hamp S, Nyman S, Lindhe J. Periodontal treatment of multirooted teeth: Results after 5 years. J Clin Periodontol 1976;2:126.

Lekovic V, Kenney EB, Carranza FA, et al. Treatment of grade II furcation defects using porous hydroxylapatite in conjunction with a polytetrafluoroethylene membrane. J Periodontol 1990;61:575.

Mellonig JT. Freeze dried bone allografts in periodontal reconstructive surgery. Dent Clin North Am 1991;35:505.

Pontoriero R, Lindhe J, Nyman S, et al. Guided tissue regeneration in the treatment of furcation defects in man. J Clin Periodontol 1987;14:619.

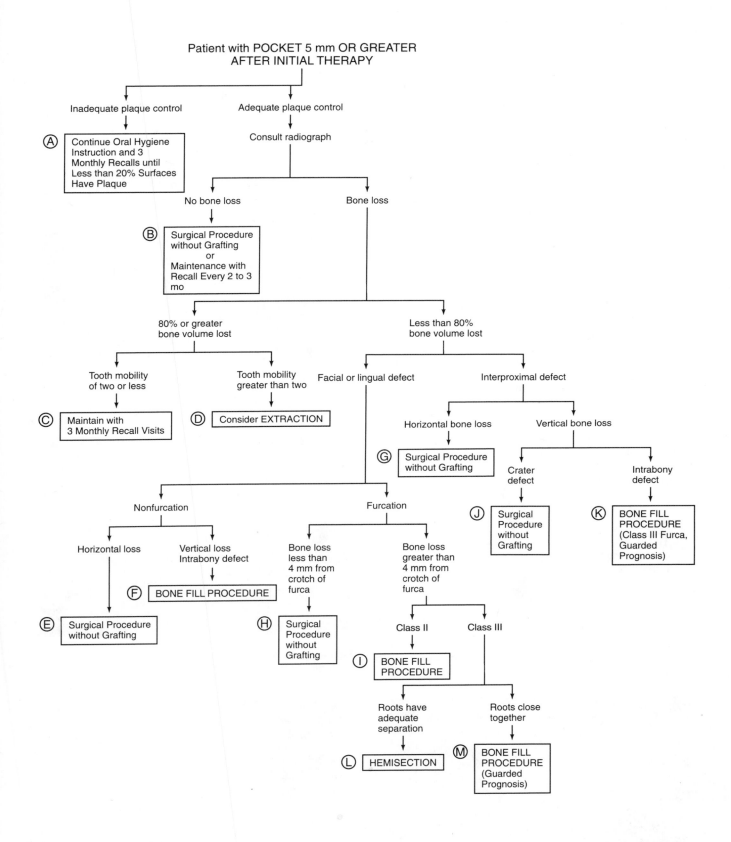

Patient with POCKET 5 mm OR GREATER
AFTER INITIAL THERAPY

Inadequate plaque control

Adequate plaque control

Ⓐ Continue Oral Hygiene Instruction and 3 Monthly Recalls until Less than 20% Surfaces Have Plaque

Consult radiograph

No bone loss

Bone loss

Ⓑ Surgical Procedure without Grafting or Maintenance with Recall Every 2 to 3 mo

80% or greater bone volume lost

Less than 80% bone volume lost

Tooth mobility of two or less

Tooth mobility greater than two

Facial or lingual defect

Interproximal defect

Ⓒ Maintain with 3 Monthly Recall Visits

Ⓓ Consider EXTRACTION

Horizontal bone loss

Vertical bone loss

Ⓖ Surgical Procedure without Grafting

Crater defect

Intrabony defect

Nonfurcation

Furcation

Ⓙ Surgical Procedure without Grafting

Ⓚ BONE FILL PROCEDURE (Class III Furca, Guarded Prognosis)

Horizontal loss

Vertical loss Intrabony defect

Bone loss less than 4 mm from crotch of furca

Bone loss greater than 4 mm from crotch of furca

Ⓕ BONE FILL PROCEDURE

Ⓔ Surgical Procedure without Grafting

Ⓗ Surgical Procedure without Grafting

Class II

Class III

Ⓘ BONE FILL PROCEDURE

Roots have adequate separation

Roots close together

Ⓛ HEMISECTION

Ⓜ BONE FILL PROCEDURE (Guarded Prognosis)

THE APPLICATION OF BONE FILL–REGENERATIVE PROCEDURES

E. Barrie Kenney

A number of procedures have proved to be clinically successful in the treatment of intrabony defects with a bone fill approach. Intraoral sites for autogenous bone grafts continue to be the primary sources for bone fill material. Extraoral sites such as iliac crest have had limited application because of the complexities involved in performing an additional surgical procedure outside the mouth. Decalcified freeze-dried bone obtained postmortem from human donors has provided a substitute for autogenous bone that ensures sufficient volume of graft material. The processing of decalcified freeze-dried bone makes the risk of transfer of disease from the donor to the recipient to be one in over a million.

Porous hydroxylapatite (PHA) is a synthetic bone substitute that can facilitate bone regeneration, but it is not so predictable in stimulating new cementum formation.

Guided tissue regeneration (GTR) techniques using polytetrafluoroethylene membranes have resulted in significant new cementum formation. In furcation regions, however, they apparently do not result in new bone deposition.

The coronally repositioned flap has been successful in treating Class II furcations in lower molars, where bone defects have shown evidence of fill 6 months after surgery.

Combinations of bone fill–regeneration procedures also have value, but additional controlled studies are needed before these applications can be clearly ascertained.

A. The presence of a furcation involvement is based on discovering the furcation on clinical examination with curved probes and by evaluation of radiographs.

B. A Class II furcation can be treated with autogenous bone if sufficient material is readily available at an intraoral site. If no suitable intraoral donor site is available, the defect can be treated with porous hydroxylapatite, either alone or in conjunction with a barrier membrane. There may be a small measurable advantage in the combination approach in terms of

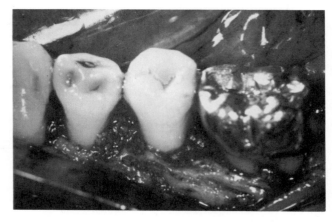

Figure 2. The defect on the distal of the second premolar has been filled with porous hydroxylapatite; the defect on the first premolar has been filled with decalcified freeze dried bone.

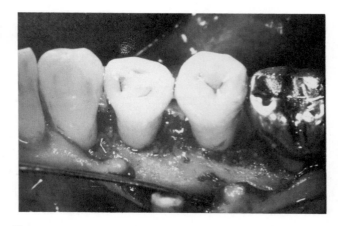

Figure 3. Six months later at surgical reentry the defects on the premolars have been resolved.

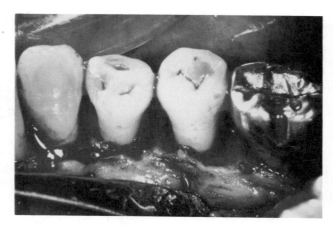

Figure 1. Intrabony defects on distal of both first and second premolars at time of flap surgery.

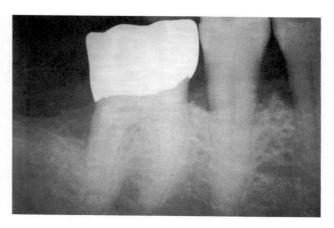

Figure 4. Presurgical radiographs between premolars and on the distal of second premolar.

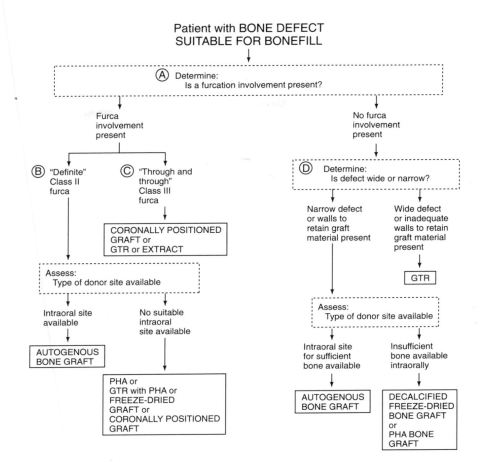

Patient with BONE DEFECT
SUITABLE FOR BONEFILL

Ⓐ Determine:
Is a furcation involvement present?

Furca involvement present — No furca involvement present

Ⓑ "Definite" Class II furca

Ⓒ "Through and through" Class III furca

CORONALLY POSITIONED GRAFT or GTR or EXTRACT

Assess:
Type of donor site available

Intraoral site available — No suitable intraoral site available

AUTOGENOUS BONE GRAFT

PHA or
GTR with PHA or
FREEZE-DRIED
GRAFT or
CORONALLY POSITIONED
GRAFT

Ⓓ Determine:
Is defect wide or narrow?

Narrow defect or walls to retain graft material present — Wide defect or inadequate walls to retain graft material present

GTR

Assess:
Type of donor site available

Intraoral site for sufficient bone available — Insufficient bone available intraorally

AUTOGENOUS BONE GRAFT

DECALCIFIED
FREEZE-DRIED
BONE GRAFT
or
PHA BONE
GRAFT

gain of attachment, but this will involve a second procedure to remove the barrier membrane. Coronally repositioned flaps require an additional measure to acid etch a suture support to the tooth, and this is complicated if a restoration covers the tooth surface.

C. Class III furcations are difficult to resolve with bone fill–regenerative procedures. Although minimally involved Class III lesions can be managed with guided tissue regeneration, it is unlikely that bone fill can be expected. Treatment of more advanced Class III lesions with coronally repositioned flaps is unpredictable, but current clinical experience suggests that it offers the best opportunity for some bone fill.

D. The treatment of choice for nonfurcation defects is determined by the geometry of the lesion. If the defect has sufficient walls to retain graft material, intraoral sites may be used to harvest autogenous bone to fill these defects. Many patients do not have acceptable donor sites, and in these cases excellent clinical results have been obtained with porous hydroxylapatite and decalcified freeze-dried bone. Guided tissue regeneration procedures may be used in these defects but will involve the patient in a second procedure, so they should be used in those cases in which simpler bone fill techniques are unpredictable (i.e., defects where there are inadequate walls to retain a graft material).

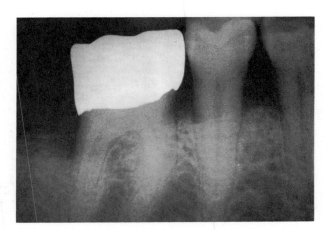

Figure 5. Radiograph 6 months after surgery showing reduction of the intrabony defects.

References

Gantes BG, Garrett S. Coronally displaced flaps in reconstructive periodontal therapy. Dent Clin North Am 1991; 35:495.

Gottlow J, Nyman S, Lindhe J. New attachment formation in the human periodontium by guided tissue regeneration: Case reports. J Clin Periodontol 1986;13:604.

Oreamuno S, Lekovic V, Kenney EB, et al. Comparative clinical study of porous hydroxylapatite and decalcified freeze-dried bone in human periodontal defects. J Periodontol 1990; 61:399.

Schallhorn RG, McClain PK. Combined osseous composite grafting, root conditioning and guided tissue regeneration. Int J Periodont Restor Dent 1988;8:9.

ONE-WALLED OSSEOUS DEFECT

Walter B. Hall

A one-walled osseous defect may be detected by careful probing and evaluation of radiographs. Radiographs alone are not sufficient to diagnose such defects but, in conjunction with careful probing, are helpful in conceptualizing such defects (Figs. 1 and 2). The one osseous wall of such a defect is always supporting the adjacent tooth; therefore, the interproximal pocket depth on the affected tooth will be several millimeters deeper than that on the adjacent tooth. At the line angles of the affected tooth, the probing will not indicate a lesser degree of bone loss than interproximally (as would be the case with a three-walled defect).

A. A tooth with a one-walled defect may be an essential tooth or it may not be important to a treatment plan for the patient. For example, canine teeth usually are essential to a restorative treatment plan; therefore, even therapy with a relatively low predictability of success should be employed to save a canine with a one-walled defect. By comparison, maxillary lateral incisors usually are not so important. Their root form and size make them less reliable as abutment teeth. If such a tooth has a deep, one-walled defect, procedures with poor likelihood of success, such as bone regeneration procedures, rarely are advisable on affected maxillary lateral incisors. If the two teeth adjacent to a tooth with a deep one-walled defect both have good bone support, removal of the badly involved tooth and its replacement with a fixed bridge may be the most sensible treatment plan. In such a case, the badly involved tooth would not be an important one. If the tooth with a deep one-walled defect is only one of many badly involved teeth, it is unlikely to be an important tooth. The treatment plan options that the dentist envisions for a patient will determine whether the tooth is essential.

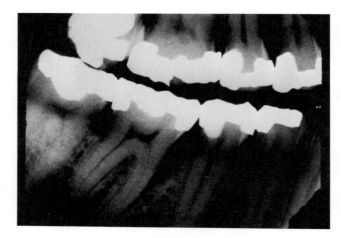

Figure 2. A one-walled defect (hemiseptum) on the mesial aspect of the first molar.

B. When the dentist has decided that a tooth is not an essential one, he should assess the risk to adjacent teeth by keeping the badly involved tooth. When good abutments on adjacent teeth are available or when the affected tooth may be easily replaced with a removable device, extraction of that tooth often is the best approach. A patient who has decided to retain the tooth should be made aware of the need for frequent planing and of the signs and symptoms of a periodontal abscess so that immediate dental treatment can be sought when they appear.

C. If keeping the affected tooth jeopardizes adjacent teeth that are potentially good abutments, it should be extracted. If the adjacent teeth are themselves potentially poor abutments, maintaining the affected tooth and its neighbors may be an acceptable alternative.

D. If the tooth with the one-walled osseous defect is an essential tooth (i.e., a canine), the depth of the defect is important in deciding among treatment alternatives.

E. For essential teeth with shallow-to-moderate one-walled defects (i.e., 1–3 mm from osseous crest to maximum depth), osseous resection on the adjacent tooth (or teeth) is a reasonable approach to eliminating the defect. The importance of the adjacent tooth could be such that removing any bone from its support would create a greater overall problem (i.e., the tooth is an abutment for an existing bridge). Attempting maintenance of the tooth could be a more reasonable approach. If an aesthetic problem would result from a resective approach, a modified Widman flap approach with one-time good access to plane the root of the affected tooth would be reasonable.

F. If the one-walled defect on an essential tooth is a deep one (i.e., 4 mm or more), extraction might be the best

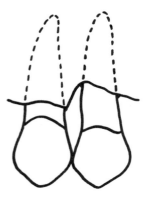

Figure 1. A hemiseptum is half of an interdental septum. The bone remaining against the adjacent, less-involved tooth constitutes the one remaining osseous wall.

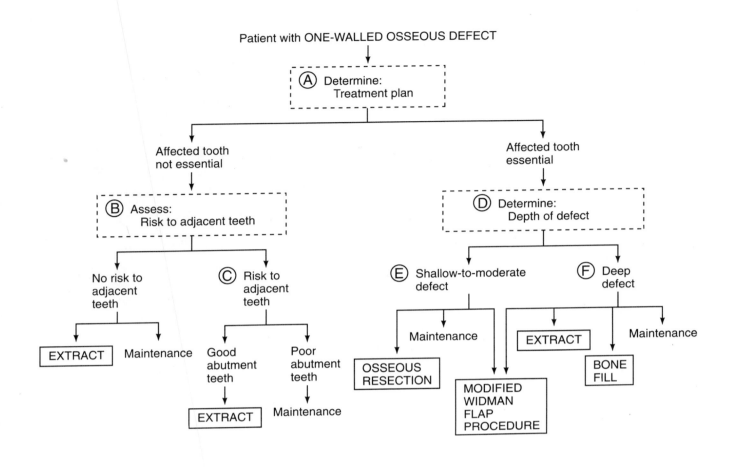

Patient with ONE-WALLED OSSEOUS DEFECT

(A) Determine:
Treatment plan

Affected tooth not essential

Affected tooth essential

(B) Assess:
Risk to adjacent teeth

(D) Determine:
Depth of defect

No risk to adjacent teeth

(C) Risk to adjacent teeth

(E) Shallow-to-moderate defect

(F) Deep defect

EXTRACT   Maintenance

Good abutment teeth

Poor abutment teeth

Maintenance

EXTRACT   Maintenance

OSSEOUS RESECTION

MODIFIED WIDMAN FLAP PROCEDURE

EXTRACT

BONE FILL

EXTRACT   Maintenance

alternative for maintaining other natural teeth. A bone fill (regenerative) approach might be attempted despite its low predictability of success if the affected tooth is very important. Maintenance or a modified Widman flap approach might be attempted, but the patient should be forewarned of the likelihood of losing the tooth to an abscess at any time.

References

Carranza FA, Jr. Glickman's clinical periodontology. 7th ed. Philadelphia: WB Saunders, 1990:833.

Friedman N. Periodontal osseous surgery: Osteoplasty and ostectomy. J Periodontol 1955; 26:257.

Genco RJ, Goldman HM, Cohen DW. Contemporary periodontics, St. Louis: CV Mosby, 1990:569.

Heins PS. Osseous surgery: An evaluation after twenty-five years. Dent Clin North Am 1960; 4:75.

Ochsenbein C. Rationale for periodontal osseous surgery. Dent Clin North Am 1960; 4:27.

Schluger S, Yuodelis R, Page RC, Johnson RH. Periodontal diseases. 2nd ed. Philadelphia: Lea & Febiger, 1990:522.

TWO-WALLED OSSEOUS DEFECT: CRATER TYPE

Walter B. Hall

A two-walled osseous defect may be detected by careful probing and evaluation of radiographs. The most common two-walled defects, craters, made up of the facial and lingual cortical plates (Figs. 1 and 2) are easily misinterpreted on radiographs. Superimposed cortical plates often hide defects. Slight angulation changes can suggest two-walled defects when none are present. Careful probing, however, can detect interproximal defects of similar depth on adjacent teeth and shallow readings at all line angles, where the cortical plates have not been resorbed. Another, less common type of two-walled defect, the non-crater type, occurs when one cortical plate has been resorbed and the other remains along with an osseous wall against one of the adjacent teeth. Radiographs can only suggest such defects. Probing can detect a shallow depth on one tooth and a deeper one on the other with no shallow depth on one line angle of the affected tooth.

A. The more common, two-walled osseous defects, on which both cortical plates remain, may be divided into those of shallow-to-moderate depth (i.e., 1–3 mm from osseous crest to maximum depth) and those that are deeper.

B. Shallow-to-moderate defects are readily eliminated by osseous resection with minimal removal of facial and lingual bone on adjacent teeth, thus providing the advantage of ease of access for cleaning by the patient or dentist as compared with the alternative procedures of maintenance or the modified Widman flap in which cleansing to the bottom of the pockets with oral hygiene devices is impossible and instrumentation at the angles at which the cortical plates meet the floor of the defects is difficult or impossible to achieve.

C. Deep defects are not good candidates for osseous resection, because too much facial and lingual bone must be sacrificed to achieve "positive" architecture. With molar teeth, uninvolved furcations may be

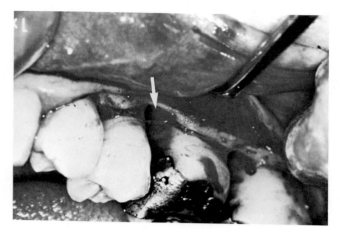

Figure 2. Two-walled, infrabony defect (crater).

exposed in the process. Deep craters may be amenable to guided tissue regeneration (GTR) (see p 158). When GTR is possible and the patient is willing to undergo such surgery, it is a predictable means of building back lost attachment and minimizing or eliminating Class II furca involvements. Successful GTR is the least expensive and most readily maintainable approach to managing the problems of deep craters.

D. Guided tissue regeneration is not feasible in all deep crater situations. If the roots of the adjacent involved teeth are only 1–2 mm apart, a root proximity problem may make barrier design impossible as the "isthmus" portion will be too narrow to act as an effective epithelial barrier. In such a case, extraction of the most badly involved tooth would be a sound approach if good abutments remain or an implant is feasible (see p 250). If either of the adjacent teeth has a Class III (through and through) furca involvement (see p 180), extraction of the involved tooth would be a good approach if satisfactory abutments remain or an implant is feasible. Alternatively, root resection (see p 138) can be employed, possibly with GTR, if poor abutments would remain if extraction were to be used. Maintenance of a "hopeless" situation might be a necessary last resort.

If the patient is unable or unwilling to proceed with these approaches, either one tooth can be extracted or the area can be maintained with a "hopeless" prognosis.

References

Carranza FA, Jr. Glickman's clinical periodontology. 7th ed. Philadelphia: WB Saunders, 1990:828.

Genco RJ, Goldman HM, Cohen DW. Contemporary periodontics. St. Louis: Mosby–Year Book, 1990:569.

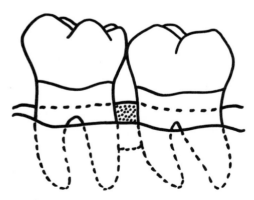

Figure 1. A crater is the type of two-walled infrabony defect in which facial and lingual cortical plates remain as the two osseous walls.

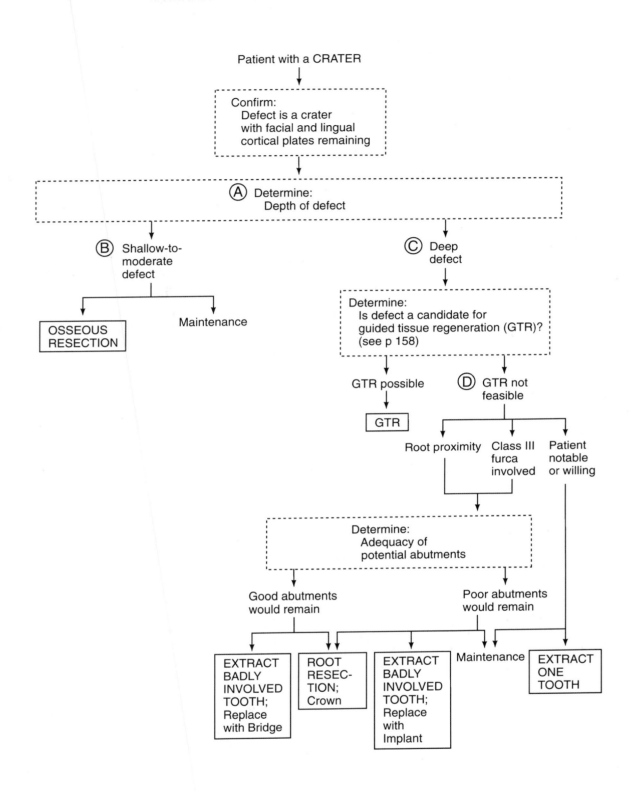

Patient with a CRATER

Confirm:
  Defect is a crater
  with facial and lingual
  cortical plates remaining

(A) Determine:
  Depth of defect

(B) Shallow-to-moderate defect

OSSEOUS RESECTION

Maintenance

(C) Deep defect

Determine:
  Is defect a candidate for
  guided tissue regeneration (GTR)?
  (see p 158)

GTR possible

GTR

(D) GTR not feasible

Root proximity

Class III furca involved

Patient notable or willing

Determine:
  Adequacy of
  potential abutments

Good abutments would remain

Poor abutments would remain

EXTRACT BADLY INVOLVED TOOTH; Replace with Bridge

ROOT RESECTION; Crown

EXTRACT BADLY INVOLVED TOOTH; Replace with Implant

Maintenance

EXTRACT ONE TOOTH

Ochsenbein C, Bohannon HM. Palatal approach to osseous surgery. I. Rationale. J Periodontol 1963; 34:60. II. Clinical application. J Periodontol 1964; 35:54.

Schluger S, Yuodelis R, Page RC, Johnson RH. Periodontal diseases. 2nd ed. Philadelphia: Lea & Febiger, 1990:513.

THREE-WALLED OSSEOUS DEFECT

Walter B. Hall

A three-walled osseous defect is detected best by careful probing; however, radiographs often are useful in suggesting the presence of such defects (Figs. 1 and 2). An interproximal, three-walled defect will have a deep interproximal reading with shallow facial and lingual readings at line angles where cortical plates remain intact. The interproximal depth on any adjacent teeth would be shallow too. Palatal, three-walled defects will elicit a deep reading with shallower readings on both sides. If the palate is flat, the presence of a third wall palatally can be assumed. In other areas, "sounding" (probing to bone with anesthetic) may be necessary to detect a third wall situated away from the tooth. Despite their depth, many three-walled defects are amenable to regenerative procedures.

A. Because such defects often occur on an endodontically involved tooth or a "cracked tooth," testing to assure that these problems do not coexist is necessary before proceeding with periodontal treatment (see p 64). If the tooth is endodontically involved but does not have a long vertical crack, endodontics should be utilized and the periodontal status reassessed after an appropriate interval. If endodontics cannot be performed, extract the tooth. If a vertical crack is present and is extensive, the tooth should be extracted or maintained with a hopeless prognosis.

B. Narrow defects, meaning ones in which the crest of the bone is 1 mm or less from the tooth at the widest point of the coronal aspect of the defect, are treated with predictable success by complete debridement and readaptation of the flap to cover the defect. Such regenerative osseous procedures are among the most successful means of adding lost support to a tooth. Such surgery, therefore, is far preferable to attempts to maintain such areas in which curettes cannot be placed or manipulated easily. Regenerative procedures in the case of narrow, three-walled defects (less

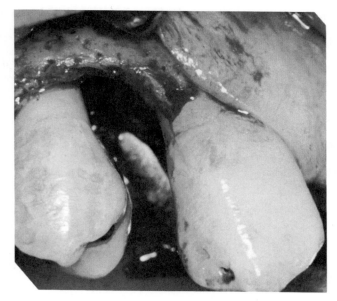

Figure 2. A three-walled infrabony defect mesial to the first premolar.

than 1 mm from tooth to crest of bone horizontally) have a very high predictability of successful regeneration with new attachment.

C. Shallow three-walled defects, 1–2 mm deep are amenable to osseous resection for pocket elimination. Some moderately deep, wide three-walled defects (2–3 mm deep) may be treated by eliminating the wider three-walled portion by osseous resection and treating the deeper, narrow portion as a narrow defect where new attachment is predictable.

D. Wide, deep three-walled osseous defects are excellent candidates for guided tissue regeneration (GTR) (see p 152). So strong is the likelihood of regeneration with new attachment that GTR always should be stressed as the treatment of choice. There are numerous three-walled defects on the distal of second molars, where an impacted or partially-erupted third molar which lay close to the root of the second molar has been extracted. These are among the most predictably successful situations in which to employ GTR. Similar defects on isolated abutment teeth may be treated routinely with GTR. Palatal three-walled defects also have high predictability for successful restoration of support by GTR. Because this approach is highly predictable and very inexpensive when compared with alternatives such as maintenance or extraction and replacement with a bridge or implant, GTR should be employed routinely for treating deep, wide three-walled defects.

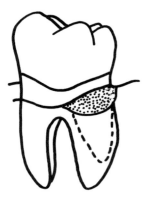

Figure 1. A wide, three-walled infrabony defect amenable to guided tissue regeneration.

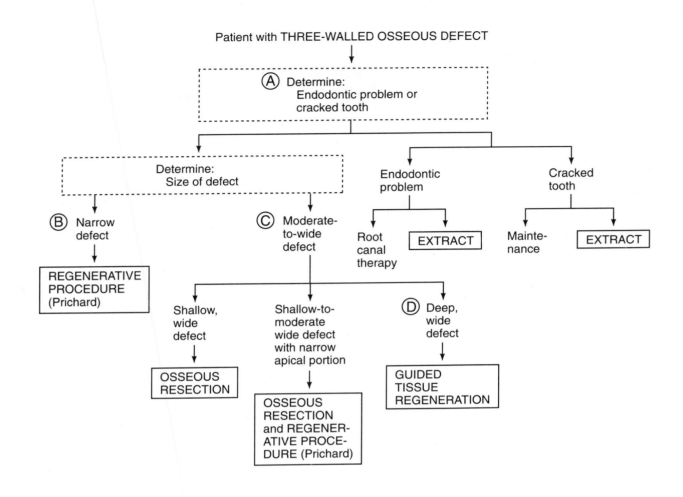

Patient with THREE-WALLED OSSEOUS DEFECT

A Determine:
Endodontic problem or
cracked tooth

Determine:
Size of defect

Endodontic
problem

Cracked
tooth

B Narrow
defect

C Moderate-
to-wide
defect

Root
canal
therapy

EXTRACT

Mainte-
nance

EXTRACT

REGENERATIVE
PROCEDURE
(Prichard)

Shallow,
wide
defect

Shallow-to-
moderate
wide defect
with narrow
apical portion

D Deep,
wide
defect

OSSEOUS
RESECTION

GUIDED
TISSUE
REGENERATION

OSSEOUS
RESECTION
and REGENER-
ATIVE PROCE-
DURE (Prichard)

References

Becker W, Becker B, Berg L, et al. New attachment after treatment with root isolation procedures: Report for treated Class III and Class II furcations and vertical defects. Int J Periodont Restor Dent 1988; 3:9.

Gottlow J, Nyman S, Karring T, Wennstrom J. New attachment formation in human periodontics by guided tissue regeneration. J Periodontol 1986; 57:727.

Lindhe J. Textbook of clinical periodontology. 2nd ed. Copenhagen: Munksgaard, 1989:450.

Prichard JF. The infrabony technique as a predictable procedure. J Periodontol 1957; 28:202.

Schallhorn RG, McClain PK. Combined osseous composite grafting, root conditioning and guided tissue regeneration. Int J Periodont Restor Dent 1988; 8:9.

APPROACHES TO THE DISTAL RIDGE POCKET

Walter B. Hall

Deep pockets on the distal surface of the most posterior teeth in either arch present unique options for treatment planning. Such defects are common to distal second molars where impacted or partially erupted third molars have been removed (see p 232). Difficulty in cleaning the distal surfaces of the most posterior teeth make pocket formation there more likely to occur. Heavy function on distal ridges may lead to fibrotic enlargement and pocket deepening. In other situations, where a two-walled defect exists between two teeth and the most posterior tooth is extracted, an osseous defect remains distal to the remaining tooth. Pocket elimination in shallower defects or regenerative procedures (Pritchard type, guided tissue regeneration) are the treatments of choice. The development of highly predictable guided tissue regeneration (GTR) procedures has changed treatment planning for more severely involved teeth radically (see p 148). The anatomical complexities of maxillary and mandibular distal ridge areas necessitate some variations in the design of flaps to avoid vascular and nerve injuries.

A. When pocket depth is present but no osseous defect is detectable, several surgical approaches to pocket elimination exist. If an adequate band of gingiva is present on the distal line angles of the teeth so that gingival excision will not create a pure mucogingival problem, gingivectomy may be used. When a fatty retromolar pad is involved in the mandibular arch, electrosurgery (which produces a fibrotic scarring in

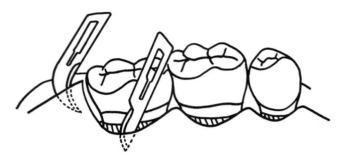

Figure 2. Distal "three-cornered tear" type of trapdoor flap used in the mandibular arch when a narrow, three-walled defect is present on the most posterior tooth.

healing) is preferable to a surgical approach. In all other areas of this type, the surgical approach is easier and less complicated to perform. If no osseous defect is present but gingivectomy would produce a pure mucogingival problem on a distal line angle of the most posterior tooth, a distal wedge or trap-door approach (Figs. 1 and 2) will permit pocket elimination without creating pure mucogingival problems.

B. If an osseous defect is present distal to the most posterior tooth, gingivectomy or electrosurgery are not appropriate approaches. The type of osseous defect which is present should be determined by probing and radiographic evaluation (see p 34). If a one-walled or two-walled non-crater type defect is present, guided tissue regeneration may not be appropriate unless the defect is an extremely deep two-walled one where the tooth is critically important to the treatment plan. Pocket elimination by osseous resection and apical positioning of the flap is the treatment of choice. As the osseous defect will have been eliminated by ostectomy, either a distal wedge or a trap-door approach may be used, because the positioning of the suture closing the flaps will be of minimal importance. Occasionally, a one-walled or two-walled non-crater type defect distal to the most posterior tooth will be so deep that the tooth should be extracted or maintained with frequent root planing. Should such a tooth have severe furcation problems or severe defects on its other surfaces, it also might be untreatable.

C. If a three-walled osseous defect is present distal to the most posterior tooth, the width of the defect from the osseous crest to the root will determine the approach to be used. A narrow, three-walled defect (1 mm or less in width) has a high predictability of success with a bone regeneration approach (see p 180).

D. If the defect is wider than 1 mm from root to osseous crest measured horizontally, the vertical depth of the three-walled defect will determine the surgical approach. If the defect is relatively shallow, 1–3 mm, at

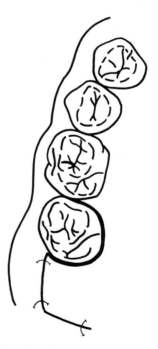

Figure 1. Distal trap-door flap for the maxillary arch when a narrow, three-walled defect is present on the most posterior tooth.

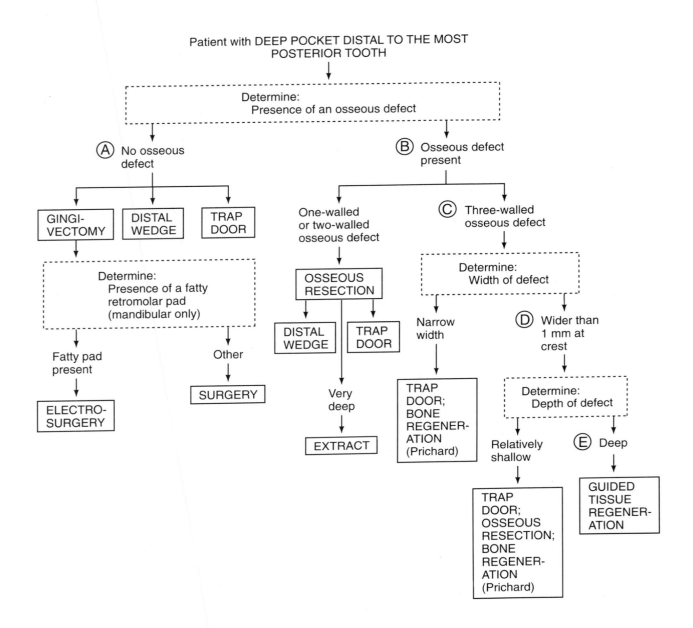

least some of its apical portion will be a narrow defect (1 mm or less from root to osseous crest measured horizontally). In such cases, osseous resection may be utilized to eliminate the wider, coronal portion and a Prichard-type regenerative approach can be utilized to gain back lost attachment in the deeper portion (see p 180). The trap-door flap design should be employed so that the suture used to close the flap does not lie over the defect to be filled.

E. If a three-walled defect is deep (more than 3 mm measured vertically) and wide (more than 1 mm from root to bone crest measured horizontally), GTR is a highly predictable approach unless the tooth has a Class III (through and through) furcation involvement, a vertical crack making it untreatable (see p 64) or severe defects on other surfaces that make it hopeless. In hopeless cases, extraction or maintenance would

be the options. When GTR is employed, the distal wedge flap design is preferred because the position of the suture is not a factor and the distal wedge holds the barrier in position better.

References

Braden BE. Deep distal pockets adjacent to terminal teeth. Dent Clin North Am 1969; 13:161.

Carranza FA, Jr. Glickman's clinical periodontology. 7th ed. Philadelphia: WB Saunders, 1990:821.

Genco RJ, Goldman HM, Cohen DW. Contemporary periodontics. St. Louis: Mosby—Year Book, 1990:563.

Robinson RE. The distal wedge operation. Periodontics 1966; 4:256.

Schluger S, Yuodelis R, Page RC, Johnson RH. Periodontal diseases. 2nd ed. Philadelphia: Lea & Febiger, 1990:493.

RIDGEPLASTY

Kenneth W. Karn

Partially edentulous ridge areas present unique problems of both a periodontal and prosthetic nature. A partially edentulous ridge is defined here as one with distal and mesial abutment teeth. The choice of therapy involves an assessment of the primary problem to be solved (either periodontal or prosthetic) as well as discussion of how to effect a compromise if both concerns are present. Study models are a valuable diagnostic aid (in addition to radiographs and a thorough clinical exam) in treatment planning to solve these problems.

A. To simplify treatment planning, one must determine whether the given situation is primarily a periodontal or prosthetic problem. The main criterion for establishing the area as primarily of periodontal concern is the presence of attachment loss with significant pocket depth. Pure mucogingival problems on adjacent teeth (inadequate attached gingiva, gingival clefts) are also considered, but they do not demand significant compromise to the prosthetic concerns and are de-emphasized during the initial assessment. Prosthetic concerns would include excess or poorly contoured ridge tissue, inadequate ridge bulk, or inadequate keratinized tissue.

B. Excessive or poorly contoured ridge tissue simply requires recontouring of the existing tissue. The ridge tissue can be used to solve mucogingival problems on adjacent teeth (even if the ridge does not require recontouring) provided adequate donor tissue is present. Keratinized tissue on the ridge may be used as donor material for a free gingival graft or for a pedicle graft if coverage of exposed root surface is desired. The recontouring process may be accomplished by gingivectomy/gingivoplasty or flap surgery. If bone is to be removed or bone fill attempted, a flap approach is recommended.

C. An inadequate bulk of ridge tissue may be present if teeth are lost because of trauma or severe periodontitis. This can be a problem aesthetically, especially for anterior fixed bridges. The ridge bulk may be augmented by means of an overlay graft using gingiva from the tuberosity or other edentulous area. Another method is to create a pouch within the connective tissue of the ridge into which synthetic bone, sclera, or fibrous tissue from another intraoral site is implanted to create the desired bulk and contour. Occasionally, the ridge has adequate bulk but lacks a broad band of keratinized tissue. This situation can be either an aesthetic problem in an anterior area where a fixed bridge is contemplated or a functional problem in a saddle area where a removable partial denture is tissue-bearing. A free gingival graft is the recommended solution.

D. Pocket reduction surgery often requires some compromises in esthetics. Plan surgery carefully (with the help of study models) to avoid such problems. Because teeth are missing, usually there is more flexibility in partially edentulous areas. If the existing keratinized tissue is ample, a gingivectomy/gingivoplasty may be used. Use apically positioned flap surgery with internal beveled resection when preservation of the existing keratinized tissue is desired or if access to bone for recontouring is necessary. Flap surgery is more comfortable for the patient during healing and is often the treatment of choice, even though the technique is more demanding than gingivectomy/gingivoplasty.

E. Intrabony pocket treatment depends on the topographic nature of the osseous defect. Narrow intrabony defects have varying degrees of regenerative potential based on the size of the defect in relation to the surrounding bony walls. Surgery for osseous regenerative procedures is more exacting and requires careful planning to assure that incisions are not placed directly over the area where regeneration is desired. The results of regenerative therapy are less predictable than pocket reduction surgery using apically positioned flaps with osseous contouring; however, the resective surgical approach often requires removal of sound bone and/or soft tissue from adjacent areas to achieve the desired result.

F. Orthodontic treatment (such as molar uprighting) may be used to deal with some of the aforementioned problems, especially pockets adjacent to drifted or tipped teeth (see p 128).

References

Genco RJ, Goldman HM, Cohen DW. Contemporary periodontics. St. Louis: CV Mosby, 1990:629.

Miller PD. Ridge augmentation under existing fixed prosthesis-simplified technique. J Periodontol 1986; 57:742.

Rosenberg S. Use of ceramic material for augmentation of the partially edentulous ridge: A case report. Compend Contin Ed 1984; 77(3):29.

Schluger S, Yuodelis R, Page RC, Johnson RH. Periodontal diseases. 2nd ed. Philadelphia: Lea & Febiger, 1990:599.

Seibert R. Reconstruction of the deformed partially edentulous ridges using full-thickness overlay grafts. Parts 1 and 2. Compend Contin Dent Ed 1983; 4(5):437; 4(6):549.

Patient with an EDENTULOUS RIDGE REQUIRING PERIODONTAL MODIFICATION

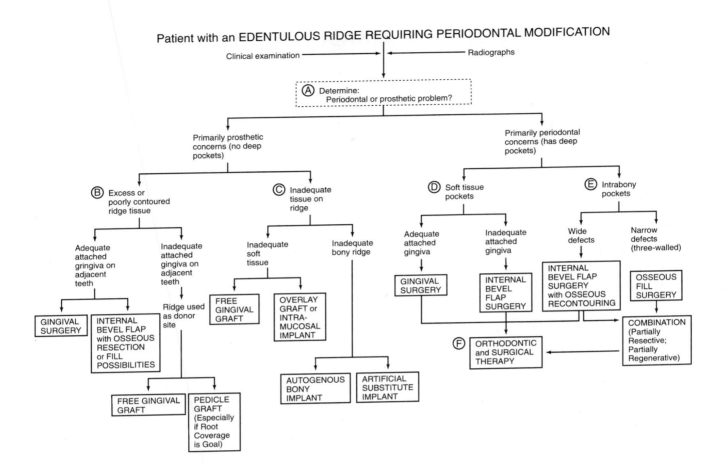

Clinical examination ⟶ ⟵ Radiographs

(A) Determine:
Periodontal or prosthetic problem?

Primarily prosthetic concerns (no deep pockets)

(B) Excess or poorly contoured ridge tissue

Adequate attached gringiva on adjacent teeth
- GINGIVAL SURGERY
- INTERNAL BEVEL FLAP with OSSEOUS RESECTION or FILL POSSIBILITIES

Inadequate attached gingiva on adjacent teeth
Ridge used as donor site
- FREE GINGIVAL GRAFT
- PEDICLE GRAFT (Especially if Root Coverage is Goal)

(C) Inadequate tissue on ridge

Inadequate soft tissue
- FREE GINGIVAL GRAFT
- OVERLAY GRAFT or INTRA-MUCOSAL IMPLANT

Inadequate bony ridge
- AUTOGENOUS BONY IMPLANT
- ARTIFICIAL SUBSTITUTE IMPLANT

Primarily periodontal concerns (has deep pockets)

(D) Soft tissue pockets

Adequate attached gingiva
- GINGIVAL SURGERY

Inadequate attached gingiva
- INTERNAL BEVEL FLAP SURGERY

(E) Intrabony pockets

Wide defects
- INTERNAL BEVEL FLAP SURGERY with OSSEOUS RECONTOURING

Narrow defects (three-walled)
- OSSEOUS FILL SURGERY

- COMBINATION (Partially Resective; Partially Regenerative)

(F) ORTHODONTIC and SURGICAL THERAPY

SUTURING FOLLOWING PERIODONTAL SURGERY

Walter B. Hall

Many innovative types of sutures may be used to close periodontal surgical wounds; however, only a small number of suture techniques that are adequate to close such surgical sites are discussed here. Mastery of these techniques will permit the dentist to manage just about all contingencies. The type of suturing to be used depends upon the surgery performed.

A. For pure mucogingival procedures such as pedicle grafts and free gingival grafts, simple interrupted sutures usually are all that is required. Suturing in these cases usually involves the use of 4.0 or 5.0 gut or 5.0 Ethibond (braided Dacron-coated Teflon) suture material and a small round, maleable, needle such as the V5 needle by Ethicon.

B. For mucogingival—osseous surgery, a wider armamentarium of sutures is needed. Usually 4.0 black silk with a back-cutting, needle is used here.

C. For modified Widman flap procedures, in which flaps are reflected only minimally before replacement in much the same coronoapical position, simple interrupted sutures approximating facial and lingual flaps at each interdental papilla usually are used.

D. For distal wedge or trap-door procedures, surgical sites usually can be completely closed with one to several simple interrupted sutures.

E. Ridgeplasty procedures always involve the use of some simple interrupted sutures. Occasionally, single-sling sutures around abutment teeth are used as well.

F. For apically positioned flap procedures in which only one to three teeth are included, single-sling sutures (Fig. 1) are an excellent choice for use in approximating palatal or lingual flaps closely to the teeth at the level of the crest of bone. On the facial flap, a single sling can be used as a suspensory suture; however, skillful architects of the osseous form often use no sutures on the facial flap. If a full sextant of teeth is treated by means of apically repositioned flaps, a continuous-sling suture (Fig. 1) is the best choice to adapt closely palatal and lingual flaps to the teeth. If the tissue is thin or needs to be stretched to gain full closure, a mattress type of continuous-sling suture may be necessary. In routine cases, a simple continuous sling will suffice. The facial flap may be suspended with a single-sling suture or, if well adapted, no sutures.

G. When vertical releasing incisions are used to permit adequate reflection or positioning of a flap, simple interrupted sutures are used to approximate the flap in its new position in relation to adjacent tissue.

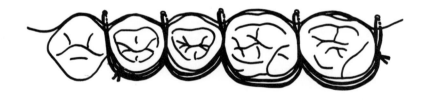

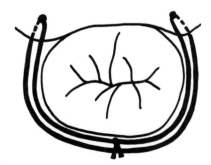

Figure 1. Continuous or single-sling sutures may be used to close posterior areas of mucogingival-osseous surgery.

Patient for SUTURING FOLLOWING PERIODONTAL SURGERY

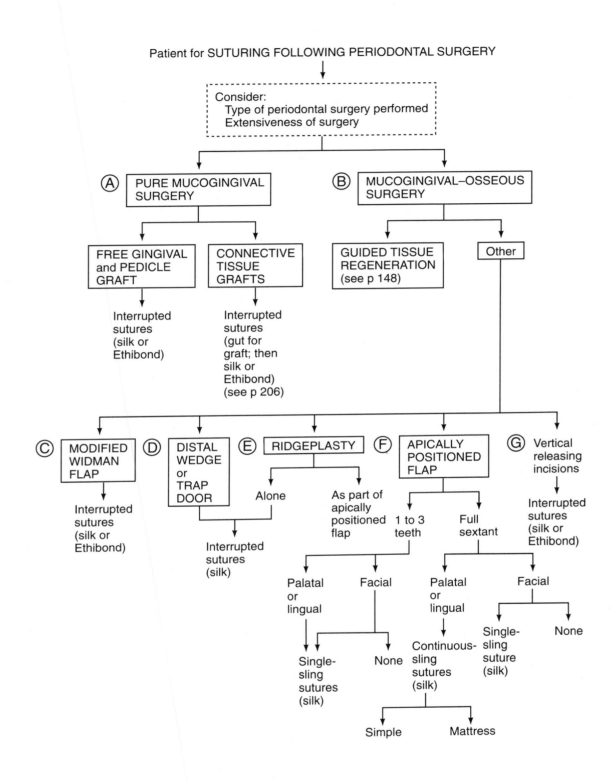

References

Carranza FA Jr. Glickman's clinical periodontology. 7th ed. Philadelphia: WB Saunders, 1990:800.

Dahlberg WH. Incisions and suturing: Some basic considerations about each in periodontal flap surgery. Dent Clin North Am 1969; 13:149.

Lindhe J. Textbook of clinical periodontology. 2nd ed. Copenhagen: Munksgaard, 1989:416.

Schluger S, Yuodelis R, Page RC, Johnson RH. Periodontal diseases. 2nd ed. Philadelphia: Lea & Febiger, 1990:479.

DRESSING FOLLOWING MUCOGINGIVAL–OSSEOUS SURGERY

Walter B. Hall

After completion of a segment of mucogingival surgery, the dentist must decide what dressing, if any, should be placed in the area. The purposes of using dressings include better control of postoperative bleeding, better patient comfort while eating, and some stabilization of loose teeth during early healing. The disadvantages of using dressings may relate to esthetics and delay in healing after the first few postoperative days. Great variability in deciding upon the need for dressings and selection of the appropriate one exists; this author offers conservative guidelines that should work well for most dentists.

A. Anterior segments of mucogingival–osseous surgery may present esthetic problems that should be considered in deciding whether to dress the wound and what dressings to use. In the maxillary anterior region, this is especially true. Because these areas lend themselves to full closure with suturing, not placing a dressing is a reasonable option. Placing a Stomahesive bandage, which dissolves in 8 to 24 hours (depending upon the activity of the tongue against it), will minimize early postoperative bleeding and further stabilize the flaps. It is simple to place, requiring only a minute or two.

B. Mandibular anterior segments usually do not present aesthetic problems, but the mandibular incisors are often quite mobile and have considerable bone loss; therefore, Coe Pak or another nondissolvable "pack" often is a good choice (Fig. 1). If a mandibular anterior segment of mucogingival–osseous surgery can be completely closed with sutures and the teeth have little mobility, Stomahesive bandage or no dressing may be sufficient; however, if closure is incomplete, leaving exposed areas, and/or mobility is significant, Coe Pak or an alternative pack is preferable.

C. In posterior segments of mucogingival–osseous surgery, the objectives of surgery and the scope of the area to be treated vary more. Tuberosity or retromolar pad surgery may be the only surgery to be performed in a posterior region. With these distal ridge procedures, when the procedure is done alone, good closure of the flaps is attainable. A dressing may be unnecessary, or Stomahesive bandage may be used to further stabilize the wound and to minimize bleeding as healing begins. If a distal ridge procedure is performed as part of surgery on adjacent posterior teeth, Coe Pak or an alternative usually is used.

D. Ridgeplasty and crown lengthening may be performed in any part of the mouth but are performed more frequently as isolated procedures in posterior segments. In anterior segments, they usually are dressed with Stomahesive bandage. In posterior segments, if good closure of the flaps can be attained with sutures, Stomahesive bandage or no dressing works well. If good closure cannot be obtained, as under existing bridges, Coe Pak or an alternative is preferable. If adjacent areas are treated along with the ridgeplasty areas or if gingivectomy is used, Coe Pak or an alternative is preferred.

E. If routine mucogingival–osseous surgery is performed in a posterior segment, two basic approaches are used most widely. When the modified Widman flap approach is used, good closure with sutures often is attainable when the flaps are replaced. In these cases, Stomahesive bandage or no dressing will suffice. When the closure is incomplete, especially between molar teeth, Coe Pak or an alternative is preferred to control bleeding and to stabilize the flaps. When pocket elimination surgery (apically positioned flap, gingivectomy) is used in posterior segments, Coe Pak or an alternative is preferred to minimize bleeding, to help stabilize teeth, to minimize sensitivity to initial temperature change, and to improve comfort in eating.

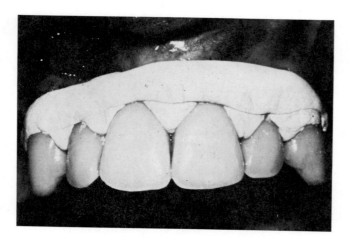

Figure 1. A Coe Pak dressing in place.

References

Carranza FA Jr. Glickman's clinical periodontology. 7th ed. Philadelphia: WB Saunders, 1990:767.

Grant DA, Stern IB, Listgarten MA. Periodontics. 6th ed. St. Louis: CV Mosby, 1988:731.

Hall WB. Pure mucogingival problems. Berlin: Quintessence Publishing, 1984:107.

Lindhe J. Textbook of clinical periodontology. 2nd ed. Copenhagen: Munksgaard, 1989:418.

O'Neil TCA. Antibacterial properties of periodontal dressings. J Periodontol 1975; 46:469.

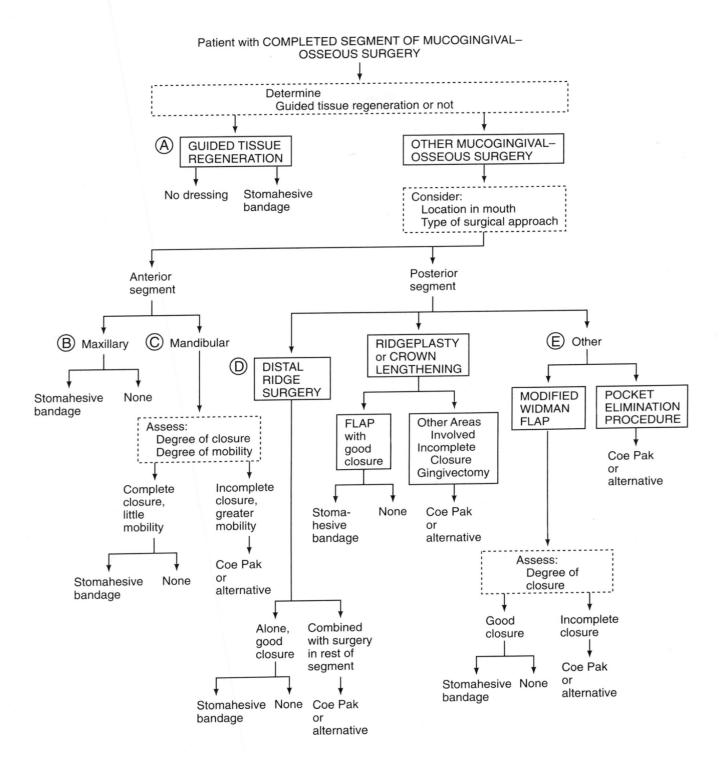

Patient with COMPLETED SEGMENT OF MUCOGINGIVAL–
OSSEOUS SURGERY

Determine
Guided tissue regeneration or not

(A) GUIDED TISSUE
REGENERATION

No dressing   Stomahesive
bandage

OTHER MUCOGINGIVAL–
OSSEOUS SURGERY

Consider:
Location in mouth
Type of surgical approach

Anterior
segment

Posterior
segment

(B) Maxillary   (C) Mandibular

Stomahesive   None
bandage

(D) DISTAL
RIDGE
SURGERY

RIDGEPLASTY
or CROWN
LENGTHENING

(E) Other

MODIFIED
WIDMAN
FLAP

POCKET
ELIMINATION
PROCEDURE

Coe Pak
or
alternative

Assess:
Degree of closure
Degree of mobility

Complete
closure,
little
mobility

Incomplete
closure,
greater
mobility

Coe Pak
or
alternative

FLAP
with
good
closure

Other Areas
Involved
Incomplete
Closure
Gingivectomy

Stomahesive   None
bandage

Stoma-   None
hesive
bandage

Coe Pak
or
alternative

Assess:
Degree of
closure

Good
closure

Incomplete
closure

Stomahesive   None
bandage

Coe Pak
or
alternative

Alone,
good
closure

Combined
with surgery
in rest of
segment

Stomahesive   None
bandage

Coe Pak
or
alternative

189

POSTSURGICAL MEDICATION

Walter B. Hall

When a segment of periodontal surgery has been completed, the dentist must decide whether postoperative medication will be needed by the patient and, if so, what should be taken. Postsurgical pain may vary in degree with different procedures and different individuals. By the time any periodontal surgical treatment is initiated, the dentist should know the patient well from the relationship developed during initial therapy. This experience will help the dentist decide whether the patient needs stronger pain control than an over-the-counter type of medication can provide. Some periodontal surgical procedures, however, require the use of prescription pain-controlling drugs, often enough that a prescription should be provided routinely. Antibiotic prescriptions, however, are rarely needed.

A. When pure mucogingival procedures are used, postsurgical pain usually is not great; therefore, over-the-counter medications, such as aspirin, Tylenol, or ibuprofen, usually suffice. Pedicle grafts and Gore-Tex regenerative root coverage procedures involve only one localized site, so prescriptions are not given routinely. Free gingival grafts and connective tissue procedures involve a donor and a receptor site. The donor site usually is from the palate, an area that is continually disturbed by tongue movement; therefore, for a tense or apprehensive patient, a prescription such as Tylenol with codeine no. 3 often is given to the patient. The patient is instructed to fill the prescription if needed; usually, the prescription is not filled.

B. Mucogingival—osseous surgery procedures usually are followed by a greater degree of postoperative pain; therefore, a prescription for Tylenol with codeine no. 3 is provided routinely, but with the admonition not to fill the prescription unless needed. Stronger medications are almost never needed unless more than one segment of surgery is performed at one visit or very extensive osseous recontouring or denudation is performed. The following guidelines may be helpful.

C. After placing an apically positioned flap with osseous recontouring, routinely prescribe a pain-controlling medication. The patient usually uses the medication. If denudation is employed to create more gingiva, the patient's need for pain control will be greater.

D. After placing an apically positioned flap with osseous fill or guided tissue regeneration, routinely prescribe a pain-controlling medication. The patient usually uses the medication. If a localized, narrow, three-walled defect is treated for bone regeneration, or larger defects are treated by guided tissue regeneration, a postsurgical antibiotic regimen should not be needed; routinely, however, if a bone fill material is used, especially if it is a commercial one, antibiotic treatment should be used for a week or more. Penicillin is the most common choice for this purpose.

E. After performing a modified Widman flap procedure, routinely prescribe a pain-controlling medication. The patient often uses the medication. Because no osseous recontouring is performed and the flaps are not fully reflected, the patient's postoperative discomfort should be less. Because new attachment is not anticipated with this procedure, an antibiotic need not be prescribed routinely.

F. After crown lengthening or distal trap-door (wedge) procedures, because these are smaller, isolated areas of surgery that usually involve some osseous recontouring, a prescription for a pain-controlling drug is given routinely but often is not used. Only if bone regeneration is attempted with a wide distal defect is there a need for antibiotics.

G. Some ridgeplasty procedures involve exposure of a large area of ridge and extensive osseous recontouring. In these cases, a prescription for a pain-controlling medication usually will be needed and used. If the area is small and can be completely closed, the prescription may not be needed.

H. Ridge augmentation may be sufficiently traumatic to require prescription pain medications; however, smaller areas, gentler techniques such as guided bone augmentation or inlay approaches, may be managed with ibuprofen or Tylenol. Antibiotics are utilized frequently.

References

Dal Pra DJ, Strohan JD. A clinical evaluation of the benefits of a course of oral penicillin following periodontal surgery. Aust Dent J 1972; 17:219.

Hall WB. Pure mucogingival problems. Berlin: Quintessence Publishing, 1984:140.

Holroyd SV. Control of pain and infection. Dent Clin North Am 1973; 17:417.

Murphy NC, DeMarco TJ. Controlling pain in periodontal patients. Dent Survey 1979; 55:46.

Strohan JD, Glenwright HD. Pain experience in periodontal surgery. J Periodont Res 1967; 1:163.

Patient with COMPLETED SEGMENT OF PERIODONTAL SURGERY

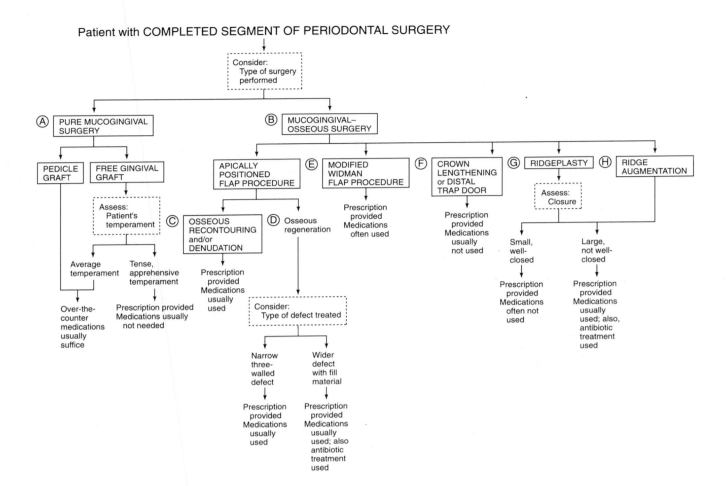

RESTORATION FOLLOWING MUCOGINGIVAL—OSSEOUS SURGERY

Walter B. Hall

The timing of restorations following mucogingival—osseous surgery depends upon what types of treatment have been done, both presurgically and surgically. A patient who has been splinted presurgically, generally speaking, can wait a longer time before deciding upon permanent restorations than one who has not been splinted. If procedures that have a lower predictability of success have been used surgically (i.e., osseous regeneration, new attachment), a longer time should be allowed before making decisions upon the restorative plan than if a more definitive approach were employed.

A. When temporary splinting or provisional splinting has been used before periodontal surgery, the teeth involved usually are so loose that the dentist has decided that splinting is necessary for comfort and function during the surgical period. Provisional splinting is done for periods up to 2 years in cases that will ultimately require extensive reconstruction and in which some of the teeth have a guarded prognosis. Temporary splinting often is extracoronal (such as a nightguard, or wire and composite splint); in these cases, restorative decisions can be made 3 months or more after the last surgery, unless a new attachment or bone regeneration approach was used, in which case a 6-month wait would be indicated. If intracoronal temporary splinting or provisional splinting was used, a minimal waiting period of 6 months after surgery, before reevaluation, is necessary. If the provisionally splinted case is an extensive one, a waiting period up to 2 years after surgery may be indicated before reevaluation and permanent restoration.

B. If a patient who has had mucogingival—osseous surgery and has not required splinting has had pocket elimination surgery (apically positioned flap with osseous recontouring or gingivectomy) or a modified Widman flap surgery, reevaluation prior to restoration can be performed as early as 1 month after the last surgery. Healing following such surgery usually is clinically completed this soon; however, if there are any significantly compromised teeth, the reevaluation should be delayed until 3 to 6 months after surgery, so that a more reliable prognostication can be made.

C. If a new attachment procedure or an osseous regenerative procedure has been used, reevaluation prior to restoration should not be performed sooner than 6 months after the last surgery. Restoration should be delayed in these cases until the long-term prognoses for these teeth are clearly established. With new attachment and osseous regeneration approaches, extensive, expensive restorations should not be placed unless the teeth have a reasonable prognosis 6 months after surgery.

References

Carranza FA Jr. Glickman's clinical periodontology. 7th ed. Philadelphia: WB Saunders, 1990:915.

Donaldson D. Gingival recession associated with temporary crowns. J Periodontol 1973; 44:691.

Nyman S, Lindhe J. A longitudinal study of combined periodontal and prosthetic treatment of patients with advanced periodontal disease. J Periodontol 1979; 50:163.

Schluger S, Yuodelis R, Page RC, Johnson RH. Periodontal diseases. 2nd ed. Philadelphia: Lea & Febiger, 1990:612.

Seibert JS, Cohen DW. Periodontal considerations in preparation for fixed and removable prosthodontics. Dent Clin North Am 1987; 31:529.

Patient with completed MUCOGINGIVAL–OSSEOUS SURGERY

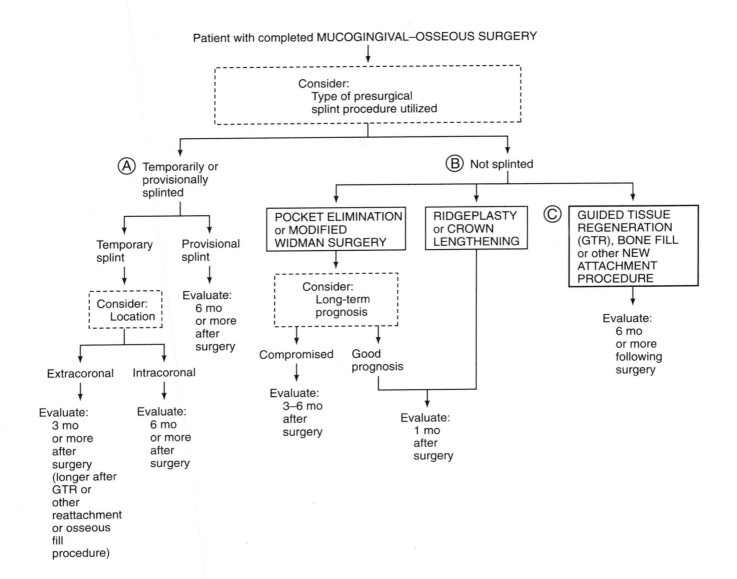

Consider:
Type of presurgical
splint procedure utilized

Ⓐ Temporarily or
provisionally
splinted

Temporary
splint

Consider:
Location

Extracoronal

Evaluate:
3 mo
or more
after
surgery
(longer after
GTR or
other
reattachment
or osseous
fill
procedure)

Intracoronal

Evaluate:
6 mo
or more
after
surgery

Provisional
splint

Evaluate:
6 mo
or more
after
surgery

Ⓑ Not splinted

POCKET ELIMINATION
or MODIFIED
WIDMAN SURGERY

Consider:
Long-term
prognosis

Compromised

Evaluate:
3–6 mo
after
surgery

Good
prognosis

RIDGEPLASTY
or CROWN
LENGTHENING

Evaluate:
1 mo
after
surgery

Ⓒ GUIDED TISSUE
REGENERATION
(GTR), BONE FILL
or other NEW
ATTACHMENT
PROCEDURE

Evaluate:
6 mo
or more
following
surgery

DEHISCENCE AND FENESTRATION

Walter B. Hall

When a tooth is in a prominent position in the arch, its root may not have bone covering its facial or lingual surface to the normal height, 1 to 1.5 mm from the cementoenamel junction (Fig. 1). The term *dehiscence* refers to the bursting through bone of a root as the tooth erupts so that bone never does, or did, extend to its normal proximity to the cementoenamel junction. The term *fenestration* refers to a circumscribed defect that creates a "window" through the bone over the prominent root. Perhaps too much effort is expended in differentiating between the two, because the consequences of having a thin "bridge" of cortical bone coronal to the circumscribed defect (a *fenestration*) and not having that bone (a dehiscence) is of little clinical consequence. True, that bone must be resorbed before loss of attachment can occur, but the ease with which the thin bridge of bone can be destroyed by inflammation makes its existence of little consequence. Various tests can be used to determine which is present and the possible therapeutic implications.

A. Radiographs will not be useful in detecting or differentiating between these two bone defects. Because the defect overlies the root in the radiograph, it cannot be seen on typical films.

B. The simplest test, but one that requires considerable experience, is to run a finger over the prominent root in apicocoronal and mesiodistal directions. The crest of the bone at the apical extent of the defect often can be felt, as can the lateral borders. As the finger is moved coronally, the "bridge" of bone can be felt at the coronal aspect of a fenestration but not in the coronal portion of a dehiscence.

C. Probing is of limited usefulness but can be important in planning treatment. A fenestration cannot be probed. A dehiscence may be probed if attachment has been lost, but it cannot be probed when attachment to the root is intact.

D. Sounding, pushing the probe through the anesthetized soft tissue over the root (Fig. 1), can be used to differentiate between the two types of defects. When an apparent fenestration or dehiscence has been located digitally, the probe is positioned over the defect and pressed into contact with the tooth. The sensation transmitted to the dentist on touching the tooth rather than bone is a "quick," "sharp," or "solid" one, whereas bone gives a mushy or softer sensation. If the sensation is one of touching the tooth, the probe is moved halfway to the free margin and is pressed through the soft tissue. If bone is touched, the defect is a fenestration; if not, it probably will prove to be a dehiscence.

E. The clinical importance of these determinations relates to the consequences of raising a flap or preparing a receptor bed for a gingival graft. If the defect is a fenestration, soft tissue will be capable of "reattaching" to the exposed surface with high predictability. If the defect is a dehiscence, reattachment to the level of the most apical aspect of the pocket or crevice depth also is likely to be successful. If the root has been exposed by inflammatory periodontal disease, only a "new attachment" (see p 254) could occur where attachment has been lost.

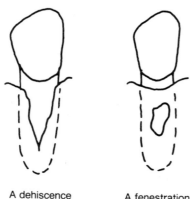

A dehiscence   A fenestration

Figure 1. A dehiscence is a bursting through bone of the tooth root whereas a fenestration is a window in the bone.

References

Elliott JR, Bowers GM. Alveolar dehiscence and fenestration. Periodontics 1963; 1:245.

Gartrell JR, Mathews DP. Gingival recession: The condition, process and treatment. Dent Clin North Am 1976; 20:199.

Hall WB. Present status of soft-tissue grafting. J Periodontol 1977; 48:587.

Hall WB. Pure mucogingival problems. Berlin: Quintessence Publishing, 1984:36.

Patient's tooth with a PROMINENT ROOT AND SOME MISSING BONE OVER IT

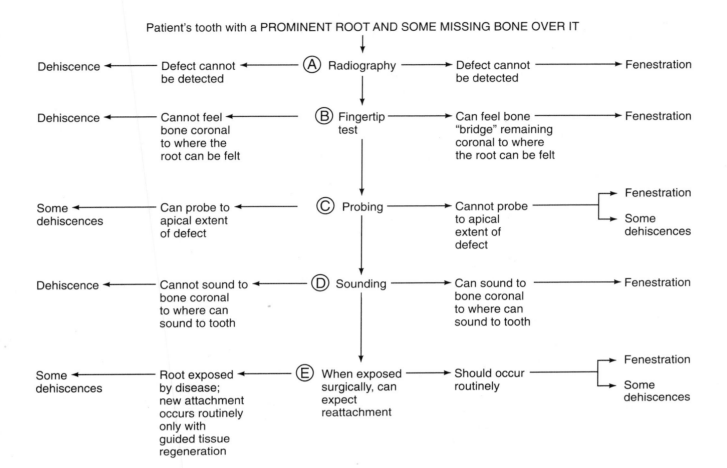

Dehiscence ← Defect cannot be detected ← Ⓐ Radiography → Defect cannot be detected → Fenestration

Dehiscence ← Cannot feel bone coronal to where the root can be felt ← Ⓑ Fingertip test → Can feel bone "bridge" remaining coronal to where the root can be felt → Fenestration

Some dehiscences ← Can probe to apical extent of defect ← Ⓒ Probing → Cannot probe to apical extent of defect → Fenestration / Some dehiscences

Dehiscence ← Cannot sound to bone coronal to where can sound to tooth ← Ⓓ Sounding → Can sound to bone coronal to where can sound to tooth → Fenestration

Some dehiscences ← Root exposed by disease; new attachment occurs routinely only with guided tissue regeneration ← Ⓔ When exposed surgically, can expect reattachment → Should occur routinely → Fenestration / Some dehiscences

CHARACTERISTICS OF A GOOD DONOR SITE FOR A PEDICLE GRAFT

Walter B. Hall

A tooth with inadequate attached gingiva and root exposure is a candidate for root coverage by means of a pedicle graft, especially if the recession is active and an aesthetic problem exists. A pedicle graft is the best approach to resolving such a problem, as the likelihood of root coverage is greater with a pedicle graft than with a free gingival graft. Also, the color match of adjacent gingiva with the gingiva in the area to be covered is more likely to be better than is that of gingiva from the palate, which is used in free gingival grafting.

A. If one of the adjacent teeth or an adjacent bridge has attached gingiva that is 1.5 times the width of root to be covered, or 2 to 3 mm tall and about 1 mm thick,

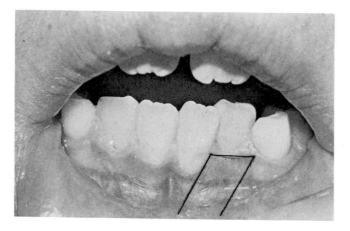

Figure 1. A good donor site on the lateral incisor for a pedicle graft to the central incisor.

a pedicle graft from that site may be laterally positioned to cover the exposed root surface, creating an adequate band of attached gingiva (Fig. 1). If neither adjacent site has attached gingiva of these dimensions, a different approach must be sought.

B. If no adequate donor site for a laterally positioned graft exists but an adjacent papilla is wide enough to create an adequate band of attached gingiva on the tooth to be treated when rotated 90 degrees, an obliquely positioned pedicle graft may be used (see p 200). If such a wide, tall, thick papilla does not exist, seek an alternative approach.

C. If the two adjacent papillae, when combined in width, will create an adjacent papillae to cover the exposed root to be treated, the double-papilla graft approach may be used (see p 202). If the two papillae together would not be adequate to cover the exposed root to be treated, a free gingival graft approach is the only one possible.

References

Carranza FA Jr. Glickman's clinical periodontology. 7th ed. Philadelphia: WB Saunders, 1990:896.

Hall WB. Pure mucogingival problems. Berlin: Quintessence Publishing, 1984:101.

Schluger S, Yuodelis R, Page RC, Johnson RH. Periodontal diseases. 2nd ed. Philadelphia: Lea & Febiger, 1990:564.

Seibert JS. Soft tissue grafts in periodontics. In: Robinson PJ, Guernsey LH, eds. Clinical transplantation in dental specialties. St. Louis: CV Mosby, 1980:107.

Patient's tooth with ROOT EXPOSURE REQUIRING A PEDICLE GRAFT

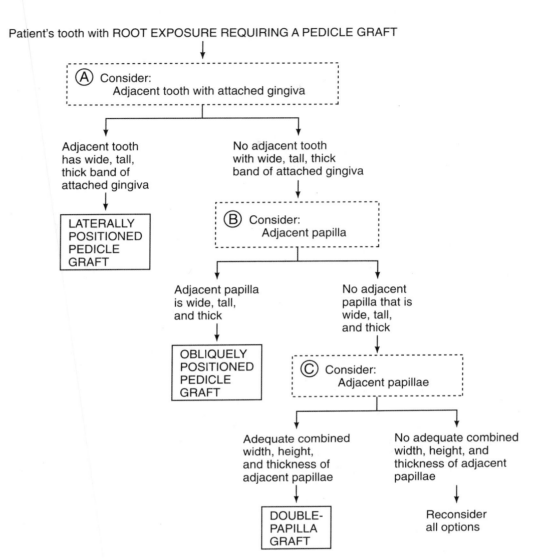

LATERALLY POSITIONED PEDICLE GRAFT PROCEDURE

Walter B. Hall

The rationale, indications, and contraindications for using the laterally positioned pedicle graft have been described (see p 104). Once a patient who meets these criteria has been identified and has agreed to the surgery, (knowing that it has a relatively low predictability of success) the procedure can be performed (Fig. 1). Several decisions must be made during and after the procedure.

A. A laterally positioned pedicle graft, performed to create a broader band of attached gingiva, may be performed with or without root coverage as a goal. Esthetic concerns particularly indicate a need to attempt root coverage, the success of which is not highly predictable. When root exposure has not occurred, root coverage is not a goal; when no aesthetic concerns exist, root coverage is not of overriding concern if a broader band of gingiva can be created to permit adequate plaque control efforts without precipitating further recession. If the patient's incidence of caries is high, the need to attempt root coverage would be greater. Esthetic and root sensitivity concerns indicate the need to attempt root coverage.

B. If root coverage is not a requirement, prepare the receptor and donor sites as described in any standard text. Suture the graft in place and, after applying pressure to drive out hemorrhage between the graft and the receptor bed, cover with Stomahesive bandage. Postoperative medication with aspirin or Tylenol is usually all that is needed, but caution the patient to avoid placing tension on, or disturbing, the graft during such activities as eating, brushing teeth, and kissing. Remove sutures a week or so later and evaluate the success of the procedure. Pedicle grafts placed on a receptor bed of periosteum and connective tissue usually are successful. If such a pedicle graft is unsuccessful (i.e., the graft sloughs or retracts from its intended position), repeat treatment is indicated but should be delayed until 1 month more after the first attempt, so that the potential donor site is adequately healed for use again.

C. If root coverage is the goal, especially to meet esthetic demands, the receptor bed is prepared as described in any standard text. The important decision to be made here relates to the possible need for reduction of a prominent root. If the root to be covered is quite prominent, it can be reduced with a back-action chisel (or rotating diamond bur) followed by root planing. This act will minimize blood pooling around the periphery of the area of root exposure (which would interfere with pedicle adaptation). It also reduces the dimensions of the area to be covered and eliminates root substance contaminated by invasive bacteria or endotoxin, which might decrease the success of the root coverage attempt. If the root is not very prominent, it need only be planed to remove the superficial "contaminated" root substance and to create a smooth surface where blood pooling would be minimized. The graft donor site is prepared, sutured, and bandaged in the standard manner. Postoperative instructions are the same as described in note B. At 1 week or so, sutures are removed and the success of the procedure is evaluated. If the graft has not been successful in obtaining adequate root coverage and a broad band of attached gingiva adequate to minimize chances of renewed root exposure (recession), the pedicle graft procedure should be repeated 1 month or more following the first surgery.

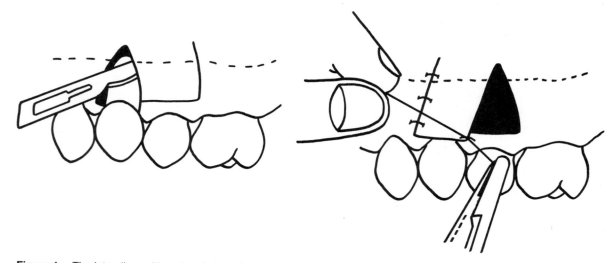

Figure 1. The laterally positioned pedicle graft procedure

Patient for a LATERALLY POSITIONED PEDICLE GRAFT

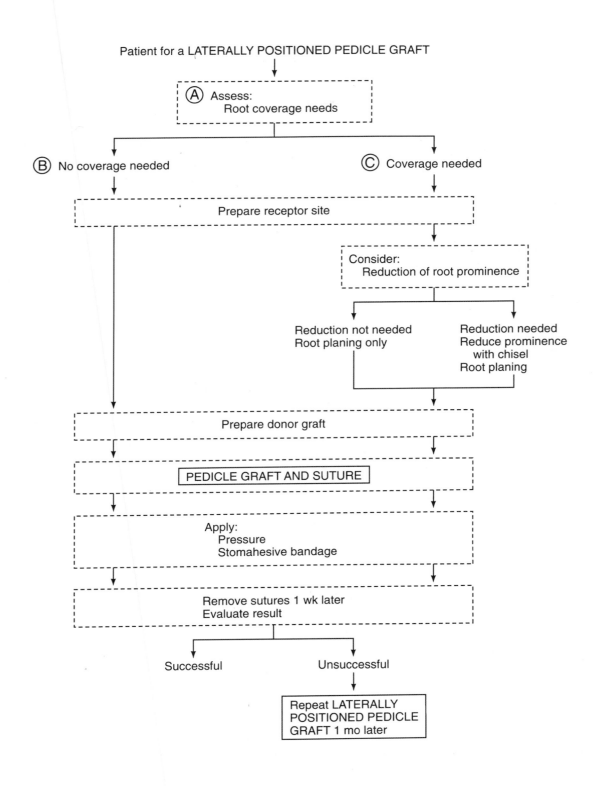

Ⓐ Assess:
Root coverage needs

Ⓑ No coverage needed   Ⓒ Coverage needed

Prepare receptor site

Consider:
Reduction of root prominence

Reduction not needed   Reduction needed
Root planing only   Reduce prominence
                              with chisel
                              Root planing

Prepare donor graft

PEDICLE GRAFT AND SUTURE

Apply:
Pressure
Stomahesive bandage

Remove sutures 1 wk later
Evaluate result

Successful   Unsuccessful

Repeat LATERALLY
POSITIONED PEDICLE
GRAFT 1 mo later

References

Carranza FA Jr. Glickman's clinical periodontology. 7th ed. Philadelphia: WB Saunders, 1990:896.

Grupe HE. Modified technique for the sliding flap operation. J Periodontol 1966; 37:491.

Hall WB. Pure mucogingival problems. Berlin: Quintessence Publishing, 1984:100.

McFall WT. The laterally repositioned flap: Criteria for success. Periodontics 1968; 5:89.

Robinson RE. Utilizing an edentulous area as a donor site in the lateral repositioned flap. Periodontics 1964; 2:79.

Schluger S, Yuodelis R, Page RC, Johnson RH. Periodontal diseases. 2nd ed. Philadelphia: Lea & Febiger, 1990:564.

OBLIQUELY POSITIONED PEDICLE GRAFT PROCEDURE

Walter B. Hall

The rationale, indications, and contraindications for using the obliquely rotated pedicle graft procedure have been described (see p 104). Once a patient who meets these criteria has been identified and has agreed to the surgery (knowing that it has a relatively low predictability of success), the procedure can be performed (Fig. 1). Several decisions must be made during and after the procedure that are quite similar to those for laterally positioned pedicle grafts.

A. An obliquely rotated pedicle graft, performed to create a broader band of attached gingiva, almost always is performed with root coverage as a goal. Esthetic concerns, including gingival color-match requirements, are key indications for using this technique. Rarely, no esthetic concerns exist, and the presence of a large adjacent papilla to serve as a donor site may permit this procedure to be used with creation of a broader band of attached gingiva as its only goal.

B. When root coverage is not a goal, prepare the receptor site and then obtain the donor graft from the adjacent papilla as described in any standard text. Suturing is difficult with such small pieces of tissue. It is very important to apply pressure to drive out hemorrhage and to apply Stomahesive bandage to stabilize the graft better during its first few hours. Postoperative discomfort usually is minimal and can be handled with over-the-counter medications. Tell the patient that it is imperative to avoid placing tension on, or disturbing, the graft during activities such as eating, brushing teeth, and kissing. One week or more later, remove sutures and evaluate the success of the graft. A graft placed on a periosteal bed usually is successful. Should it slough or pull away, re-treat a month or more later when the donor papilla is fully healed.

C. When root coverage is the goal, prepare the receptor site as described in any standard text. Usually reduction of the root prominence is required with this procedure. Reducing the area to be covered by the graft by flattening the bulge of the root will create a situation in which the height of the papillae will be better able to reach beyond the root further for suturing the donor papilla tip over the opposite adjacent papilla bed. Perform the reduction with a back-action chisel or a rotating diamond bur. Plane smooth to minimize peripheral blood pooling (which would interfere with graft adaptation) and to eliminate root substance contaminated by invasive bacteria and their products. Next, prepare the donor papilla graft and suture in place. Apply pressure and then place Stomahesive bandage to stabilize the graft better during initial healing. Postsurgical instructions are the same as described in B. Remove sutures a week or more later, and evaluate the success of the graft. If the graft has not been successful in creating a broader band of attached gingiva and adequate root coverage, repeat the obliquely rotated pedicle graft procedure a month or more following the first surgery.

References

Grant DA, Stern IB, Listgarten MA. Periodontics. 6th ed. St. Louis: CV Mosby, 1988:899.

Hall WB. Pure mucogingival problems. Berlin: Quintessence Publishing, 1988:113.

Leis HJ, Leis SN. The papilla rotation flap. J Periodontol 1978; 49:400.

Pennel BM, Higson JD, Downer JD, et al. Oblique rotated flap. J Periodontol 1965; 36:305.

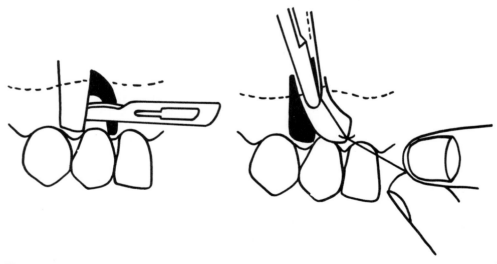

Figure 1. The obliquely positioned pedicle graft procedure.

Patient for an OBLIQUELY ROTATED PEDICLE GRAFT

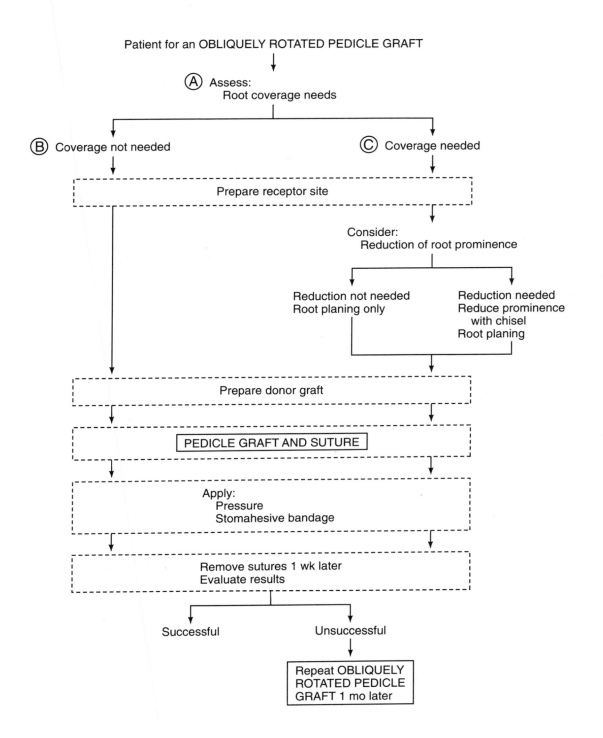

Ⓐ Assess:
Root coverage needs

Ⓑ Coverage not needed

Ⓒ Coverage needed

Prepare receptor site

Consider:
Reduction of root prominence

Reduction not needed
Root planing only

Reduction needed
Reduce prominence
with chisel
Root planing

Prepare donor graft

PEDICLE GRAFT AND SUTURE

Apply:
Pressure
Stomahesive bandage

Remove sutures 1 wk later
Evaluate results

Successful

Unsuccessful

Repeat OBLIQUELY
ROTATED PEDICLE
GRAFT 1 mo later

DOUBLE-PAPILLA PEDICLE GRAFT PROCEDURE

Walter B. Hall

The rationale, indications, and contraindications for using the double-papilla pedicle graft procedure are described (see p 104). Once a patient who meets these criteria has been identified and has agreed to the surgery (knowing that it has the lowest degree of predictability of success of the pedicle graft procedures), the procedure can be performed (Fig. 1). Several decisions must be made during and after surgery.

A. The double-papilla pedicle graft procedure as a means of increasing the band of attached gingiva is designed as a root coverage procedure; however, with a variation in design, it can be used where recession has not occurred and where a broader band of attached gingiva is needed that will have good color match with adjacent gingiva when esthetics are a prime concern. In almost all reported cases of the use of the double-papilla approach, root exposure is the prime reason to consider surgery.

B. When only a broader band of attached gingiva is needed and root coverage will not be attempted, prepare the receptor site by making a superficial incision at the mucogingival junction or at least 1 to 2 mm apical to the free margin of the soft tissue around the receptor tooth. Expose a periosteal bed for 4 to 5 mm apically to accommodate the pedicle grafts. Prepare the pedicle grafts in the usual manner but rotate 90 degrees into position so that their most coronal edges abut one another. Suture the grafts, apply pressure, and place a Stomahesive bandage over the surgical site. Discomfort is minimal following the procedure and can be managed with over-the-counter medication. Caution the patient to avoid placing tension on, or disturbing, the graft during activities such as eating, brushing teeth, and kissing. Remove sutures 1 week or more following surgery, and evaluate the success of the procedure. Pedicle grafts placed on a periosteal bed usually succeed

unless grossly disturbed during healing. If the graft is not successful, consider a free graft, but a repeat double-papilla graft usually is indicated 1 month or more after the initial surgery.

C. If root coverage is the goal, as it usually is with this procedure, prepare the receptor bed as described in any standard text. Reduction of root prominence usually is needed to minimize the area to be covered by the graft. It can be done with a back-action chisel or rotating diamond bur. In some cases, however, all that is needed is root planing to remove invasive bacteria and their products and to create a smooth surface to which the grafts are adapted. Prepare the papillary donor pedicle grafts. Suture them together and cover the prepared root surface. Apply pressure to drive out hemorrhage beneath the graft, and place a Stomahesive bandage to cover the surgical site. Postoperative medications and precautions are the same as those described in B. One week or more later, remove sutures and evaluate the success of the procedure. If the graft has not been successful in creating adequate root coverage and a broad band of attached gingiva, repeat the double-papilla pedicle graft procedure 1 month or more after the first surgery.

References

Cohen DW, Ross SE. The double-papilla repositioned flap in periodontal therapy. J Periodontol 1968; 39:65.

Goldman HM, Cohen DW. Periodontal therapy. 6th ed. St. Louis: CV Mosby, 1980:907.

Hall WB. Pure mucogingival problems. Berlin: Quintessence Publishing, 1984:117.

Robinson PJ, Guernsey LH. Clinical transplantation in dental specialties. St. Louis: CV Mosby, 1980:117.

Schluger S, Yuodelis R, Page RC, Johnson RH. Periodontal diseases. 2nd ed. Philadelphia: Lea & Febiger, 1990:567.

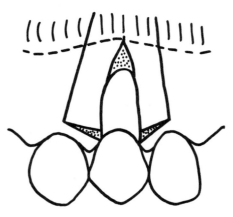
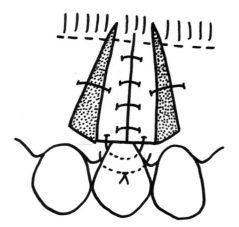

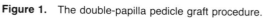
Figure 1. The double-papilla pedicle graft procedure.

Patient for an DOUBLE-PAPILLA PEDICLE GRAFT

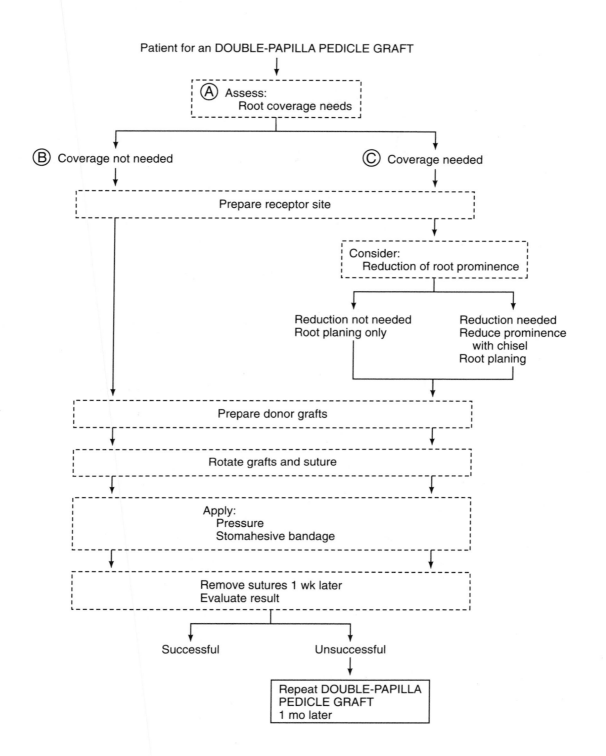

(A) Assess:
Root coverage needs

(B) Coverage not needed   (C) Coverage needed

Prepare receptor site

Consider:
Reduction of root prominence

Reduction not needed   Reduction needed
Root planing only   Reduce prominence
                              with chisel
                              Root planing

Prepare donor grafts

Rotate grafts and suture

Apply:
Pressure
Stomahesive bandage

Remove sutures 1 wk later
Evaluate result

Successful   Unsuccessful

Repeat DOUBLE-PAPILLA
PEDICLE GRAFT
1 mo later

FREE GINGIVAL GRAFT PROCEDURE

Walter B. Hall

The free gingival graft is perhaps the most predictable of periodontal surgical procedures. The indications for its use have been described (see p 104). The relative ease of mastering this technique and the mystique of plastic surgical procedures have led to more widespread use of the procedure than some clinicians believe is merited. This surgical procedure, nevertheless, has many important uses: to prevent or control loss of attachment resulting from recession, to prevent or control esthetic problems, and to permit restorative or orthodontic treatment without iatrogenic root exposure (loss of attachment). When a patient has a problem of minimal attached gingiva, with or without recession, and the dentist and patient agree that treatment is indicated, a series of decisions in proceeding with this surgery will be needed.

A. Whether root coverage is a goal will determine how the receptor site is prepared. When root exposure has not occurred, the technique is performed one way. When root exposure has occurred, root coverage may become the goal if aesthetic or restorative indications exist. Most often these indications are present in maxillary anterior and maxillary premolar areas. Often some teeth will need more attached gingiva, whereas an adjacent one may require root coverage. Modify the surgical procedure to meet these individual needs.

B. When root coverage is to be attempted, remove all sulcus epithelium and skim the superficial epithelium and connective tissue from adjacent papillae to the level of the cementoenamel junction (CEJ). More apically, separate the alveolar mucosa from the gingiva by an incision immediately coronal to the CEJ and reflect apically to expose a 5- to 6-mm bed. Should the root coverage fail, an adequate band of attached gingiva will have to be created to minimize the likelihood of further recession.

C. When root coverage is not a goal, prepare the receptor bed with an incision slightly coronal to the mucogingival junction. Expose a bed 5 to 6 mm in height by reflecting the alveolar mucosa with a periosteal elevator. Make a periosteal fenestration at the apical extent of the bed to ensure that the graft will not be mobile.

D. A combination approach may be indicated when only an occasional tooth within a segment to be grafted requires root coverage.

E. When root coverage is to be performed, reduce the prominent root with a back-action chisel so that hemorrhage will not pool peripherally. Reduce the root to keep the dentin free of bacteria or endotoxin. The reduced dimension of the root will make new attachment more likely to occur.

F. Once the graft is taken, if root coverage is the goal, suture the graft, stretched tightly between the de-epithelialated papillae, with interrupted or single-sling sutures. When root coverage will not be attempted, use single, interrupted sutures in the area of each papilla to stabilize the graft.

G. Once the graft is placed, apply pressure with wet gauze for 3 to 4 minutes, place a Stomahesive bandage covering the graft, and provide postoperative instructions on ways to avoid disturbing the graft.

References

Carranza FA Jr. Glickman's clinical periodontology. 7th ed. Philadelphia: WB Saunders, 1990:883.

Hall WB. Pure mucogingival problems. Berlin: Quintessence Publishing, 1984:127.

Matter J. Creeping attachment of free gingival grafts: A five-year follow-up study. J Periodontol 1981; 51:681.

Miller PD. Root coverage using free soft-tissue autograft following citric acid application. Part I: Technique. Int J Periodont Restor Dent 1982; 2:65.

Nabers JM. Extension of the vestibular fornix utilizing a gingival graft—case history. Periodontics 1966; 4:77.

Rateitschak KH, Rateitschak EM, Wolf HF, Hassell JM. Color atlas of periodontology. Stuttgart: Georg Thieme Verlag, 1985:230.

Schluger S, Yuodelis R, Page RC, Johnson RH. Periodontal diseases. 2nd ed. Philadelphia: Lea & Febiger, 1990:567.

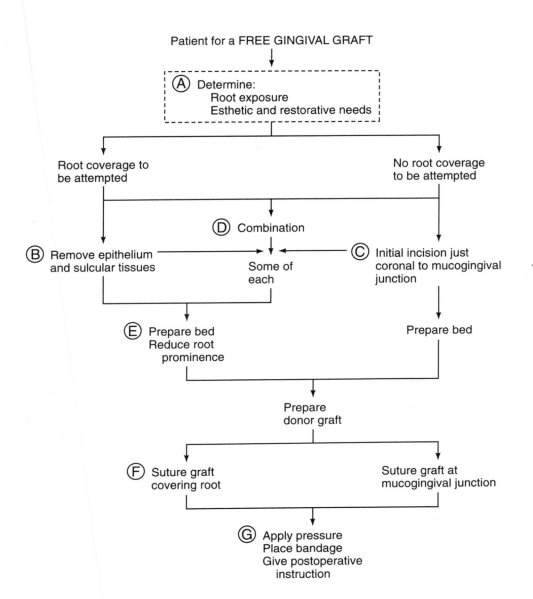

Patient for a FREE GINGIVAL GRAFT

Ⓐ Determine:
    Root exposure
    Esthetic and restorative needs

Root coverage to be attempted

No root coverage to be attempted

Ⓓ Combination

Ⓑ Remove epithelium and sulcular tissues

Some of each

Ⓒ Initial incision just coronal to mucogingival junction

Ⓔ Prepare bed
Reduce root prominence

Prepare bed

Prepare donor graft

Ⓕ Suture graft covering root

Suture graft at mucogingival junction

Ⓖ Apply pressure
Place bandage
Give postoperative instruction

THE INTERPOSITIONAL CONNECTIVE TISSUE GRAFT

W. Peter Nordland

The interpositional connective tissue graft should be considered in instances in which augmentation of gingiva is needed for root coverage or ridge augmentation is indicated to correct aesthetic or poorly cleansible edentulous ridge areas.

Root coverage is more predictable in areas where root exposure has occurred if this technique is utilized rather than gingival grafting, because the donor graft is surrounded by sources of nutritious supply from the flap side as well as the periosteal side, thus ensuring greater nutrition sources to maintain the transplanted tissue. Esthetic results are better than those obtained with a free gingival graft, where color match often is a problem. Generally, patients experience less discomfort from the donor site for an interpositional corrective tissue graft than with a free gingival graft, because the donor area is sutured closed rather than being left to heal by secondary intent, as is true with the free gingival graft.

Root coverage procedures are especially important when esthetic concerns are great or when root sensitivity or root caries are problems. The interpositional connective tissue graft is especially useful when tissue color match is critical, when multiple adjacent teeth require coverage, or when ridge plumping is needed (see p 214).

A. If a patient has inadequate attached gingiva and resultant root exposure, the primary concern would be esthetic. If esthetics are not a concern, other (p 104) mucogingival surgical procedures may suffice. When esthetics are important, the connective tissue graft may still be the better approach.

B. Next, determine the number of adjacent teeth with similar requirements. If the problem is a localized one, the various pedicle graft approaches (see p 104) may suffice and have the advantage of not requiring surgical entry of a distant donor site. If multiple adjacent teeth are involved or if a pedicle graft donor site is not available, the interpositional connective tissue graft is the technique of choice because a large enough donor site to cover several adjacent roots usually is available.

C. An adequate donor site for a connective tissue graft usually exists in the fatty submucosal area beneath the anterior palatal/ridge area; occasionally, however, no fatty submucosal area can be detected by palpation of the potential donor site with the index finger. When an adequate site is present, the interpositional connective tissue graft technique is the one of choice. In the recessional case, in which no adequately fatty donor site is available, the guided tissue regeneration (GTR) for root coverage approach (see p 254) is the best alternative.

References

Cole R, Crigger M, Bogle G, et al. Connective tissue regeneration to periodontally diseased teeth: A histologic study. J Periodontol Res 1980; 15:1.

Langer B, Cologna LJ. Subepithelial graft to correct ridge concavities. J Prosthet Dent 1980; 44:363.

Langer B, Langer L. Subepithelial connective tissue graft technique for root coverage. J Periodontol 1985; 56:715.

Nordland WP. Periodontal plastic surgery: Aesthetic gingival regeneration. J Calif Dent Assoc 1989; 17:11.

Patient with INADEQUATE ATTACHED GINGIVA AND ROOT EXPOSURE

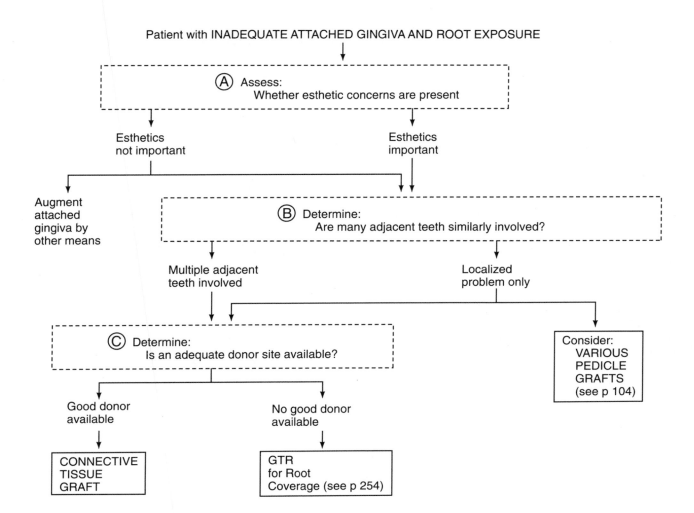

Ⓐ Assess:
Whether esthetic concerns are present

Esthetics
not important

Esthetics
important

Augment
attached
gingiva by
other means

Ⓑ Determine:
Are many adjacent teeth similarly involved?

Multiple adjacent
teeth involved

Localized
problem only

Ⓒ Determine:
Is an adequate donor site available?

Consider:
VARIOUS
PEDICLE
GRAFTS
(see p 104)

Good donor
available

No good donor
available

CONNECTIVE
TISSUE
GRAFT

GTR
for Root
Coverage (see p 254)

CORONALLY POSITIONED PEDICLE GRAFT

Craig Gainza

The coronally positioned flap technique was popularized in the 1970s by Bernimoulin. The indications for it have diminished in recent years owing to the success of single-stage root coverage procedures; however, the coronally positioned flap continues to remain a popular therapy. The advantage to this procedure (similar to that for the pedicle graft) is maintenance of a continuous blood supply during healing. Frequently, this procedure is combined with root conditioning to expose dentinal collagen, detoxify endotoxin, and encourage new tissue attachment. Adequate attached gingiva is necessary for successful coronal positioning of a flap. This procedure requires 3 to 5 mm of keratinized tissue apicocoronally. The tissue should be 1.5 mm in thickness.

After determining the adequacy of attached gingiva, address the aesthetic needs of the patient. A simple evaluation of the lip posture at rest and during a relaxed smile will provide adequate exposure of recessed tissue. The patient's comments and own perception of esthetics are critical in determining the next stage of treatment planning.

A. If there are no esthetic needs, and adequate attached gingiva exists, implement restorative therapy as needed and place the patient on a maintenance program.

B. If there are esthetic concerns and adequate attached tissue is present, a coronally positioned flap will provide tissue reattachment to cover the exposed root surfaces. If Class V caries and/or sensitivity is present, a coronally positioned flap with root conditioning (root planing and citric acid) can resolve the recession and dental pathology without a restoration.

C. Patients who present with inadequate attached gingiva and request esthetic improvement will require evaluation for root caries (their removal if present) and determination of sufficient or insufficient adjacent donor tissue. If there is insufficient donor tissue, free graft procedures are suggested. Miller, using free soft-tissue autografts, has been successful at complete coverage of wide and deep wide recession. The predictability of free graft procedures has further improved with the interpositional approach to soft-tissue grafting, as described by Langer. The advantage to both techniques is that they involve only a single surgical procedure. Occasionally, complete root coverage cannot be achieved by the free graft procedure alone; however, adequate attached tissue may exist. When incomplete coverage has occurred in the presence of adequate attached gingiva, the coronally positioned flap can be employed as a second-stage surgical procedure.

D. If there is inadequate gingiva and no esthetic requirements, as occurs frequently in the premolar/molar region, a simple free gingival graft can create an adequate band of attached gingiva. If there are shallow root caries and/or sensitivity, a Class V

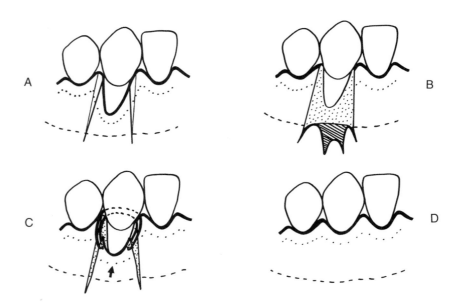

Figure 1. A, Flap design for root coverage with a coronally positioned pedicle graft. **B,** Pedicle graft reflected. Side flaps removed. **C,** Pedicle graft being coronally positioned with a single sling suture. **D,** Root coverage completed.

Patient with GINGIVAL RECESSION

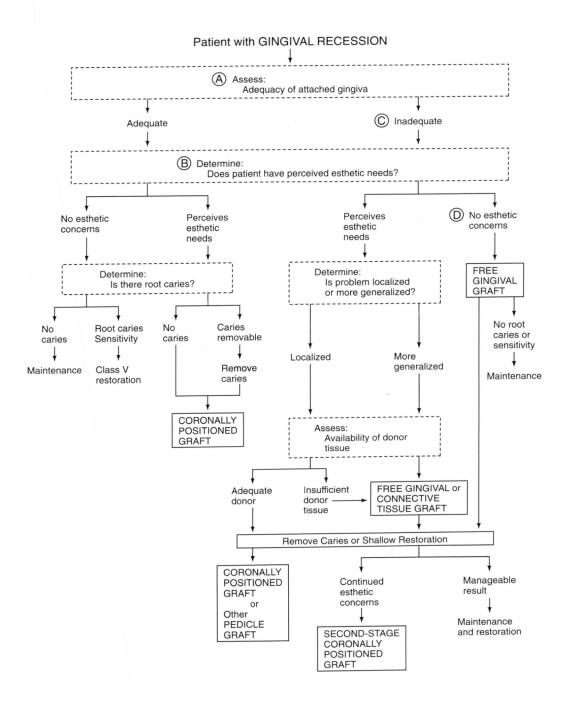

restoration can be placed and the patient placed on maintenance. To avoid a Class V restoration altogether and to correct the gingival recession, a subepithelial connective tissue graft, a large free gingival graft, or two-stage free graft/coronally positioned flap may be employed.

References

Allen EP. Use of mucogingival surgical procedures to enhance esthetics. Dent Clin North Am 1988; 32:2.

Bernimoulin OJ, Luscher B, Muhleman HR. Coronally repositioned flap: Clinical evaluation after one year. J Clin Periodontol 1975; 2:1.

Langer B, Calagna L. The subepithelial connective tissue graft. J Prosthet Dent 1980; 44:363.

Miller PD. Root coverage using a free soft-tissue autograft following citric acid application. I. Technique. Int J Periodont Restor Dent 1982; 2:65.

Miller PD. Root coverage using the free soft-tissue autograft following citric acid application. III. A successful and predictable procedure in areas of deep-wide recession. Int J Periodont Restor Dent 1985; 5:15.

FREE GINGIVAL GRAFT UTILIZING THE STRIP TECHNIQUE

Henry Takei

The strip graft technique is a useful supplement to the numerous other techniques (e.g., free gingival graft, pedicle grafts, etc.) used in mucogingival surgery when there is a need for additional keratinized gingiva. This technique is not utilized for root coverage, because strips of donor tissue cannot be placed over denuded root surfaces and still survive. This technique has the following advantages:

1. Large areas can be grafted with minimal donor tissue because slender strips of donor tissue are used instead of large pieces of donor palatal tissue.
2. Postsurgical discomfort and complications such as bleeding are minimized at the donor site. Epithelialization of the donor wound occurs within 7 to 10 days.
3. It is useful for periodontal–prosthetic surgery, which entails vestibular deepening along with the addition of keratinized tissue.

The use of this technique has greatly enhanced the ability of the clinician to increase both vestibular depth and keratinized tissue in large areas with minimal trauma to the donor site.

A. If a patient requires additional attached gingiva, the need for root coverage must be decided first. If root coverage is possible and desirable, a connective tissue graft, a free gingival graft, or a pedicle graft would be the treatment of choice (see p 104).

B. Root coverage may be possible, but not desirable (e.g., full-coverage restorations are planned and root exposure is minimal), or root coverage may not be possible. In such cases, assess the extent of the area requiring more attached gingiva to determine which type of graft should be employed.

C. If the area to be augmented is small or localized, a free gingival graft or pedicle graft would be the treatment of choice.

D. If the area needing additional attached gingiva is extensive, a strip graft is the treatment of choice, because a large area can be grafted with a donor site half the size of that employed in the free gingival graft technique. The technique is technically demanding and should be employed by skillful, experienced practitioners only.

References

Carranza FA Jr. Glickman's clinical periodontology. 7th ed. Philadelphia: WB Saunders, 1990:886.

Rateitschak KH, Rateitschak EM, Wolff HF, Hassell TM. Color atlas of periodontology. New York: Thieme, 1985:242.

Takei HH, Carranza FA, et al. The free mucosal autograft—new technical variants. Int J Periodont Restor Dent (in press).

Patient in NEED OF ADDITIONAL ATTACHED GINGIVA

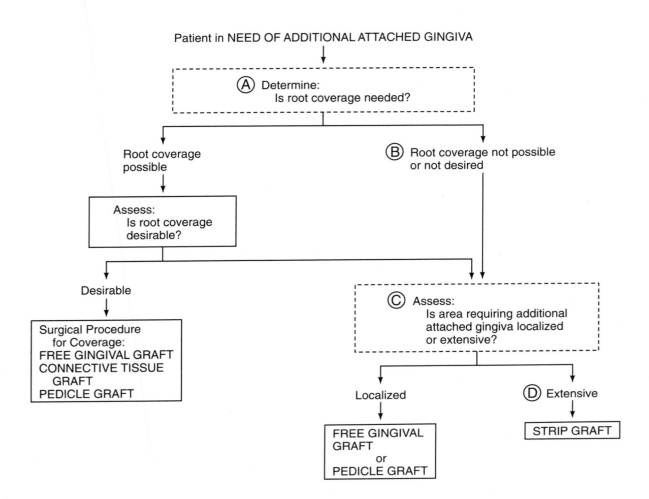

Ⓐ Determine:
Is root coverage needed?

Root coverage
possible

Ⓑ Root coverage not possible
or not desired

Assess:
Is root coverage
desirable?

Desirable

Surgical Procedure
for Coverage:
FREE GINGIVAL GRAFT
CONNECTIVE TISSUE
 GRAFT
PEDICLE GRAFT

Ⓒ Assess:
Is area requiring additional
attached gingiva localized
or extensive?

Localized

Ⓓ Extensive

FREE GINGIVAL
GRAFT
or
PEDICLE GRAFT

STRIP GRAFT

DENUDATION

Walter B. Hall

Denudation is the exposure of bone that is left denuded to heal by secondary intention as additional gingiva. The procedure is of limited usefulness because of its reputation as an uncomfortable procedure associated with slow healing and further bone loss. Nevertheless, the procedure has a place in the armamentarium of any accomplished therapist as a means of creating more attached gingiva predictably when used judiciously.

A. When a patient has a pure mucogingival problem, a problem of inadequate attached gingiva that is not associated with pocket formation and bone loss (periodontitis), the locale of the problem will determine whether gingival grafting or denudation is the appropriate surgical approach. If the problem is on the facial aspect of a mandibular second or third molar, denudation is a logical approach. In this area, the vestibule often is shallow and the facial cortical plate is thick. In such cases, gingival grafting is unlikely to be successful. If the vestibule is shallow and the cortical plate is dense, more gingiva can be created by deepening the vestibule. In such cases, gingival grafting is unlikely to be successful. If the vestibule is shallow and the cortical plate is dense, more gingiva can be created by deepening the vestibule with osseous recontouring and apically positioning the soft tissue so that 4 to 5 mm of bone are left denuded to heal by secondary intention as a broader band of attached gingiva. If the vestibule is sufficiently deep already, the soft tissue can be displaced 4 to 5 mm apically and the bone is left to heal by secondary intention as a broader band of attached gingiva.

B. If the pure mucogingival problem is in the same area as a mucogingival—osseous problem (periodontitis), two approaches are possible. The flap may be apically positioned following osseous recontouring to eliminate osseous defects and enough bone left exposed to heal by secondary intention as gingiva. Alternatively, a two-surgery approach can be used; place a free gingival graft first and then apically position it following osseous recontouring, or apically position the flap and place a free gingival graft later. For most patients, the single-surgery approach that involves denudation is preferable to a two-surgery approach that includes free gingival grafting and apical positioning of a flap at separate visits.

References

Bohannon HM. Studies in the alterations in vestibular depth. 1. Complete denudation. J Periodontol 1962; 33:120.

Carranza FA Jr. Glickman's clinical periodontology. 7th ed. Philadelphia: WB Saunders, 1990:890.

Hall WB. Pure mucogingival problems. Berlin: Quintessence Publishing, 1984:161.

Lindhe J. Textbook of clinical periodontology. 2nd ed. Copenhagen: Munksgaard, 1989:433.

Schluger S, Yuodelis R, Page RC, Johnson RH. Periodontal diseases. 2nd ed. Philadelphia: Lea & Febiger, 1990:563.

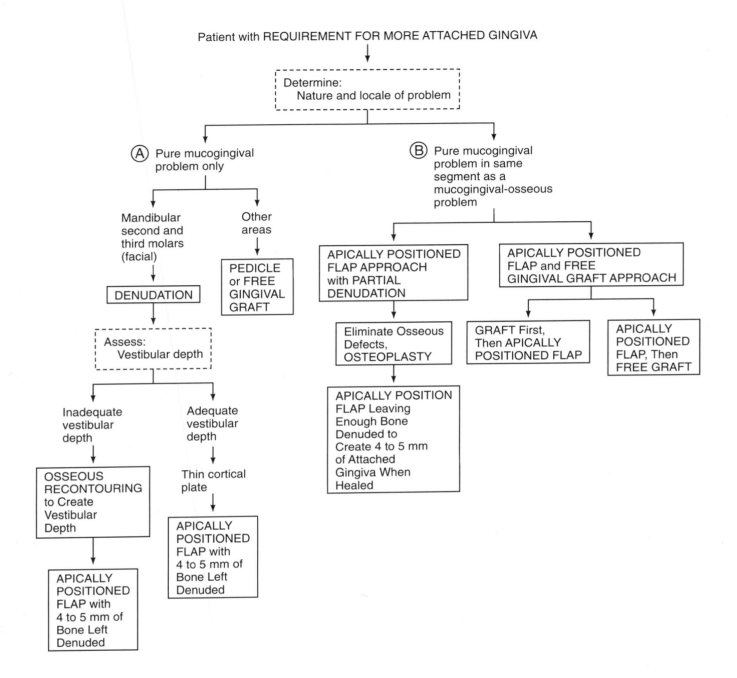

Patient with REQUIREMENT FOR MORE ATTACHED GINGIVA

Determine:
Nature and locale of problem

(A) Pure mucogingival problem only

(B) Pure mucogingival problem in same segment as a mucogingival-osseous problem

Mandibular second and third molars (facial)

Other areas

PEDICLE or FREE GINGIVAL GRAFT

DENUDATION

Assess:
Vestibular depth

Inadequate vestibular depth

Adequate vestibular depth

OSSEOUS RECONTOURING to Create Vestibular Depth

Thin cortical plate

APICALLY POSITIONED FLAP with 4 to 5 mm of Bone Left Denuded

APICALLY POSITIONED FLAP with 4 to 5 mm of Bone Left Denuded

APICALLY POSITIONED FLAP APPROACH with PARTIAL DENUDATION

APICALLY POSITIONED FLAP and FREE GINGIVAL GRAFT APPROACH

Eliminate Osseous Defects, OSTEOPLASTY

GRAFT First, Then APICALLY POSITIONED FLAP

APICALLY POSITIONED FLAP, Then FREE GRAFT

APICALLY POSITION FLAP Leaving Enough Bone Denuded to Create 4 to 5 mm of Attached Gingiva When Healed

RIDGE AUGMENTATION

Walter B. Hall

Periodontal surgery may be used to improve the form of an edentulous ridge to permit placement of a more esthetic and cleansible fixed bridge on an area where the loss of teeth has resulted in a grossly deficient or grotesquely malformed ridge. Such problems often occur when teeth are lost due to an accident or severe abscessing. Fracture of a cortical plate during extraction of teeth also may create such defects. Either the ridge may be contorted in a manner that makes the bridge construction difficult to clean and unaesthetic, or the ridge may be so deficient that excessively long, ugly pontics have been or would be placed in fixed-bridge construction.

A. When a patient presents with an edentulous ridge area, both adequate proximal and distal abutment teeth must be present for ridge augmentation to be necessary.

B. Determine the amenability of the site for fixed-bridge construction. If the edentulous area is too lengthy to permit fixed-bridge construction, either a removable denture approach or implants are indicated (see pp 242, 244).

C. If the edentulous site is amenable to fixed-bridge construction, assess the form of the edentulous ridge area to decide whether an aesthetic, cleansible bridge can be constructed utilizing the ridge as it exists. If no augmentation is needed, but the ridge is grotesquely formed or so shaped that an aesthetic, cleansible bridge cannot be constructed, one should consider ridge augmentation.

D. The approach to ridge augmentation is selected by assessing the availability of a soft-tissue donor site for an inlay or overlay approach. If a good donor site is available, that approach may be offered to the patient. When no adequate donor site is available, only the grinded bone augmentation (GBA) approach or use of a synthetic bone fill material can be presented to the patient.

References

Abrams L. Augmentation of the deformed residual edentulous ridge for fixed prosthesis. Compend Contin Ed Dent 1980; 1:205.

Genco RJ, Goldman HM, Cohen DW. Contemporary periodontics. St. Louis: CV Mosby, 1990:643.

Rosenberg S. Use of ceramic material for augmentation of the practically edentulous ridge: A case report. Compend Contin Ed Dent. 1984; 77(3):20.

Schluger S, Yuodelis R, Page RC, Johnson RH. Periodontal diseases. 2nd ed. Philadelphia: Lea & Febiger, 1990:632.

Seibert J. Reconstruction of the deformed partially edentulous ridges using full-thickness overlay grafts. Parts 1 and 2. Compend Contin Ed Dent. 1983; 4(5):437.

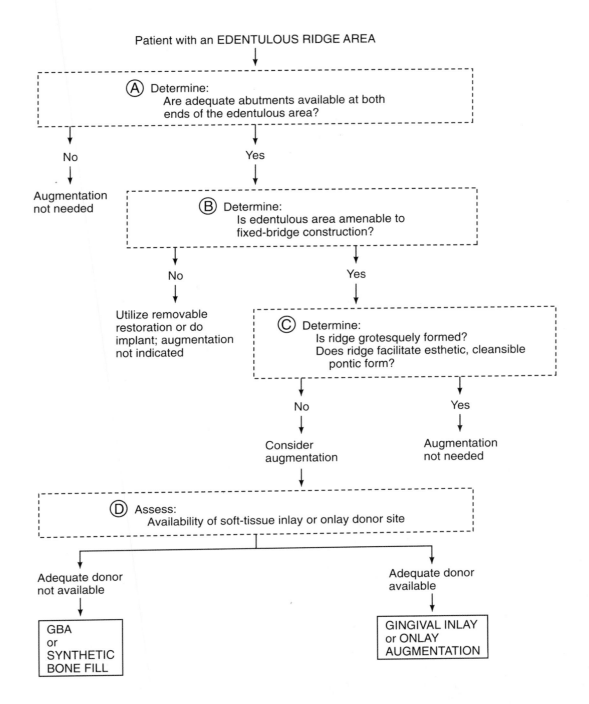

Patient with an EDENTULOUS RIDGE AREA

(A) Determine:
Are adequate abutments available at both
ends of the edentulous area?

No

Augmentation
not needed

Yes

(B) Determine:
Is edentulous area amenable to
fixed-bridge construction?

No

Utilize removable
restoration or do
implant; augmentation
not indicated

Yes

(C) Determine:
Is ridge grotesquely formed?
Does ridge facilitate esthetic, cleansible
pontic form?

No

Consider
augmentation

Yes

Augmentation
not needed

(D) Assess:
Availability of soft-tissue inlay or onlay donor site

Adequate donor
not available

GBA
or
SYNTHETIC
BONE FILL

Adequate donor
available

GINGIVAL INLAY
or ONLAY
AUGMENTATION

DRESSING FOLLOWING PURE MUCOGINGIVAL SURGERY

Walter B. Hall

The dentist who has completed a pure mucogingival surgical procedure must decide whether a dressing is necessary and, if so, which one. The best dressing for a gingival graft is one that will not move during the time it is present and one that will not require removal when it could tug on sutures. It should provide stability for the graft and minimize bleeding and should not permit blood to collect between the graft and the donor site. Cyanoacrylate dressings such as isobutyl cyanoacrylate or trifluor isopropyl cyanoacrylate are excellent for these purposes but are not approved for use in the United States. In some other countries, however, they are available and will work well.

A. Pedicle grafts and free gingival graft receptor sites present similar problems. If the pure mucogingival graft procedure has been done alone, a dressing may not be necessary; however, Stomahesive bandage has the distinct advantages of maintaining the adaptation of the graft to the receptor bed and minimizing bleeding or blood pooling (Fig. 1). The simplicity of placement of Stomahesive bandage and its gradual dissolvability make it the dressing of choice (in the opinion of this author). Coe Pak or an alternative has the disadvantages of difficulty of stabilization when

papillae completely fill interproximal spaces and the probability that movement of the pack during healing will disrupt the tenuous, developing union of graft and receptor site. If the pure mucogingival procedure is part of a mucogingival–osseous procedure, Coe Pak or an alternative becomes the selection of choice, because the opening of interproximal spaces will permit solid, stable pack application.

B. The donor site for a free gingival graft also must have a dressing placed to minimize bleeding and to protect the donor area from the tongue and from food. Isobutyl cyanoacrylate or trifluor isopropyl cyanoacrylate works well for this purpose and should be used in countries where they are legal. Otherwise, the selection of a dressing seems to be the dentist's choice. The author favors the use of Stomahesive bandage, which lasts only 6 to 8 hours in the palate because of tongue activity and which must be replaced by the patient several times in the first few days. Others may favor placement of Colycote or Surgicel, which minimize bleeding but not as well as Stomahesive bandage does. Others may favor placing Coe Pak and suturing it in place. This is a tedious process that results in poorer control of bleeding, but the Coe Pak does not require replacement.

C. When denudation is used to produce a broader band of attached gingiva, it is usually as part of a mucogingival–osseous procedure for pocket elimination. Coe Pak or an alternative is the dressing of choice in such cases. The pack may have to be replaced for a second week because of the slowness of healing when bone is left denuded.

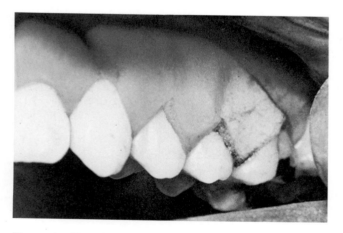

Figure 1. Stomahesive bandage covering a pure mucogingival surgical site.

References

Carranza FA Jr. Glickman's clinical periodontology. 7th ed. Philadelphia: WB Saunders, 1990:767.

Coslet JG, Rosenberg ES, Tisot R. The free autogenous gingival graft. Dent Clin North Am 1980; 24:675.

Hall WB. Pure mucogingival problems. Berlin: Quintessence Publishing, 1984:107.

Lindhe J. Textbook of clinical periodontology. 2nd ed. Copenhagen: Munksgaard, 1989:418.

Patient AFTER PURE MUCOGINGIVAL SURGERY

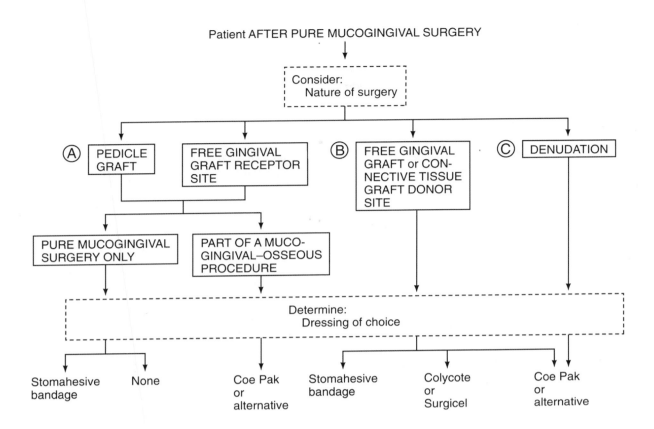

Consider:
Nature of surgery

(A) PEDICLE GRAFT

FREE GINGIVAL GRAFT RECEPTOR SITE

(B) FREE GINGIVAL GRAFT or CONNECTIVE TISSUE GRAFT DONOR SITE

(C) DENUDATION

PURE MUCOGINGIVAL SURGERY ONLY

PART OF A MUCO-GINGIVAL–OSSEOUS PROCEDURE

Determine:
Dressing of choice

Stomahesive bandage

None

Coe Pak or alternative

Stomahesive bandage

Colycote or Surgicel

Coe Pak or alternative

RESTORATION FOLLOWING PURE MUCOGINGIVAL SURGERY

Walter B. Hall

The timing of a restorative procedure following a pure mucogingival surgical procedure is crucial to maintaining a successful graft. The timing is dependent upon what restorative procedure is to be done and upon the objectives of the graft that was used (root coverage or only a broader band of attached gingiva to prevent further recession).

A. If a supragingival restoration is planned, it can be performed as soon as the success of the graft has been assured, usually no sooner than 2 weeks postsurgically. If waiting longer presents no great difficulty, a longer period for healing before the supragingival restoration is placed would be desirable.

B. When a rest-proximal plate 1 (RP1) bar type of removable partial denture or an overdenture is planned, root coverage is not an objective of pure mucogingival surgery. Grafts are done to create an adequate band of attached gingiva to underlay a "1 bar" for the partial or to provide 2 to 5 mm of attached gingiva on the overdenture teeth; nevertheless, allow a month or more before taking impressions to prepare the RP1 removable denture or the overdenture.

C. If a restoration is to be placed close to the free margin of the gingiva or subgingivally following pure mucogingival surgery, the objective of the graft procedure will influence when the restorative procedure can be performed. If root coverage has not been attempted, the restoration can be placed 2 weeks or more after the surgical procedure, although a longer period of healing would be desirable. If root coverage has been the objective of the gingival grafting procedure, allow a longer period for healing before preparing a restoration close to the new free margin of the gingiva or subgingivally. Regardless of whether the graft was a pedicle type or a free gingival type, disturbance of the new marginal gingiva too soon after surgery can result in graft retraction or failure. Allow at least a month before restorative preparation. A much longer period would be desirable in hopes of developing a more stable attachment of the grafted gingiva and root.

References

Lange DE, Bernimoulin JP. Exfoliative cytological studies in evaluation of free gingival graft healing. J Clin Periodontol 1974; 1:89.

McFall WT. The laterally repositioned flap: Criteria for success. Periodontics 1968; 5:89.

Wilderman MR, Wentz FM. Repair of a dentogingival defect with a pedicle flap. J Periodontol 1965; 36:218.

Patient's tooth with GINGIVAL GRAFT PLACED AND REQUIRING RESTORATION

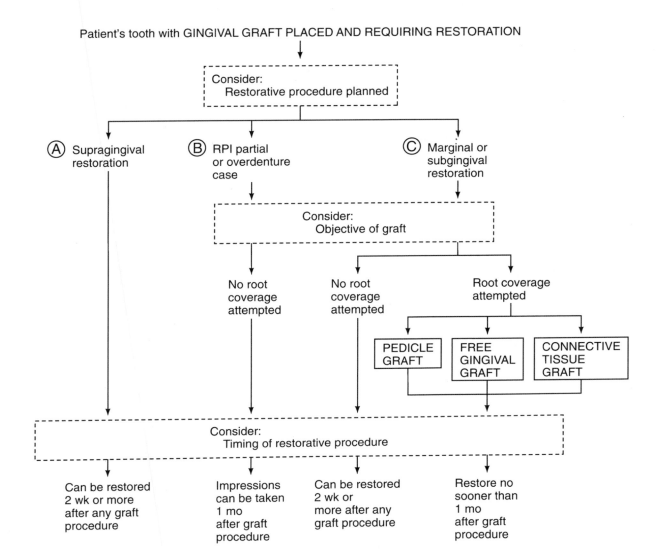

Consider:
Restorative procedure planned

Ⓐ Supragingival restoration

Ⓑ RPI partial or overdenture case

Ⓒ Marginal or subgingival restoration

Consider:
Objective of graft

No root coverage attempted

No root coverage attempted

Root coverage attempted

PEDICLE GRAFT

FREE GINGIVAL GRAFT

CONNECTIVE TISSUE GRAFT

Consider:
Timing of restorative procedure

Can be restored 2 wk or more after any graft procedure

Impressions can be taken 1 mo after graft procedure

Can be restored 2 wk or more after any graft procedure

Restore no sooner than 1 mo after graft procedure

POSTSURGICAL REEVALUATION

Walter B. Hall

When a patient's periodontal surgery has been completed, the dentist must decide when to evaluate the success of the surgery. The term usually applied to this examination is *reevaluation,* which includes visual examination and charting. Radiographic evaluation at this time is not advisable, because little if anything could be learned from the films (insurance companies should be told so if they request films), and the additional radiation exposure could not be justified. The timing of postsurgical reevaluation is dependent upon what surgical procedures have been used. Generally, the longer the period before reevaluation, the more accurate the prediction will be; however, the patient and dentist may have valid reasons to wish to proceed as soon as reasonable (e.g., splinting with fixed bridges may improve patient function and comfort).

A. After pocket elimination surgery (apically positioned flap and osseous recontouring, gingivectomy), reevaluate 1 month following the last surgery. No new attachment has been attempted, so probing will not endanger the success of the procedure.

B. New attachment procedures are dependent upon the development of a new connective tissue attachment to new cementum (cementoid). The success of these procedures is not highly predictable. Early probing can disturb a developing new attachment and can result in a less desirable "long epithelial attachment." Allow at least 6 months before the new attachment area is probed. Such areas include all bone-regeneration sites, all gingival grafts in which root coverage has been attempted, and second molar roots exposed in relation to the removal of an impacted or partially erupted third molar.

C. *Reattachment* is the term used to describe the healing together of a gingival flap and a root surface that have been separated by surgery rather than by disease. The viable root surface and the flap routinely heal to-gether. When such an approach has been used (e.g., when the retraction of a flap exposes a dehiscence or fenestration), allow 1 month or more following the surgery before performing reevaluation with probing. It should not be necessary to wait as long as when new attachment has been attempted.

D. When a replaced flap approach is used, such as the modified Widman flap or the excisional new attachment procedure (ENAP), a true new connective-tissue attachment is no longer a reasonable objective, as was stated many years ago for such procedures. A "long epithelial attachment" is now the expected result in such cases. If "new attachment" is not the goal, then, probing and reevaluation can be performed as early as 1 month after surgery, though waiting longer would be desirable.

E. When gingival grafting procedures are used to broaden the band of attached gingiva and no root coverage is attempted, reevaluation can be performed at 1 month (or possibly earlier).

References

Carranza FA Jr. Glickman's clinical periodontology. 7th ed. Philadelphia: WB Saunders, 1990:964.

Grant DA, Stern IB, Listgarten MA. Periodontics. 6th ed. St. Louis: CV Mosby, 1988:1095.

Lindhe J. Textbook of clinical periodontology. 2nd ed. Copenhagen: Munksgaard, 1989:439.

Pihlstrom BL, Ortiz-Campos C, McHugh RB. A randomized four-year study of periodontal therapy. J Periodontol 1981; 52:227.

Westfelt E, Nyman S, Socransky S, Lindhe J. Significance of the frequency of professional tooth cleaning following periodontal surgery. J Clin Periodontol 1983; 10:148.

Patient on COMPLETION OF SURGICAL THERAPY

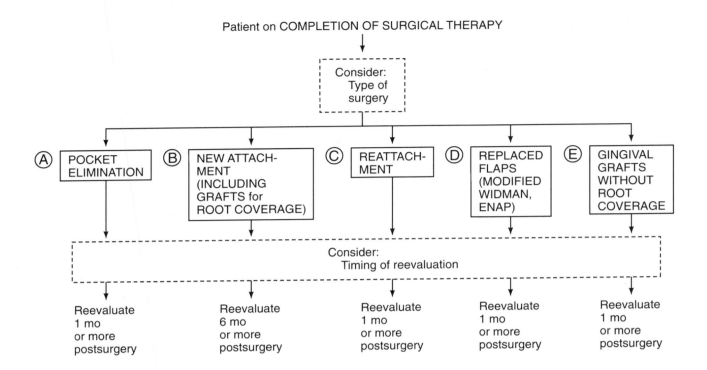

Consider:
Type of
surgery

Ⓐ POCKET
ELIMINATION

Ⓑ NEW ATTACH-
MENT
(INCLUDING
GRAFTS for
ROOT COVERAGE)

Ⓒ REATTACH-
MENT

Ⓓ REPLACED
FLAPS
(MODIFIED
WIDMAN,
ENAP)

Ⓔ GINGIVAL
GRAFTS
WITHOUT
ROOT
COVERAGE

Consider:
Timing of reevaluation

Reevaluate
1 mo
or more
postsurgery

Reevaluate
6 mo
or more
postsurgery

Reevaluate
1 mo
or more
postsurgery

Reevaluate
1 mo
or more
postsurgery

Reevaluate
1 mo
or more
postsurgery

A BEHAVIORAL APPROACH TO RECALL VISITS

Walter B. Hall

The timing of recall visits for periodontal patients can be planned in several ways. Some dentists, citing long-term studies of periodontal treatment based on a uniform recall interval, recall all their patients at 3-month intervals. They believe that they can predict their success rates with various forms of treatment more accurately on this basis, but the problem with this approach is the patient's response. For years, many dentists recalled their patients twice a year, because studies indicated that, with such recalls, caries would not develop so rapidly as to endanger many teeth. In "behavioral" terms, however, many patients "learned" that they had to return to the dentist every 6 months whether they needed it or not (i.e., whether they had made a good effort at oral hygiene or not). Patients understood this message long before dentists did, and oral hygiene and the incidence of caries improved little during that era. An approach that uses the long-term study concepts in a more behaviorally sound way is to "reward" patients depending upon the adequacy of their home care efforts between visits; thus, if a patient is doing well (based upon assessments of plaque, inflammation, and pocket depth), the time before the next recall would be extended, which offers a direct reward for individual efforts and reinforces desirable behavior. With a large group of patients, the average recall time is likely to be 3 months; however, no individual patient is likely to be recalled regularly at 3-month intervals.

The greatest advantage of the behavioral approach to timing of recall visits is that patients are given an immediate reinforcing "reward" for good or poor effort. The patients can see either that their efforts have paid off or that lack of effort has brought an appropriate reward. In the fixed-interval (every 3 months) approach, only praise or scolding is the reward or punishment available to the dentist. The more tangible reward of less cost (in time, money, and discomfort) is much more likely to prove successful. Additionally, the dentist can demonstrate how the treatment was altered to respond to patient behavior between visits, and patients must accept their own responsibility for their progress and its costs.

A. When an individual patient's first recall visit is to be scheduled, information on which to base the recall interval is not clearly defined. The patient may have remaining areas of compromise, such as individual teeth for which definitive treatment was impossible (because these teeth already had lost too much attachment), or the selection of a less definitive treatment was made for financial reasons. Some patients are compromised by the status of their health. Others may be compromised by less-than-ideal restorative work or tooth alignment. If the patient has areas of compromise, they should be annotated and the recall interval decreased. If a compromised patient has shown little motivation to develop home care skills, the first recall visit should be set at 1 to 2 months; with evidence of good oral hygiene skill development and motivation, however, the first recall could be set at 2 to 3 months. If the patient has no areas of compromise remaining, evidence of oral hygiene skill and motivation can be used to set the first recall interval. If the patient's efforts have been minimally successful, a first recall visit might be set at 2 to 3 months; with greater success, the interval could be increased to 3 months or more.

B. Further recall visits are easier to schedule in a behaviorally successful manner. At each recall visit, evaluate plaque control, gingival inflammation status, and pocket depths, and use this measure of the patient's "success" to determine the next recall interval. Patient behavior over the years is rarely consistent. Many factors in patients' lives influence their efforts at oral hygiene. Periods of stress or illness affect their ability to deal with plaque. If plaque control has been inadequate, shorten the recall interval. If much inflammation is present and/or if pocket depths are increasing, shorten the intervals even further. If the patient's efforts do not improve, alternative approaches (even extraction of poor-risk teeth that can endanger adjacent abutments) may be necessary. If efforts do improve after several recall visits, an increase in the time between recalls would be an appropriate reward. Maintain a patient whose efforts are fair or adequate at the current recall intervals. Reward a patient whose efforts have given excellent results by increasing the time between recalls.

References

Chace R. The maintenance phase of periodontal therapy. J Periodontol 1951; 22:23.

Lindhe J. Textbook of clinical periodontology. 2nd ed. Copenhagen: Munksgaard, 1989:615.

Parr RW. Periodontal maintenance therapy. Berkeley: Praxis Publishing, 1974:1.

Ramfjord SP, Knowles JW, Nissle RR, et al. Longitudinal study of periodontal therapy. J Periodontol 1973; 44:66.

Ramfjord SP, Morrison EC, Burgett FG, et al. Oral hygiene and maintenance of periodontal support. J Periodontol 1982; 53:26.

Schluger S, Yuodelis R, Page RC, Johnson RH. Periodontal diseases. 2nd ed. Philadelphia: Lea & Febiger, 1990:732.

Patient with CURRENT PERIODONTAL TREATMENT COMPLETED

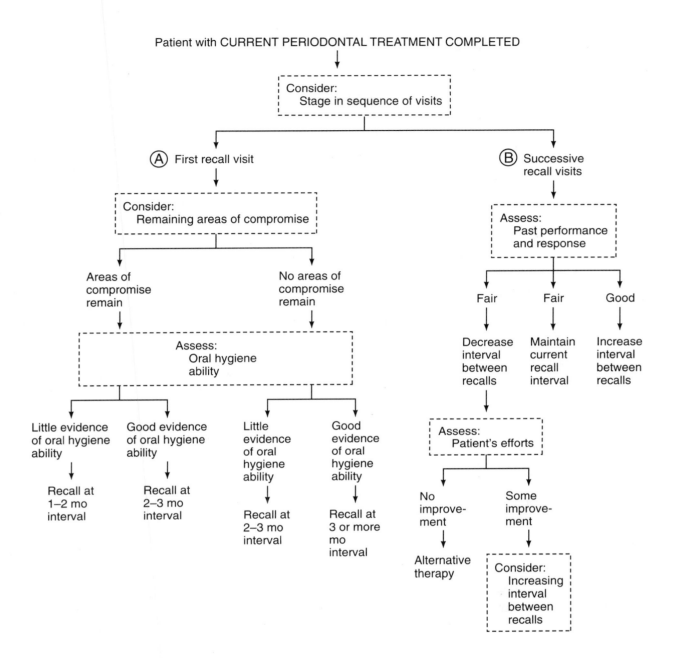

INFORMED CONSENT

Charles F. Sumner III

Dentistry has entered into the world of litigation, which demands detailed records and all-inclusive forms. Because most dental procedures are elective and risk may outweigh the benefits, we have a potential problem of informed consent. Consent need not be written. If the information is complete and conveyed to the patient in language he understands, and if the patient is given the opportunity to ask questions that are then satisfactorily answered, the duty to inform probably has been fulfilled. The courts have held that patients can give a valid consent to surgery when disclosure of risks has been made by a nurse assistant and not by the surgeon; however, the legal process tends to create fictions. In this area of informed consent, the fiction is that the patient, by signing a form, is provided usable information for a reasoned decision. A wise practitioner should not rely only upon his record of having satisfactorily informed the patient of the risk and alternatives of the pending procedure but should also have in his files a signed and witnessed consent form.

A. Although the purpose of the documented consent is to reduce the dentist's exposure to litigation, it would be well to recognize its value as a practice-building tool. Properly planned, written, and presented, the consent form could allay the patient's normal fears and apprehension; educate as to the scope and limitations of treatment and thereby avoid unrealistic expectations. There is no excuse for the failure to compose and properly present individual consent forms for general and special procedures.

B. Originally conceived as an offshoot of the law of battery, informed consent is now generally treated under a theory of negligence. The battery theory remains applicable when the treatment or procedure was completely unauthorized, whereas negligence principles apply to the more often encountered situations in which the treatment was authorized but consent was uninformed. Under negligence theory, there must be established a duty of care, a breach of that duty, and injury and proximate or legal causal relationship between the breach and the injury. A patient establishes proximate cause in an informed consent case by proof that a proper disclosure would have resulted in a decision against the proposed treatment or procedure.

  The proper disclosure in the majority of jurisdictions is the "traditional" or "professional" view with regard to scope of disclosure. The physician is required to disclose only such risks that a reasonable practitioner of like training would have disclosed in the same or similar circumstances; however, each state has its own standards for informed consent, and these standards are rapidly changing. Some states hold the "material risk and objective standard." Others take their standard from battery and have a "patient-based standard." Others require that the patient be advised in great graphic detail of all the risk and the alternatives to each procedure. In view of this variability, the dentist would be wise to learn which standard is currently being followed in his locale before finalizing his consent form in print. The better consent form would also be customized to the treatment procedure. Generalized consent forms are less likely to provide usable information for reasoned decisions. The rule is that the dentist performing the procedure, not the referring dentist, has the obligation to explain that procedure to the patient.

C. The courts have held that, as an integral part of the physician's overall obligation to the patient, there is a duty of reasonable disclosure of the available choices with respect to proposed therapy and of the dangers inherently and potentially involved in each. This holding was based upon four postulates that have become the basis of the informed consent laws. First, the knowledge of the patient and the doctor are not in parity. Second, an adult of sound mind exercises control over his own body and, in exercising this control, has the right to determine whether or not to undergo treatment. Third, the patient's consent to proposed treatment must be an informed one. Fourth, due to the nature of the physician—patient relationship, the physician has an obligation to the patient that transcends arms-length transactions. Alternative plans must be explained as thoroughly and objectively as the plan favored by the doctor.

D. When the treatment is cosmetic or when cosmetics play a large role in the patient's decision to accept therapy, there is an even greater need to communicate and gain acceptance of the limitations of proposed therapy and the alternatives available. Dentistry is both an art and a science. Treatment results will be judged by experts from among a dentist's peers. Judgment of cosmetic results will be determined by the limitations indicated in the pretreatment agreement.

E. Customized, detailed material is recommended for high-risk procedures. The complexity and extent of the description should be in proportion to the complexity and extent of the proposed procedure and the risk to the patient. When the risks are relatively minor and are known to be of low incidence, the demand for detail in disclosure is diminished. Conversely, when the risks are high but their incidence is low, or when the incidence is high but the risk is low, the fact is material and must be disclosed for a patient to arrive at a reasoned decision.

F. The essence of informed consent is that no one can agree to a treatment if he is not presented with sufficient facts and time to allow for a reasoned decision. Nevertheless, there must be some discussion and agreement as to the course to be taken when emergencies arise during treatment when time is not sufficient for deliberation and consent.

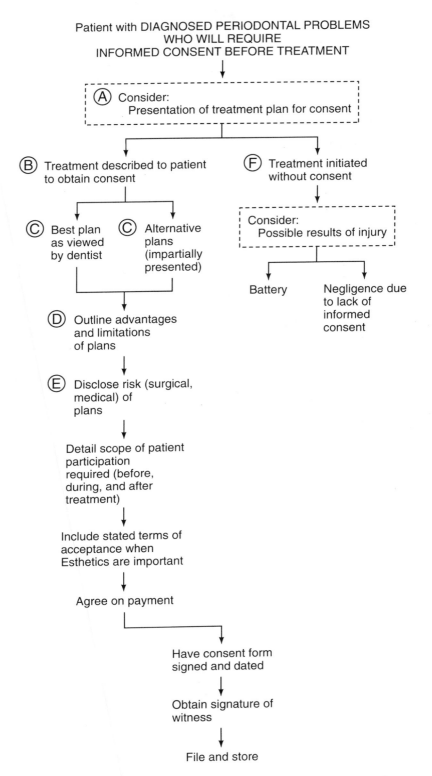

Patient with DIAGNOSED PERIODONTAL PROBLEMS
WHO WILL REQUIRE
INFORMED CONSENT BEFORE TREATMENT

(A) Consider:
Presentation of treatment plan for consent

(B) Treatment described to patient to obtain consent

(F) Treatment initiated without consent

Consider:
Possible results of injury

(C) Best plan as viewed by dentist   (C) Alternative plans (impartially presented)

Battery   Negligence due to lack of informed consent

(D) Outline advantages and limitations of plans

(E) Disclose risk (surgical, medical) of plans

Detail scope of patient participation required (before, during, and after treatment)

Include stated terms of acceptance when Esthetics are important

Agree on payment

Have consent form signed and dated

Obtain signature of witness

File and store

CAVEAT

The most complete, signed, and witnessed consent form will not excuse responsibility or mitigate against the damages when battery and/or negligence can be established by the evidence. When the question is "Whose standard is to be followed in the informed consent?" the answer may well be that no matter the standard, the jury must give their verdict and will probably use their own personal standards in doing so.

References

Canterbury v Spence 464 F2d 354 (D.C. Cir. 1972).
Cobbs v. Grant (1972) 502 p. 2d 1.
Gaskin v. Goldwasser (1988) 520 N.E. 1d 1085.
Llera v. Wisner (1976) 557 P2d 805.
Moore v Preventive Medicine Medical Group, Inc (1986) 178 Cal. App. 3d 738.
Mustacchio v. Parker (1988) 535 So. 2nd 833.
Professional Liability Committee—first line of defense in malpractice claims. JADA Feb. 1974; 88:341.
Roybal v. Bell (1989) 7878 P.2d 108.

PERIODONTAL DRESSINGS

Gerald J. DeGregori

The purpose of periodontal dressings is wound protection following periodontal surgical procedures. Additional benefits include patient comfort, hemostasis, control of granulation tissue growth, and some splinting action of mobile teeth after periodontal surgery. Generally, periodontal dressings are divided into two categories: (1) those containing zinc oxide and eugenol, and (2) those containing neither zinc oxide nor eugenol.

A. An example of a dressing containing zinc oxide and eugenol is Peridres. This material is supplied as a powder, which contains zinc oxide, kaolin, rosin, and tannic acid, and liquid, which contains eugenol and thymol (a preservative). The two are mixed together into a dough-like consistency, and either may be used immediately or may be wrapped in aluminum foil and refrigerated for up to 1 week for use later. Because the mixing process for the zinc oxide—eugenol dressing is rather messy, the feature of storage for future use is significant. The advantages of a dressing such as Peridres are a distinct splinting effect, as it sticks well to the teeth, and the action of the tannic acid, which is an active hemostatic agent. The disadvantages include a rough surface on setting, which retains plaque and debris, thus complicating oral hygiene procedures; the rock-hard consistency of the product on setting, which, if engaged into an undercut such as beneath a bridge pontic, may be very traumatic upon removal; and the distinct taste of eugenol, which may linger for days. The setting time of dressings containing zinc oxide and eugenol may be accelerated by adding a slight amount of powdered zinc acetate to the mixture. These dressings cannot adhere to mucosal surfaces.

B. An example of a dressing that does not contain eugenol is Coe Pak. This material is supplied in two tubes (an accelerator and a base). It relies on a reaction between a metallic oxide and fatty acids to bring about the setting reaction. The working time may be shortened by adding a few drops of water to the mixture, and it may be lengthened by using a retardant supplied with each box of material. Equal lengths of accelerator and base are extruded from each tube onto a mixing pad and are mixed quickly to a uniform, light-pink color. With fingers lubricated with petrolatum, form the material into small, pencil-shaped rolls to be applied to the surgical site. Advantages of this material include the pleasing color, acceptable taste, and a certain pliability on setting that facilitates removal, especially from undercut areas. Its disadvantages include its minimal splinting ability; the fact that, if it is not securely locked into undercut areas, such as the interproximal space, it most probably will be lost prematurely; and the absence of an active hemostatic agent within the pack material. It does not have the ability to adhere to mucosal surfaces.

C. Some operators take advantage of the features of both types of dressing materials by combining the powder portion of the dressing containing zinc oxide and eugenol with the mixture that does not contain zinc oxide and eugenol. The rosin enhances the adhesive capability of the material, and the tannic acid contributes to the hemostatic properties of the dressing.

D. Often, additional hemostasis is needed for the donor site of a free gingival graft. Surgical absorbable hemostat is a gauze-like material that may be placed directly over the palatal wound. It provides a matrix for clotting over which the periodontal dressing may be placed. Care should be taken not to overlap the Surgicel onto tooth structure, as it may interfere with the retention of the periodontal dressing.

E. Should the dressing be required to adhere to mucosal surfaces for a short time (24—36 hours), Stomahesive bandage may be used. It is a gelatin-like material with an adhesive surface protected by a paper coating. Once the paper is removed, the product may be placed on mucosal surfaces and will adhere, provided it is slightly warmed by the operator's finger and the warm environment of the oral cavity. Longevity of this dressing is minimal. Some operators find it acceptable to protect the donor and recipient sites of a free gingival graft or to protect localized areas of gingivoplasty.

References

Carranza FA Jr. Glickman's clinical periodontology. 7th ed. Philadelphia: WB Saunders, 1990:767.

Grant DA, Stern IB, Listgarten MA. Periodontics. 6th ed. St. Louis: CV Mosby, 1988:731.

Hall WB. Pure mucogingival problems. Berlin: Quintessence Publishing, 1984:107.

Rateitschak KH, Rateitschak EM, Wolf HF, Hassell TM. Color atlas of periodontology. Stuttgart: Georg Thieme Verlag, 1985:162.

Patient for PERIODONTAL DRESSING

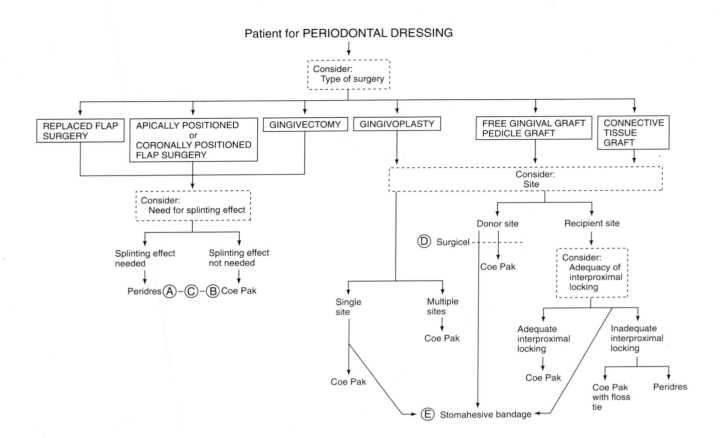

Consider:
Type of surgery

REPLACED FLAP SURGERY

APICALLY POSITIONED or CORONALLY POSITIONED FLAP SURGERY

GINGIVECTOMY

GINGIVOPLASTY

FREE GINGIVAL GRAFT PEDICLE GRAFT

CONNECTIVE TISSUE GRAFT

Consider:
Need for splinting effect

Splinting effect needed

Splinting effect not needed

Peridres Ⓐ – Ⓒ – Ⓑ Coe Pak

Consider:
Site

Donor site

Recipient site

Ⓓ Surgicel

Coe Pak

Consider:
Adequacy of interproximal locking

Single site

Multiple sites

Coe Pak

Adequate interproximal locking

Inadequate interproximal locking

Coe Pak

Coe Pak with floss tie

Peridres

Coe Pak

Ⓔ Stomahesive bandage

DENTIN HYPERSENSITIVITY

William P. Lundergan

Dentin hypersensitivity affects about one out of every seven dental patients. Furthermore, with the aging of the populace and increased tooth retention, the number of dental patients with sensitive teeth will no doubt increase. Dentin hypersensitivity can occur whenever fresh dentin is exposed to thermal, tactile, evaporative, or chemical stimuli. The term *root hypersensitivity* is commonly used to describe dentin hypersensitivity associated with gingival recession, abrasion, erosion, root planing, or periodontal flap surgery. Root hypersensitivity can present a perplexing and frustrating problem for both the patient and the dentist during definitive periodontal treatment and subsequent maintenance therapy.

A. The first steps in treating dentin hypersensitivity are to identify the sensitive area and to establish an etiology. Caries, a fractured tooth or restoration, occlusal trauma, recent restorative therapy, gingival recession, abrasion, erosion, and recent root planing or periodontal flap surgery should be evaluated as possible causes. Treatment should be appropriate for the identified etiology. If an evaluation of tooth vitality shows irreversible pulpal inflammation, endodontic therapy will be required. If the tooth is fractured, an endodontic and periodontal evaluation may be required to establish a prognosis. Severe fractures usually require extraction of the tooth.

B. Treatment for root hypersensitivity begins with meticulous plaque control and the use of a desensitizing toothpaste. (Toothpastes containing potassium nitrate or strontium chloride have been shown to be effective desensitizers. Several commercial products have been evaluated and accepted by the American Dental Association's Council on Dental Therapeutics.) Root hypersensitivity associated with severe abrasion or erosion may require restorative procedures in conjunction with instructions on proper brushing technique (abrasion cases) and/or dietary counseling (erosion cases). Should the patient experience no relief following 2 weeks of meticulous home care with a densensitizing toothpaste, or if the patient is too sensitive to practice proper plaque control, office procedures should be combined with the home regimen.

C. A multitude of agents and methods have been used in the treatment of root hypersensitivity, but no one therapy has proved to be universally effective. It is prudent to use the most conservative treatment that is effective for a particular patient. Multiple office procedures, often combining more than one method, may be required for best results. In some instances, local anesthesia may be necessary before initiating the desensitizing procedure. Commonly used agents include fluoride, calcium hydroxide, potassium oxalate, ferric oxalate, restorative resins, and varnishes. Iontophoresis, a method of delivering charged molecules or medicaments via an electrical current, has been used successfully with a 1% to 2% sodium fluoride solution. In severe cases that do not respond to more conservative treatment, endodontic therapy may be required.

Reference

Curra FA. Tooth hypersensitivity. Dent Clin North Am 1990; 34(3).

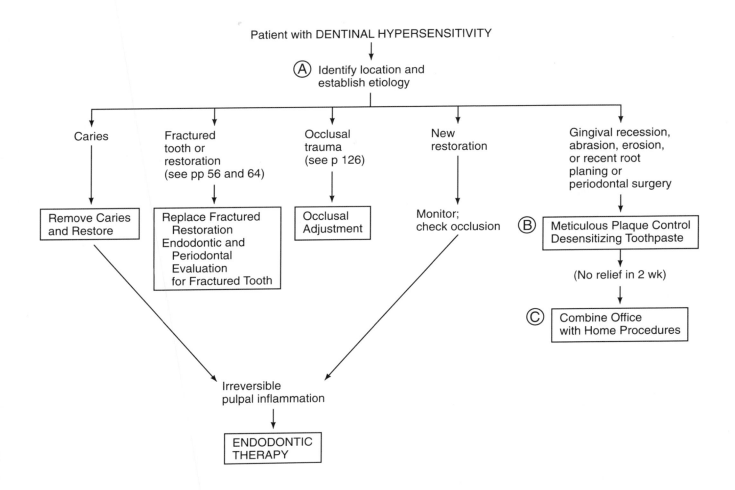

Patient with DENTINAL HYPERSENSITIVITY

(A) Identify location and establish etiology

Caries

Fractured tooth or restoration (see pp 56 and 64)

Occlusal trauma (see p 126)

New restoration

Gingival recession, abrasion, erosion, or recent root planing or periodontal surgery

Remove Caries and Restore

Replace Fractured Restoration Endodontic and Periodontal Evaluation for Fractured Tooth

Occlusal Adjustment

Monitor; check occlusion

(B) Meticulous Plaque Control Desensitizing Toothpaste

(No relief in 2 wk)

(C) Combine Office with Home Procedures

Irreversible pulpal inflammation

ENDODONTIC THERAPY

IMPACTED THIRD MOLARS

Walter B. Hall

Impacted third molars often create serious periodontal problems on adjacent teeth or become involved with periodontal problems on adjacent teeth as they develop. Early extraction of developing third molars may prevent some of these problems from occurring; however, patients often hesitate over treatment of potential problems that are not symptomatic. As an impacted third molar develops, it may grow increasingly closer to the second molar root (Fig. 1). Once it is close, removal of the third molar may result in pocket depth distal to the second molar. Such surgically related pockets usually are accompanied by a three-walled residual osseous defect. If the defect is narrow, it may be amenable to a bone regeneration procedure. The decision as to residual pocket depth and the possibility of bone regeneration should be delayed for 6 months or more following the extraction.

A. If the impacted third molar is not close to the root of the second molar and the third molar is fully formed, the decision to retain or extract is not a periodontal one. If the third molar is still developing and appears unlikely to become close to the root of the second molar, the decision to retain or extract is not a periodontal one; however, if further development of the third molar is likely to result in its crown approaching the second molar root, the prompt extraction of the third molar is desirable periodontally.

B. If the impacted third molar already is close to, or touching, the root of the second molar, the existing periodontal status of the second molar will influence decisions regarding the third molar.

C. If the second molar is not periodontally involved, prompt extraction of the third molar is desirable periodontally. Do not probe the distal surface of the second molar for 6 months. Then, if a pocket exists, and the osseous defect appears to be a three-walled one, its narrow portion would be amenable to osseous regeneration (see p 182). If the distal furcation of a maxillary second molar is involved significantly, the molar may be a good candidate for bone regeneration; however, ostectomy may be preferable if it is a shallowed effect.

D. If the crown of an impacted third molar is close to a second molar root that is periodontally involved, the degree of bone loss on the second molar will influence treatment planning. If the bone loss is early to moderate and the third molar could erupt to replace the second molar, consider extraction of the second molar. If a probe placed in the distal defect on the second molar can touch the third molar crown (this requires especially careful probing), extract the second molar promptly. If the crown of the third molar cannot be touched, the extraction may be delayed but is still periodontally desirable. If the third molar is unlikely to erupt to adequately replace the second molar, extract the third molar promptly, if its crown can be touched, or later, if it cannot be touched. If the second molar has advanced bone loss but the third molar could erupt into an adequate position to replace it, extract the second molar promptly. If the third molar is unlikely to erupt to replace the second molar, the patient may consider extraction of the third molar and an attempt to maintain the second (possibly with a modified Widman flap approach initially). Extraction of both molars would be a sounder approach.

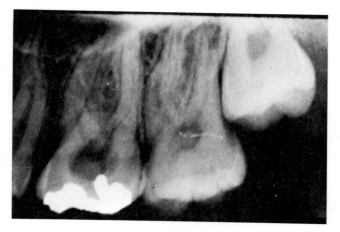

Figure 1. An impacted third molar appearing to contact the root of the adjacent second molar.

References

Ash MM, Costich ER, Hayward JR. Study of periodontal hazards of third molars. J Periodontol 1962; 33:209.

Ash MM. Third molars as periodontal problems. Dent Clin North Am 1964; 8:51.

Friedman JW. The case for preservation of third molars. J Calif Dent Assoc 1977; 5:50.

Hall WB. Removal of third molars: a periodontal viewpoint. In: McDonald RL, ed. Current therapy in dentistry. St. Louis: CV Mosby, 1980:225.

Laskin DM. Indications and contraindications for removal of impacted third molars. Dent Clin North Am 1969; 13:919.

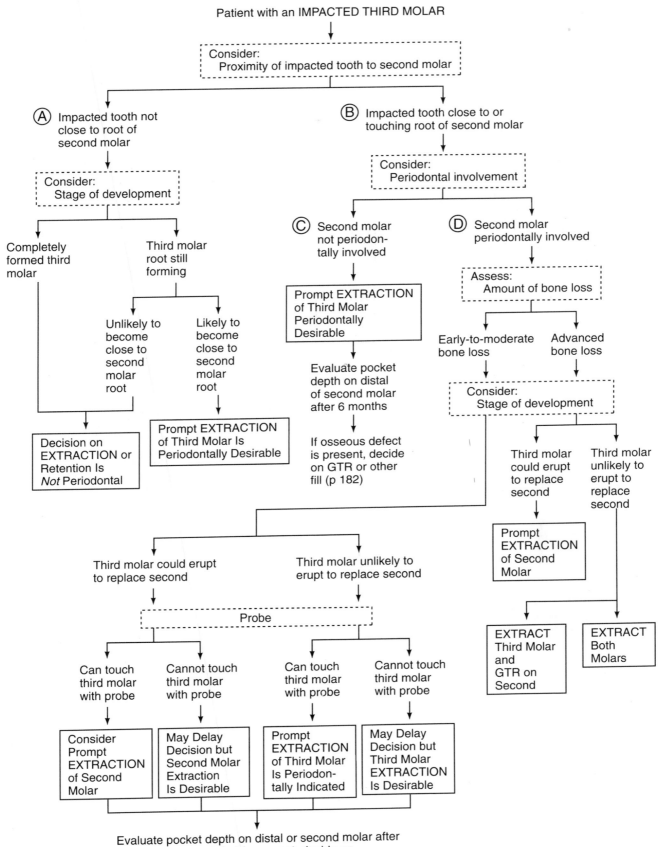

Patient with an IMPACTED THIRD MOLAR

Consider:
Proximity of impacted tooth to second molar

(A) Impacted tooth not close to root of second molar

(B) Impacted tooth close to or touching root of second molar

Consider:
Stage of development

Consider:
Periodontal involvement

Completely formed third molar

Third molar root still forming

(C) Second molar not periodontally involved

(D) Second molar periodontally involved

Unlikely to become close to second molar root

Likely to become close to second molar root

Prompt EXTRACTION of Third Molar Periodontally Desirable

Assess:
Amount of bone loss

Early-to-moderate bone loss

Advanced bone loss

Decision on EXTRACTION or Retention Is *Not* Periodontal

Prompt EXTRACTION of Third Molar Is Periodontally Desirable

Evaluate pocket depth on distal of second molar after 6 months

Consider:
Stage of development

If osseous defect is present, decide on GTR or other fill (p 182)

Third molar could erupt to replace second

Third molar unlikely to erupt to replace second

Third molar could erupt to replace second

Third molar unlikely to erupt to replace second

Prompt EXTRACTION of Second Molar

Probe

EXTRACT Third Molar and GTR on Second

EXTRACT Both Molars

Can touch third molar with probe

Cannot touch third molar with probe

Can touch third molar with probe

Cannot touch third molar with probe

Consider Prompt EXTRACTION of Second Molar

May Delay Decision but Second Molar Extraction Is Desirable

Prompt EXTRACTION of Third Molar Is Periodontally Indicated

May Delay Decision but Third Molar EXTRACTION Is Desirable

Evaluate pocket depth on distal or second molar after 6 mo; if osseous defect is present, decide on guided tissue regeneration or other fill (p 152)

231

PARTIALLY ERUPTED THIRD MOLAR

Walter B. Hall

Partially erupted third molars present a unique set of periodontal problems. A partially erupted third molar has pocket depth at least to its cementoenamel junction. Although this is only a pseudopocket initially, it can lead to loss of attachment on the third molar and to pocket formation on the adjacent second molar. Extraction of the third molar before significant periodontal problems occur is desirable; however, if the third molar is impacted against the root of the second molar, a residual defect on the distal of the second molar is likely to occur following the extraction. This defect is more likely to occur than with fully impacted third molars, because insufficient gingiva to permit primary closure of the wound following third molar extraction is more likely to exist around partially erupted than around fully impacted teeth.

A. A third molar can be partially erupted but not in close proximity to the second molar (i.e., a vertical impaction in the ramus of the mandible). If the second molar is healthy or has had little bone loss, consider extraction of the third molar eventually. If the second molar has moderate-to-severe bone loss and the partially erupted third molar could be moved into good position following extraction of its neighbor, one may consider extracting the second molar and moving the third molar orthodontically into its position or uprighting it for use as an abutment.

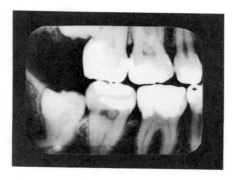

Figure 1. Partially erupted third molar appearing to be in close contact with the second molar.

B. If the partially erupted third molar is close to, or touching, the second molar (Fig. 1), other options apply. If the third molar is close to, or touching, the crown of the second molar only and the second molar has little or no bone loss, prompt extraction of the third molar is periodontally advisable before significant pocketing occurs distal to the second molar. If the second molar has moderate-to-advanced bone loss and the third molar has adequate remaining support, the second molar should be removed and the third molar moved orthodontically into its place or uprighted for use as an abutment.

C. If the partially erupted third molar is close to, or touching, the root of the second molar, several possibilities exist. If the second molar has little or no bone loss and the third molar has little remaining support, prompt extraction of the third molar and evaluation of the pocket status distal to the second molars, no sooner than 6 months after the extraction, are indicated. A residual, narrow, three-walled defect may be amenable to bone regeneration surgery. If the third molar has little or no bone loss and the second molar has moderate-to-advanced bone loss, the second molar could be extracted and the third molar moved orthodontically either into its place or uprighted to serve as an abutment. If both molars are badly involved, both should be extracted; they are prone to abscess formation because of difficulty of cleaning by either the patient or the dentist.

References

Ash MM, Costich ER, Hayward JR. Study of periodontal hazards of third molars. J Periodontol 1962; 33:209.

Ash MM. Third molars as periodontal problems. Dent Clin North Am 1964; 8:51.

Braden BE. Deep distal pockets adjacent to terminal teeth. Dent Clin North Am 1969; 13:161.

Hall WB. Removal of third molars: A periodontal viewpoint. In: McDonald RL, ed. Current therapy in dentistry. St. Louis: CV Mosby, 1980:225.

Patient with a PARTIALLY ERUPTED THIRD MOLAR

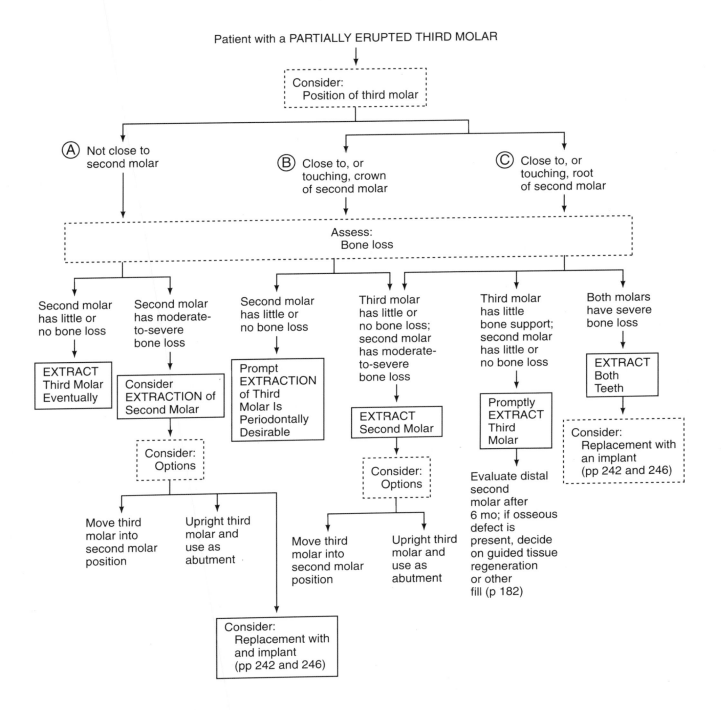

Consider:
Position of third molar

(A) Not close to second molar

(B) Close to, or touching, crown of second molar

(C) Close to, or touching, root of second molar

Assess:
Bone loss

Second molar has little or no bone loss

Second molar has moderate-to-severe bone loss

Second molar has little or no bone loss

Third molar has little or no bone loss; second molar has moderate-to-severe bone loss

Third molar has little bone support; second molar has little or no bone loss

Both molars have severe bone loss

EXTRACT Third Molar Eventually

Consider EXTRACTION of Second Molar

Prompt EXTRACTION of Third Molar Is Periodontally Desirable

EXTRACT Second Molar

Promptly EXTRACT Third Molar

EXTRACT Both Teeth

Consider: Options

Consider: Options

Evaluate distal second molar after 6 mo; if osseous defect is present, decide on guided tissue regeneration or other fill (p 182)

Consider: Replacement with an implant (pp 242 and 246)

Move third molar into second molar position

Upright third molar and use as abutment

Move third molar into second molar position

Upright third molar and use as abutment

Consider: Replacement with and implant (pp 242 and 246)

CROWN LENGTHENING

Wilbur Hughes

When the crown of a tooth is badly broken down because of caries, a fracture, or a combination of the two, the dentist may be able to build up the crown with a restorative material and pins or to increase the length of the crown surgically. If a crown build-up would create an unstable base for a restoration (i.e., the tooth is a canine or a bridge abutment), consider crown lengthening. The procedures are essentially similar to various periodontal surgical procedures. The periodontal status of the tooth will affect selection of the appropriate periodontal procedure (Fig. 1).

A. If the tooth is periodontally healthy or affected only by gingivitis, the problem may be one of excess gingiva or one in which the bone level is normal and no excess gingiva is present. If the problem is excess gingiva only, decide whether cutting away the excess will create a problem of inadequate attached gingiva. A tooth that is going to be crowned needs 2 to 3 mm of attached gingiva to prevent recession following the restorative procedure. If enough will remain, perform gingivectomy surgically or electrosurgically (the dentist's choice). If sufficient attached gingiva would remain, use an apically positioned flap approach, which would save the gingiva but change its position apically and, thus, lengthen the crown.

B. If the bone level is normal and no fracture extends to the root, use mucogingival—osseous surgery to expose 2 to 3 mm of root beyond where the crown margin will be placed. This amount of additional root exposure is necessary to meet physiologic minimum requirements for 1 mm of connective attachment and 1 mm of epithelial attachment apical to the crown margin. If a fracture extends into the root, perform mucogingival—osseous surgery to expose the fracture area and possibly involve adjacent teeth (to avoid large discrepancies in gingival height). If the fracture extends apical to the crest of the bone, essentially creating a defect similar to a narrow three-walled defect, treat the defect for bone regeneration (see pp 152 and 180).

C. If the tooth requiring crown lengthening has periodontal pockets and no fracture is present, use mucogingival—osseous surgery to eliminate the periodontal pockets and to lengthen the crown. If a fracture extends to the crest of the bone, use the same approach; however, if a fracture extends apical to the bone crest and creates an osseous defect similar to a narrow, three-walled defect resulting from periodontitis, treat that portion for bone regeneration as part of the pocket elimination procedure to accomplish crown lengthening. Consider crown lengthening in cases in which perforations can be made suprabony, in which longer crown preparations are needed for retention, or in which existing tissue prohibits one from obtaining impressions for restoration.

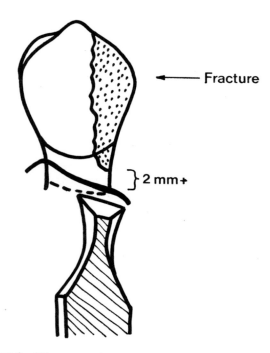

Figure 1. When crown lengthening is performed where a fracture extends apically into the root, bone must be removed to expose a minimum of 2 mm of root structure apical to the ultimate margin of the restoration.

References

Carranza FA Jr. Glickman's clinical periodontology. 7th ed. Philadelphia: WB Saunders, 1990:921.

Genco RJ, Goldman HM, Cohen DW. Contemporary periodontics. St. Louis: CV Mosby, 1990:626.

Hall WB. Periodontal preparation of the mouth for restoration. Dent Clin North Am 1980; 24:207.

Schluger S, Yuodelis RA, Page RC, Johnson RH. Periodontal diseases. 2nd ed. Philadelphia: Lea & Febiger, 1990:619.

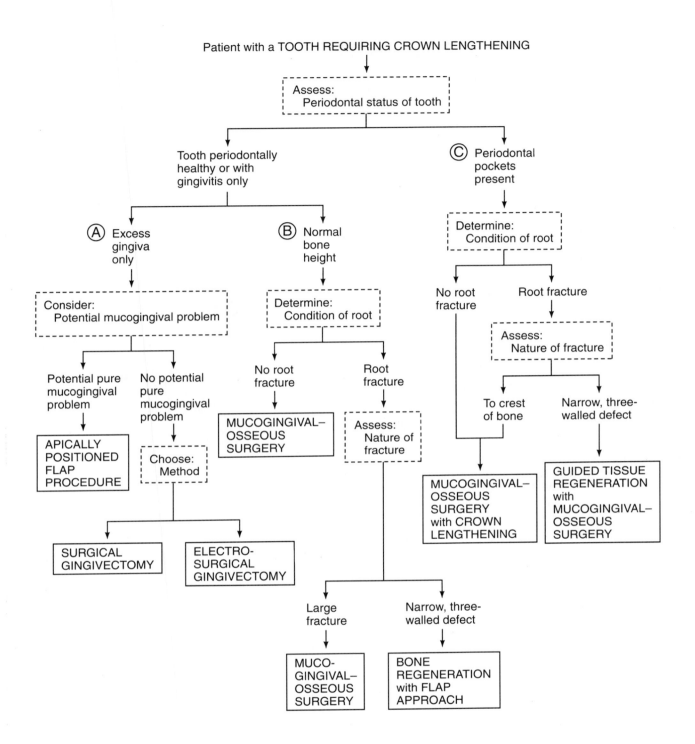

Patient with a TOOTH REQUIRING CROWN LENGTHENING

Assess:
Periodontal status of tooth

Tooth periodontally healthy or with gingivitis only

Ⓒ Periodontal pockets present

Ⓐ Excess gingiva only

Ⓑ Normal bone height

Determine:
Condition of root

Consider:
Potential mucogingival problem

Determine:
Condition of root

No root fracture

Root fracture

Potential pure mucogingival problem

No potential pure mucogingival problem

No root fracture

Root fracture

Assess:
Nature of fracture

APICALLY POSITIONED FLAP PROCEDURE

Choose:
Method

MUCOGINGIVAL–OSSEOUS SURGERY

Assess:
Nature of fracture

To crest of bone

Narrow, three-walled defect

SURGICAL GINGIVECTOMY

ELECTRO-SURGICAL GINGIVECTOMY

MUCOGINGIVAL–OSSEOUS SURGERY with CROWN LENGTHENING

GUIDED TISSUE REGENERATION with MUCOGINGIVAL–OSSEOUS SURGERY

Large fracture

Narrow, three-walled defect

MUCO-GINGIVAL–OSSEOUS SURGERY

BONE REGENERATION with FLAP APPROACH

CROWN LENGTHENING: A EUROPEAN VIEW

Carlo Clauser
Giovan Paolo Pini-Prato

Main indications for crown-lengthening procedures are (1) tooth fracture or caries that require a preparation apical to the gingival margin (GM); (2) an abutment tooth that is too short to provide adequate retention (e.g., an extruded tooth that has to be cut to restore a proper occlusal plane); and (3) a tooth the appearance of which is not acceptable, because it looks too short. Establish proper plaque control, rule out any periodontal pathology involving surgery before planning a crown-lengthening procedure. Figures 1 to 3 indicate the salient steps in the procedure.

A. An exposed zone of healthy dental surface coronal to the GM is required to prepare and maintain the margins of restorations properly; thus, keep the margins of the restorations extracrevicular whenever aesthetics, solder joint size, and retention are not concerns. In the anterior areas, on the buccal aspects, aesthetic needs sometimes require intrasulcular margins; on the other hand, in these areas, both restorative and maintenance procedures are easier.

B. An adequate amount of space is required for the junctional epithelium and the sulcus coronal to the connective tissue attachment. The GM on healthy teeth usually is located 1 to 2 mm coronal to the point where the tip of a gently inserted probe stops (i.e., to the clinical attachment level, or AL). This point differs only slightly (usually more apical) from the connective tissue attachment level, as determined histologically, in the absence of inflammation. The measured distance between the planned GM and the actual AL can vary around the tooth. To plan the surgical procedure, consider the site where the GM is nearest to the AL. In cases of doubt, leave a greater amount exposed.

C. Judge the thickness of the bone by inspection (prominent roots have thin buccal bone plates) and palpation. In case of doubt, choose the apically positioned flap procedure.

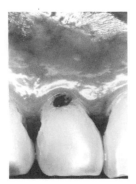

Figure 1. A lateral incisor requiring crown lengthening (preoperative view).

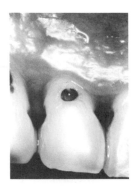

Figure 2. The same tooth following crown lengthening.

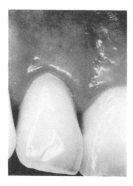

Figure 3. The same tooth restored following crown lengthening.

D. The removal of Sharpey's fibers from the root surface prevents reattachment; the position of the postoperative AL will not be coronal to the root-planed area. Evaluate the AL of the adjacent teeth, especially in cases of root proximity. If too much healthy supporting tissue has to be removed, consider extraction of the tooth that is undergoing the crown-lengthening procedure.

E. Whereas ostectomy is aimed only at making root planing feasible, osteoplasty should provide a proper profile for maintenance and guide the subsequent, spontaneous, bone resorption. If root planing prevents the reattachment of fibers coronally to the crestal bone level, some bone has to be resorbed to leave room for the supracrestal connective tissue. Remodel this bone during surgery to prevent the subsequent formation of angular defects. Thinning the crestal bone 1 mm apically to the AL means that all the thickness will be resorbed to the level that is needed for the newly formed connective tissue attachment, without any further loss of bone support.

Patient with TOOTH REQUIRING CROWN LENGTHENING

Determine:
Location of the postsurgical gingival margin

↓

Consider:
Esthetics

No esthetic problem — Esthetics Important

Determine:
Need for restoration

(A) Restoration necessary — No restoration

Locate GM apical to the restoration margin (extrasulcular)

Locate GM coronal (1 mm) to the restoration margin (intrasulcular)

Locate GM as required for esthetics

(B) Assess:
Distance between the planned GM and preoperative AL by probe

Distance < 1.5 mm — Distance > 1.5 mm

Need for thorough root planing to planned AL — Leave attachment apparatus untouched

(C) Thick crestal bone — (C) Thin crestal bone or interdental area involved

Probe under anesthesia

Probe reaches bone crest coronally to planned AL — Probe can be forced into soft tissues to planned AL

No bone surgery

Need for Surgical Exposure of Crestal Bone by a FULL-THICKNESS FLAP PROCEDURE

(D) Root Planing to the Planned AL

Retain attachment fibers apical to the planned AL

Consider:
Location of mucogingival junction (MGS)

OSTECTOMY to the Planned AL if Needed to Gain Access for Root Planing

MGJ apical to postoperative AL — MGJ coronal to postoperative AL

(D) Root Planing to the Planned AL

(E) OSTEOPLASTY to Contour Bone Apical to the Planned AL

GINGIVECTOMY GINGIVOPLASTY

Evaluate:
Amount of keratinized tissue

APICALLY POSITIONED FLAP PROCEDURE — FREE GRAFT — Partial-Thickness APICALLY POSITIONED FLAP PROCEDURE — FREE GRAFT

References

Leon AR. The periodontium and restorative procedures: A critical review. J Oral Rehabil 1977; 4:105.

Maynard GD, Wilson RD. Physiologic dimensions of periodontium fundamental to successful restorative dentistry. J Periodontol 1979; 4:170.

Proye MP, Polson AM. Effect of root surface alterations on periodontal healing. I. Surgical denudation. J Clin Periodontol 1983; 9:428.

CROWN MARGIN PLACEMENT

Kathy I. Mueller
Galen W. Wagnild

The marginal periodontium includes the area in which the fields of restorative dentistry and periodontics become intimately related. This area, although small, is operated in daily by restorative dental practitioners and requires definitive, logical decisions regarding margin location to facilitate long-term, predictable results at this junction. Although controversy exists, recent literature supports movement away from margins deep within the gingival crevice and toward shallow, intracrevicular or supragingival placement.

A. Evaluate the tooth in need of restoration on both structural and esthetic levels before determining margin location.

B. Clinical findings, such as caries, existing restoration, fractures, cervical erosion, and uncontrollable root sensitivity, may dictate restoration placement below the level of the free gingival margin. Extension of the preparation into the gingival crevice may engage enough additional tooth structure to provide the restoration with adequate retention and resistance form, to secure sufficient sound tooth structure for margin placement, and to minimize root sensitivity of nonendodontic origin. The physiologic zones or biologic width present in the area of intracrevicular margin placement must meet minimum guidelines (Fig. 1). Attempts to modify the tooth preparation by apical position of the restorative margin are limited by this fragile tissue complex. Violation of this width may result in gingival inflammation, loss of crestal bone, and pocket formation or apical migration of the marginal tissue. If structural problems cannot be solved without destroying the integrity of the biologic width, surgical lengthening of the clinical crown or orthodontic extrusion is indicated to reestablish this zone.

C. Esthetic requirements may dictate intracrevicular margin location despite other clinical findings that would allow supragingival placement. Determine margin location with respect to esthetics using a combination of factors, including tooth position, visibility of margin area during function, and the patient's understanding of the objectives of the restorative effort. When esthetics are important, the crevice should be entered minimally, with the restoration usually from 0.5 to 1 m apical to the free gingival margin. A restorative attempt to hide a metal collar within the anatomic confines of a shallow, healthy crevice is often not possible without compromising the esthetics or sacrificing the biologic width. Such conflicts between esthetics and tissue health may best be resolved by minimal entrance into the crevice and use of a porcelain shoulder margin or a margin supported by metal but without a visible metal collar. When esthetics are secondary and structural evaluation permits, locate restorative margins outside of the gingival crevice. Such margins are more accurately prepared, more predictably registered, and more accessible for evaluation, finishing, and patient maintenance. Patients who require restoration after periodontal therapy that apically repositions gingival tissue pose additional complexities. If esthetics are important, the restorative practitioner must first carefully establish that a gingival crevice has indeed reformed postsurgically; placing a restorative margin under the tissue level when no crevice exists may lead to breakdown of the tissue complex, pocket formation, or apical migration of the gingiva. Secondly, an

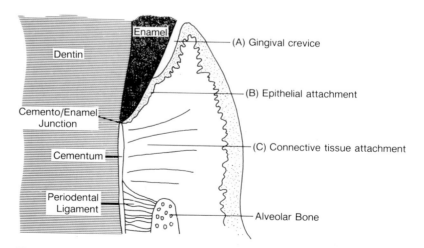

Figure 1. Restorative margins located apical to the free gingival margin must terminate in *(A)*; entry into *(B)* or *(C)* may cause breakdown of the attachment apparatus.

Patient for RESTORATIVE MARGIN LOCATION

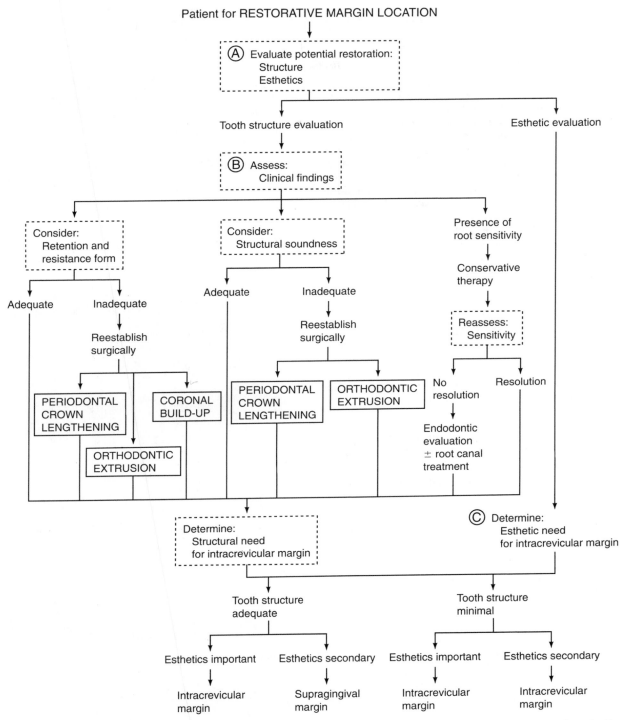

attempt to locate margins within the gingival crevice of an elongated tooth requires additional axial wall reduction with possible pulpal encroachment. If possible, postsurgical margins should be left above the treated tissue level and above exposed furcations.

References

Nevins M, Skurow HM. The intracrevicular restorative margin, the biologic width, and maintenance of the gingival margin. Int J Periodont Restor Dent 1984; 3:31.

Schluger S, Yuodelis RA, Page RC. Periodontal disease. Philadelphia: Lea & Febiger, 1977:586.

Shillingburg HT, Hobo S, Whitsett DL, Fundamentals of fixed prosthodontics. 2nd ed. Berlin: Quintessence Publishing, 1981:79.

Wilson RD, Maynard G. Intracrevicular restorative dentistry. Int J Periodont Restor Dent 1981; 4:35.

SOLITARY DEEP PERIODONTAL DEFECTS

Gonsalo Hernandez Vallejo

Isolated periodontal defects (IPD) can be defined as the loss of periodontal attachment accompanied by a notable increase in probing depth in a localized site. Isolated periodontal defects are common findings when exploring a patient, and they are usually seen in patients who are not affected by chronic periodontal disease. They appear frequently in the region of molars and incisors and, although some of them occur with an unfavorable prognosis, most of them can be successfully treated by eliminating the underlying cause once the diagnosis has been established.

Once the IPD has been detected on probing, it is crucial to determine the status of the tooth crown, independent of the clinical characteristics of the gingiva.

A. If the tooth has a filling or artificial crown, or if an active (nontreated) carious lesion is detected, the first step in diagnosis should be to assess the bone condition by radiographic examination.

B. Appearance of lateral–periapical radiolucency usually indicates the presence of causes related to endodontic problems. In these cases, one should carefully examine the root image while looking for fractures associated with intraradicular posts or root canal treatment. Horizontal fractures can easily be observed, but when the root image is normal, a lateral–periapical abscess due to defective endodontic filling, or pulpal necrosis usually is the cause. If the endodontic treatment is satisfactory, then suspect cracked tooth syndrome.

C. When the radiographic examination does not show bone involvement, check tooth vitality. If the tooth is nonvital, the presence of recently developed pulpal involvement or root crack has to be taken into account. When response to a vitality test is positive, the diagnostic course depends upon the presence of an artificial crown filling or nontreated active caries. If the tooth is filled or crowned, examination of the quality of the restoration's margin may reveal the presence of overhanging margins that may act as a local factor in promoting food impaction, chronic inflammation, and periodontal abscess accompanied by loss of attachment. If normal margins are found, the next step includes the examination of margins with respect to the gingiva, because subgingival margins facilitate the presence of an irritative environment for the periodontium and attachment loss, as occurs with microfiltration associated with the use of subgingival composites. If the margin is supragingivally located, the quality of interproximal contacts has to be assessed for conditions that favor food impaction. When the interproximal contacts are normal, the possibility of a crack or other cause described in D should be kept in mind. If a vital tooth presents caries, supra- or subgingival location has to be determined (Fig. 1). Deep subgingival caries may be associated with attachment loss in the affected aspect of the tooth. If the caries is supragingivally located, a crack due to excessive or abnormal forces, or causes described in D have to be suspected.

D. Cases in which an IPD coexists with an intact tooth crown, assess the morphology of the crown for developmental abnormalities. Enamel grooves appear frequently in the palatal aspect of lateral and central incisors; these defects sometimes continue towards the root to different depths, creating deep periodontal pockets whose location clinically coincides with the entrance of the groove (Fig. 2). Enamel projections are also responsible for IPD; they tend to appear more frequently in the furcation area of a mandibular second or third molar and are sometimes accompanied by furcation involvement (Figs. 3 and 4). If these two conditions do not appear, perform a careful probing of the defect to evaluate the root morphology; sometimes irregularities or hollows corresponding to

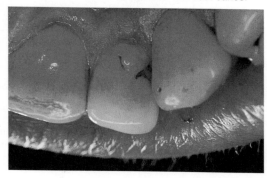

Figure 1. Periodontal defect associated with root caries.

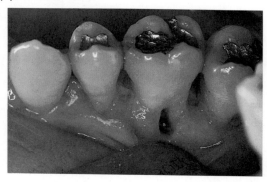

Figure 2. Palatal groove in a upper lateral incisor associated with a deep periodontal defect.

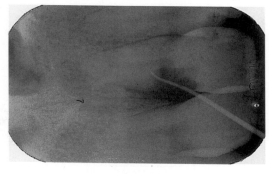

Figure 3. Periodontal defect (12 mm depth) with furcation involvement associated with enamel projection.

Patient with an ISOLATED DEEP PERIODONTAL DEFECT

Determine: Tooth crown status

- Presence of crowned/filled tooth (A) Presence of active caries
  - **Assess:** Radiographs for bone status
    - (B) Periapical/lateral radiolucency
      - **Examine:** Root image
        - Fracture
        - Normal root image
          - Periapical/lateral abscess
          - Suspect cracked tooth syndrome
    - (C) No periapical/lateral radiolucency
      - **Assess:** Tooth vitality
        - Nonvital → (Normal root image)
        - Vital
          - **Assess:** Quality of restoration margins
            - Overhanging Food impaction Periodontal abscess
            - Normal margins
              - **Assess:** Location of the margin
                - Subgingival margin
                - Supragingival
                  - **Assess:** Quality of interproximal contact
                    - Open contacts Food impaction
                    - Normal contact
          - **Assess:** Location of caries
            - Subgingival caries
              - Suspect cracked tooth syndrome
            - Supragingival caries
              - **Assess:** Causes related to D

- (D) Intact tooth crown
  - **Assess:** Morphology of the crown
    - Grooves Incisors
    - Enamel projection Molars Furcations
    - Normal external anatomy
      - Probe the defect to assess root condition
        - Root caries
        - Enamel pearl
          - Confirm by radiograph
        - Smooth/ normal root
          - **Assess:** Tooth position
            - No inclination
            - Tilted molar Second mandibular molar (mesial pocket)
              - (E) **Assess:** Radiographs
                - Enamel pearl
                - Root caries
                - Impaction of third molar
                - Third molar removed
                - Bone "cup" defect (LJP)

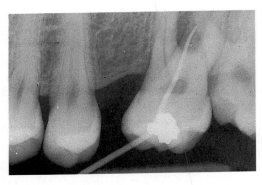

Figure 4. Periodontal defect in a second upper molar associated with an enamel projection.

cemental caries and enamel pearls can be discovered. If the root condition is normal, examination of tooth position may give information about tilted molars, which usually correspond to mandibular second molars when the first molar has been lost. This situation is frequently accompanied by IPD on the mesial aspect of the molar.

E. Teeth that show intact, normal crown/root anatomy and are positioned normally should be evaluated radiographically, which can give information about some conditions associated with IPD. Although enamel pearls and root caries may be detected upon probing, they should be confirmed by radiographs. Radiography also provides data about the periodontal defects located on the distal aspect of second molars that are usually associated with bone loss due to third molar impaction or extraction. Finally, "cup" images of bone loss associated with IPD on first molars or central incisors, which may appear isolated but affect one or two teeth, may suggest localized juvenile periodontitis.

References

Jeffcoat MK, Howell TH. Alveolar bone destruction due to overhanging amalgam in periodontal disease. J Periodontol 1980; 51:599.

Moskow BS, Martinez P. Studies on root enamel. I. Some historical notes on cervical enamel projections. J Clin Periodontol 1990; 17:29.

Moskow BS, Martinez P. Studies on root enamel. II. Enamel pearls. A review of their morphology, localization, nomenclature, occurrence, classification, histogenesis and incidence. J Clin Periodontol 1990; 17:275.

Schluger S, Yuodelis R, Page RC, Johnson RH. Periodontal diseases. 2nd ed. Philadelphia: Lea & Febiger, 1990:102.

OSSEOINTEGRATED IMPLANTS FOR THE PARTIALLY EDENTULOUS MAXILLA

Juan Pi Urgell

When the maxilla is partially edentulous, the anatomic structures that influence the possible use of implants are the maxillary sinuses, the nasal cavity, and the surrounding bone structure. The best method of evaluating the appropriateness of these structures for the use of osseointegrated implants is the computed tomography (CT) scan, although a conventional tomography scan may suffice.

A. When the CT scan or conventional tomograph indicates lack of sufficient bone or the existence of bone of poor quality (bone that is not very trabecular), which would negate the possibility of utilizing implants, the patient is advised of the necessity of employing a conventional prosthesis. At least 8 mm of bone must be present between the maxillary sinus or nasal cavity and the crest of the alveolar ridge for osseointegrated implants to be employed.

B. If there is sufficient trabecular bone, evaluate the periodontal and dental health of the remaining teeth to determine the type of implant design to be employed. If the bone is of poor quality, a conventional removable prosthesis is advisable.

C. If the remaining maxillary teeth are dentally sound, their periodontal status is the determining factor in tissue-integrated prosthesis (TIP) design. Teeth that are dentally and/or periodontally compromised require alteration in the design of the prosthesis.

D. If the remaining dentally sound teeth have been periodontally compromised, two implants and a bridge connected telescopically to the abutments would be employed so that, should a natural tooth be lost, the restoration might still be salvaged. If they are not periodontally involved, two implants and a self-retained bridge would be employed.

E. If the remaining teeth need extensive periodontal or dental treatment and will be opposing the natural teeth, two or three implants connected by interlocks to the natural abutments are used. If a removable prosthesis is present already, one implant connected by an interlock to the natural abutments could be employed as a replacement, reducing the treatment costs.

When inadequate quantity or quality of bone is present to permit the use of tissue-integrated prostheses because implants cannot be placed, conventional prostheses are the only alternative. In free-end saddle cases, removable prostheses are used. In cases with useful posterior abutments present, a conventional fixed bridge is indicated. If the natural abutments are periodontally and/or dentally badly compromised, a conventional removable prosthesis, with or without extraction of those teeth, is the alternative.

One major advance in the last 2 years when dealing with partially edentulous maxilla is the performance of sinus grafting. When there is not enough bone (minimum 10 mm because of the lack of predictability with a 7-mm fixture), a graft is performed to elevate the sinus mucosa.

Different material has been used, but the most predictable is autogenous bone or autologous bone.

In the most posterior maxilla, use pterygomaxillary fixtures to increase the predictability of success. In most cases, it is necessary to use a long fixture that is distally inclined to engage the pterygomaxillary phisurae. Very dense bone formed by the pterygoid process and vertical part of the palatine bone.

References

Boyne PJ, James RA. Grafting of the maxillary sinus floor with autogenous marrow and bone. J Oral Surg 1980; 6:613.

Damien CJ, Parson JR. Bone graft and bone graft substitutes: A review of current technology and applications. J Appl Biomaterials 1991; 2:187.

Ericsson I, Lekholm U, Branemark P, et al. A clinical evaluation of fixed bridge restoration supported by the combination of teeth and osseointegrated titanium implants. J Clin Periodontol 1986; 13:307.

Lekholm U. Clinical procedures for treatment with osseointegrated dental implants. J Prosthet Dent 1983; 50:1117.

Sullivan D. Prosthetic considerations for the utilization of osseointegrated fixtures in the partially edentulous arch. Int J Oral Maxillofac Implants 1986; 1:81.

Sullivan D, Krogh P. A solution for the prosthetic problem of the hemidentate arch with tissue integrated prosthesis. Int J Periodont Restor Dent 1986; 4:66.

Tulasne JF. Implant treatment of missing posterior dentition: The Branemark osseointegrated implant. Berlin: Quintessence Publishing, 103.

Patient with SOME POSTERIOR EDENTULOUS AREAS IN THE MAXILLA

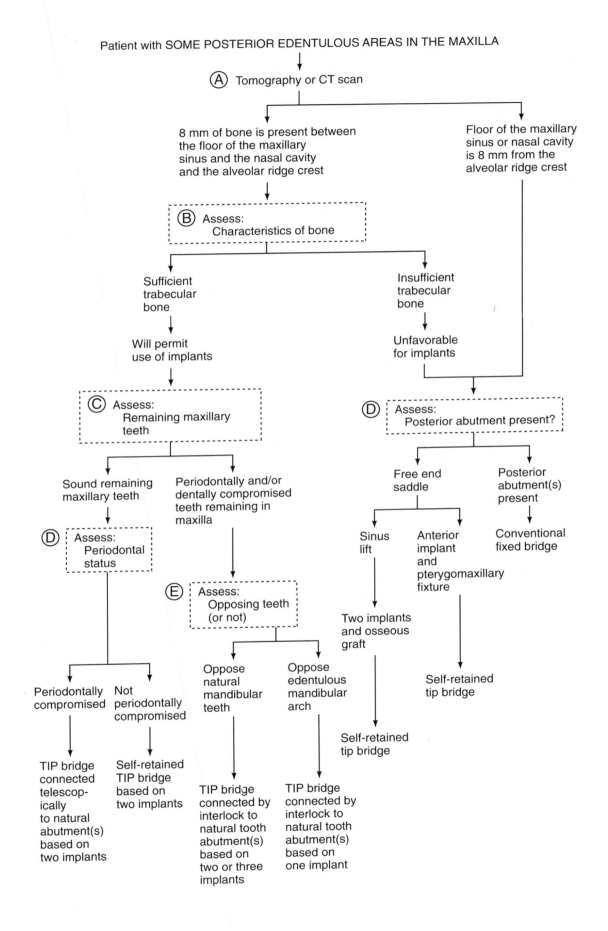

(A) Tomography or CT scan

8 mm of bone is present between the floor of the maxillary sinus and the nasal cavity and the alveolar ridge crest

Floor of the maxillary sinus or nasal cavity is 8 mm from the alveolar ridge crest

(B) Assess: Characteristics of bone

Sufficient trabecular bone

Will permit use of implants

Insufficient trabecular bone

Unfavorable for implants

(C) Assess: Remaining maxillary teeth

Sound remaining maxillary teeth

Periodontally and/or dentally compromised teeth remaining in maxilla

(D) Assess: Posterior abutment present?

Free end saddle

Posterior abutment(s) present

Sinus lift

Anterior implant and pterygomaxillary fixture

Conventional fixed bridge

(D) Assess: Periodontal status

(E) Assess: Opposing teeth (or not)

Two implants and osseous graft

Self-retained tip bridge

Periodontally compromised

Not periodontally compromised

Oppose natural mandibular teeth

Oppose edentulous mandibular arch

Self-retained tip bridge

TIP bridge connected telescopically to natural abutment(s) based on two implants

Self-retained TIP bridge based on two implants

TIP bridge connected by interlock to natural tooth abutment(s) based on two or three implants

TIP bridge connected by interlock to natural tooth abutment(s) based on one implant

OSSEOINTEGRATED IMPLANTS FOR THE TOTALLY EDENTULOUS MAXILLA

Juan Pi Urgell

When a patient has severely periodontally compromised teeth remaining in the maxilla, the possibility of removing those teeth and replacing them with a tissue-integrated prosthesis (TIP) or a conventional prosthesis must be considered along with the various options offered by the remaining teeth for conventional, natural tooth-based partial prostheses. For this reason, the bases for selecting or rejecting the TIP in an edentulous maxilla situation are discussed.

A. A most important factor to consider in deciding whether or not to use osseointegrated implants in an edentulous maxilla case is aesthetic in nature. If the patient has a short upper lip and smiling would expose the titanium posts, a fixed type of prosthesis often could not be made with acceptable aesthetic characteristics. A removable replacement becomes the only alternative.

B. If sufficient bone of a trabecular nature is present (at least 8 mm between the alveolar crest and the floor of the nasal cavity and maxillary sinuses), a TIP can be employed. Four implants and an overdenture retained by a bar or magnets would be employed; however, if sufficient bone does not exist, a conventional denture is the only option when the remaining maxillary teeth are removed.

C. If esthetic considerations do not dictate otherwise and sufficient bone of a trabecular nature is not present, a conventional denture is necessary. If sufficient bone remains, the options for placement of TIP are dependent upon the status of the dentition in the mandible.

D. If the maxillary TIP would oppose a natural dentition in the mandible, two to four implants and an overdenture would be the treatment of choice.

E. If the opposing mandibular dentition is a denture, budgetary factors are important in selecting the type of TIP to be fabricated. Fixed prostheses are considerably more expensive than removable ones. For the financially compromised patient, an overdenture may be the only option. For the financially able, a fixed-tissue integrated prosthesis based upon four to six osseointegrated implants often is a more desirable option.

When evaluating a patient with a totally edentulous maxilla, esthetics is one of the factors that will indicate the type of restoration. Not only the smile line but the lip support and the intermaxillary spaces must be explored.

When there is a severely absorbed bone, use of an onlay graft from the iliac crest is indicated in a one-stage surgery to provide stability of the graft and to avoid a second surgery for implant placement.

References

Adell R, et al. A 15-year study of osseointegrated implants in the treatment of the edentulous jaw. Int J Oral Surg 1981; 6:387.

Adell R, Branemark PI. Reconstruction of severely resorbed edentulous maxillary using osseointegrated fixtures in immediate autogenous bone grafts. Int J Oral Maxillofac Implants. 1990; 5(3):233.

Branemark PI, et al. Osseointegrated implants in the treatment of the edentulous jaw: Experience from a 10-year period. Scand J Plast Reconstruct Surg 1977; 11(suppl 16).

Jackson T. The application of rare earth magnetic retention to osseointegrated implants. Int J Oral Maxillofac Implants 1986; 1:81.

Kahnberg KE, Nystrom E. Combined use of bone grafts and Branemark fixtures in the treatment of severely resorbed maxillae. Int J Oral Maxillofac Implants 1989; 4:4.

Zarb G. Osseointegrated dental implants: Preliminary report on a replication study. J Prosthet Dent 1983; 50:271.

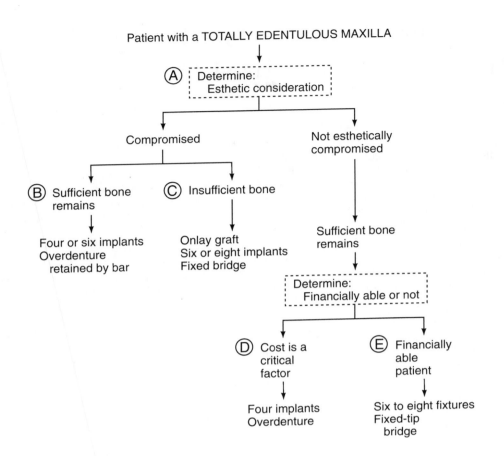

Patient with a TOTALLY EDENTULOUS MAXILLA

Ⓐ Determine:
Esthetic consideration

Compromised

Not esthetically
compromised

Ⓑ Sufficient bone
remains

Four or six implants
Overdenture
retained by bar

Ⓒ Insufficient bone

Onlay graft
Six or eight implants
Fixed bridge

Sufficient bone
remains

Determine:
Financially able or not

Ⓓ Cost is a
critical
factor

Four implants
Overdenture

Ⓔ Financially
able
patient

Six to eight fixtures
Fixed-tip
bridge

OSSEOINTEGRATED IMPLANTS FOR THE PARTIALLY EDENTULOUS MANDIBLE

Juan Pi Urgell

When the mandible is partially edentulous, consider three design options: Kennedy type 1 (bilateral posterior edentulous areas), type 2 (unilateral posterior edentulous areas), and type 3 (unilateral posterior edentulous areas with anterior and posterior abutments present).

A. Investigate the existing distance between the mandibular canal and the alveolar crest and the width of the mandibular bone. A panoramic radiograph and either a tomograph or computed tomography (CT) scan are needed for this purpose. The radiographic study shows one of the following: (1) the mandible is more than 8 mm high and 4 mm wide (in which case the patient is a candidate for osseointegrated implants), or (2) these necessary minimum requirements do not exist (in which case the patient is best served by a conventional prosthesis of either a fixed or removable variety). The patient's economic situation is considered in deciding upon the fixed (more expensive) or removable (cheaper) option.

B. If sufficient bone exists and no posterior abutment is present (a free-end saddle situation), consider the following solutions: (1) If remaining teeth need no restoration, place two implants and a free-standing TIP bridge. (2) If the remaining teeth do require restoration or root canal treatment, place one implant to support a bridge joined to the remaining teeth by means of a nonrigid anchor (a stress-broken fixed bridge).

C. When abutments remain anterior and posterior to the edentulous area (a Kennedy type 3 situation) and the remaining teeth are in good condition, place two implants to support a free-standing TIP bridge, because two implants are enough for the replacement of four to six teeth if further tooth loss should occur. If the teeth are in poor condition because of extensive caries, one implant supporting a prosthesis united to the crowns of natural anterior and posterior abutments by means of semirigid interlocks is employed. If significant periodontal problems exist and the loss of the natural abutments might occur, one or two implants, united with the natural ones by means of telescoping restorations, are utilized in order to permit the continued use of the restoration if further tooth loss occurs.

D. When tissue-integrated prostheses (TIP) cannot be considered owing to inadequate mandibular bone to allow placement of implants, conventional prostheses are the only alternative. In free-end saddle cases, conventional removable prostheses are used. In cases in which useful posterior abutments are present, a conventional fixed bridge is indicated. If the natural abutments are badly compromised periodontally and/or dentally, a conventional removable prosthesis, with or without extraction of those teeth, is the alternative.

Treatment of the partially edentulous mandible has been limited by the presence of the alveolar nerve. When there is no more than 8 mm from the mandibular canal to alveolar crest, one should consider performing nerve lateralization to allow placement of the fixture and repositioning of the alveolar nerve.

References

Ericsson I, Lekholm U, Branemark P, et al. A clinical evaluation of fixed bridge restorations supported by the combination of teeth and osseointegrated titanium implants. J Clin Periodontol 1986; 13:307.

Lekholm U. Clinical procedures for treatment with osseointegrated dental implants. J Prosthet Dent 1983; 50:1117.

Sullivan D. Prosthetic considerations for the utilization of osseointegrated fixtures in the partially edentulous arch. Int J Oral Maxillofac Implants 1986; 1:81.

Sullivan D, Krogh P. A solution of the prosthetic problem of the hemidentate arch with tissue integrated prosthesis. Int J Periodont Restor Dent 1986; 4:66.

Patient with SOME POSTERIOR EDENTULOUS AREAS IN THE MANDIBLE

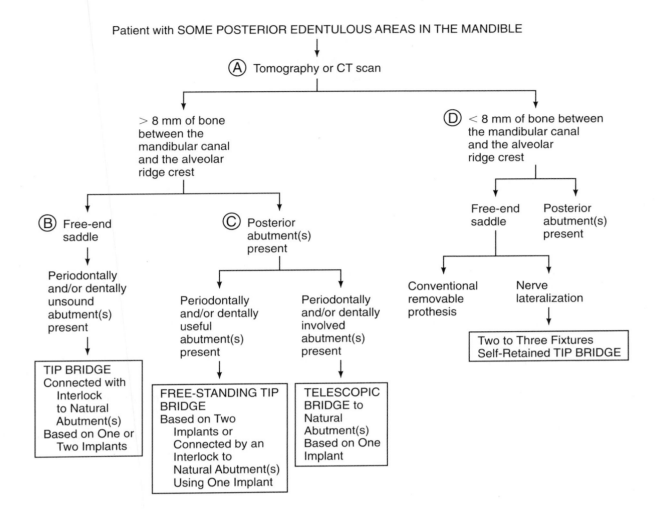

(A) Tomography or CT scan

> 8 mm of bone between the mandibular canal and the alveolar ridge crest

(D) < 8 mm of bone between the mandibular canal and the alveolar ridge crest

(B) Free-end saddle

(C) Posterior abutment(s) present

Periodontally and/or dentally unsound abutment(s) present

Periodontally and/or dentally useful abutment(s) present

Periodontally and/or dentally involved abutment(s) present

Free-end saddle

Posterior abutment(s) present

Conventional removable prothesis

Nerve lateralization

TIP BRIDGE Connected with Interlock to Natural Abutment(s) Based on One or Two Implants

FREE-STANDING TIP BRIDGE Based on Two Implants or Connected by an Interlock to Natural Abutment(s) Using One Implant

TELESCOPIC BRIDGE to Natural Abutment(s) Based on One Implant

Two to Three Fixtures Self-Retained TIP BRIDGE

OSSEOINTEGRATED IMPLANTS FOR THE TOTALLY EDENTULOUS MANDIBLE

Juan Pi Urgell

When a patient has severely periodontally compromised teeth remaining in the mandible, one must consider the possibility of removing those teeth and replacing them with a tissue-integrated prosthesis (TIP) or a conventional prosthesis. In addition, the remaining teeth offer various options for conventional natural tooth-based partial prostheses. For this reason, the bases for selecting or rejecting the TIP in an edentulous mandible situation are discussed in this text.

A. Whether the mandible is of sufficient dimension or is extremely resorbed is the key factor in determining whether a TIP can or cannot be made. In extreme cases, sufficient bone may not be present to permit placement of osseointegrated implants, and a conventional denture is the only option. If implants can be placed, the options for placing a TIP are dependent upon the status of the dentition in the maxilla.

B. If the TIP would oppose a natural dentition in the maxilla, two to four implants and an overdenture is the treatment of choice. If the prosthesis would oppose a maxillary denture, cost factors influence the design of the TIP.

C. For the financially compromised patient, two osseointegrated implants supporting an overdenture are a less expensive option. For the financially able, a fixed TIP based upon four to six implants is more desirable.

D. For the patient with a minimally resorbed mandible, cost factors are more important than the nature of the opposing dentition in the maxilla. If the cost of a fixed prosthesis based upon four to six implants is prohibitive, an overdenture based upon two implants is an option. When cost factors do not dictate treatment, the fixed prosthesis with more implants is a more satisfactory alternative.

References

Adell R, et al. A 15-year study of osseointegrated implants in the treatment of the edentulous jaw. Int J Oral Surg 1981; 6:387.

Branemark PL, et al. Osseointegrated implants in the treatment of the edentulous jaw: Experience from a 10-year period. Scand J Plast Reconstr Surg 1977; 11(suppl 16).

Jackson T. The application of rare earth magnetic retention to osseointegrated implants. Int J Oral Maxillofac Implants 1986; 1:81.

Zarb G. Osseointegrated dental implants: Preliminary report on a replication study. J Prosthet Dent 1983; 50:271.

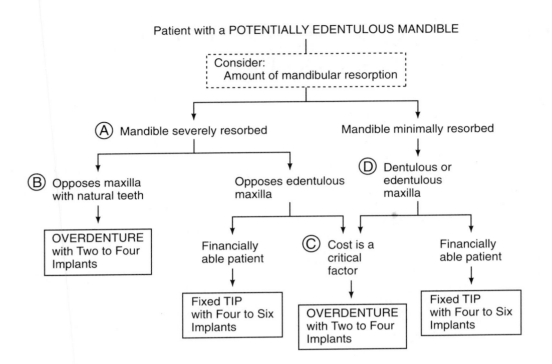

Patient with a POTENTIALLY EDENTULOUS MANDIBLE

Consider:
Amount of mandibular resorption

(A) Mandible severely resorbed

Mandible minimally resorbed

(B) Opposes maxilla with natural teeth

Opposes edentulous maxilla

(D) Dentulous or edentulous maxilla

OVERDENTURE with Two to Four Implants

Financially able patient

(C) Cost is a critical factor

Financially able patient

Fixed TIP with Four to Six Implants

OVERDENTURE with Two to Four Implants

Fixed TIP with Four to Six Implants

GUIDED BONE AUGMENTATION FOR OSSEOINTEGRATED IMPLANTS

William Becker
Burton E. Becker

The principles of guided tissue regeneration (GTR) that have been used for periodontal regeneration can be used for root form dental implants as well. The tissues involved in the healing of an extraction socket are flap connective tissue and bone. Membrane barriers may be used to exclude flap connective tissue from collapsing into an extraction socket that has received an immediately placed implant, thus allowing the necessary cells for bone formation access to the area. The barrier creates a space and protects the clot during the early healing phase, creating an environment for potential bone formation around the portion of the implant that is not fully encompassed by bone. A specially designed e-otfte membrane (Gore-Tex Augmentation Material, WJ Gore and Associates, Flagstaff, AZ) is used for this purpose. The oval-shaped material has an inner portion that is totally occlusive and a peripheral portion that allows for the ingrowth of connective tissue fibrils. The use of guided bone augmentation (GBA) with osseointegrated implants has been demonstrated in animal and human clinical studies.

A. Successful use of GBA for implants placed into extraction sockets requires careful case selection. Teeth that have advanced untreatable periodontitis, recurrent endodontic lesions, or fractures that are not exposable by crown lengthening are ideal candidates for extraction accompanied by immediate implant placement. In order to obtain maximum implant stability, there should be a minimum of 3 to 5 mm of bone apical to the root tip. Implants placed into thin edentulous ridges may result in fenestrations. These defects can be treated with GBA.

B. When the site is exposed surgically, the type of defect and site that are present are evaluated, and the stability of an implant potentially or after placement is assessed. If a stable implant cannot be placed, alternative restorative plans should be proposed.

C. Fenestration defects that result from placing the implant close to the facial surface of the implant can be treated with GBA. The implant must be completely stable. If the fenestration exposes only one or two threads, no barrier is necessary. When a large fenestration is present, exposing three or more threads of the implant, a barrier should be placed over the defect for GBA.

D. When an implant has been placed into an extraction socket, an intra-alveolar defect may exist. When implants are placed into extremely narrow sockets, as those present on mandibular anterior teeth, or into extremely wide bone and leave no exposure of the implant in the adjacent socket, no GTR is necessary. Defects that are less than 3 mm deep and do not expose more than three threads may have a barrier placed. Defects that are greater than 3 mm deep and expose more than three threads should be considered for GBA.

E. An implant that is placed into an extraction socket that is missing one or more bony walls may be treated with GBA. If two walls cannot be stabilized, the implant should be removed immediately. Many times, one or two bony walls are partially missing and the implant is stable. This is the ideal defect in which to use GBA.

F. When any of the aforementioned defects occur in conjunction with a narrow ridge, GBA may be used to attempt to augment the width of the ridge.

When barriers are used for implant augmentation, complete flap closure over the barrier should be obtained before removal; the barrier occasionally becomes exposed. If a small area becomes exposed prior to 30 days, the area may be cleansed with chlorhexidine swabs. If the barrier has a large exposed area and inflammation is present, it should be removed immediately. Ideally, the barrier should remain completely covered until its removal at 4 to 6 weeks after placement.

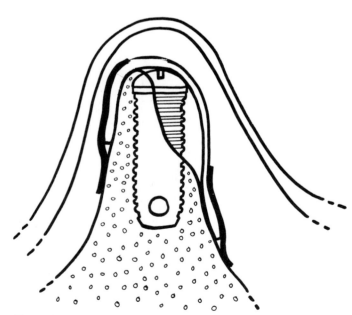

Figure 1. An implant with exposed body knurling covered with a membrane for guided bone augmentation.

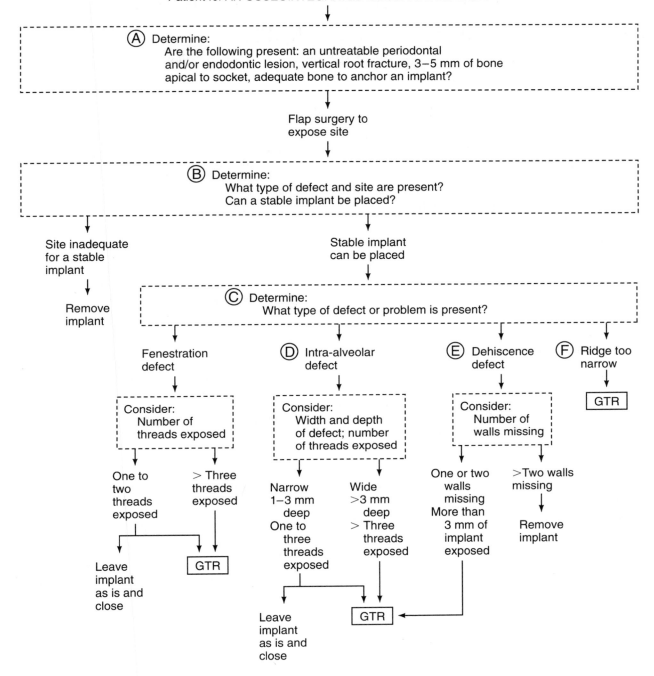

Patient for AN OSSEOINTEGRATED IMMEDIATE IMPLANT

Ⓐ Determine:
Are the following present: an untreatable periodontal and/or endodontic lesion, vertical root fracture, 3–5 mm of bone apical to socket, adequate bone to anchor an implant?

Flap surgery to expose site

Ⓑ Determine:
What type of defect and site are present?
Can a stable implant be placed?

Site inadequate for a stable implant

Remove implant

Stable implant can be placed

Ⓒ Determine:
What type of defect or problem is present?

Fenestration defect

Ⓓ Intra-alveolar defect

Ⓔ Dehiscence defect

Ⓕ Ridge too narrow

GTR

Consider:
Number of threads exposed

Consider:
Width and depth of defect; number of threads exposed

Consider:
Number of walls missing

One to two threads exposed

> Three threads exposed

Narrow 1–3 mm deep
One to three threads exposed

Wide >3 mm deep
> Three threads exposed

One or two walls missing
More than 3 mm of implant exposed

>Two walls missing

Remove implant

Leave implant as is and close

GTR

Leave implant as is and close

GTR

References

Becker W, Becker BE, Prichard J, et al. Root isolation for new attachment procedures: A surgical and suturing method: Three case reports. J Periodontol 1987; 58:819.

Becker W, Becker BE, Ochsenbein O, et al. Bone formation at dehisced dental implant sites treated with implant augmentation material: A pilot study in dogs. Int J Periodont Restor Dent 1989; 9:333.

Dahlin C, Sennerby L, Lekholm U, et al. Generation of new bone around titanium implants using a membrane technique: An experimental study in rabbits. Int J Oral Maxillofac Implants 1989; 4:19.

Gottlow J, Nyman S, Lindhe J. New attachment formation as a result of controlled tissue regeneration. J Clin Periodontol 1984; 11:494.

Lazzara RJ. Immediate implant placement into extraction sites: Surgical and restorative advantages. Int J Periodontol Restor Dent 1989; 9:333.

Nyman S, Lang NP, Buser D, Bragge U. Bone regeneration adjacent to titanium dental implants using guided tissue regeneration: A report of two cases. Int J Oral Maxillofac Implants 1990; 5:9.

PERIMPLANTITIS: ETIOLOGY OF THE AILING, FAILING, OR FAILED DENTAL IMPLANT

Mark Zablotsky
John Kwan

The discipline of implant dentistry has gained clinical acceptance owing to long-term studies that suggest very high success/survival rates in both partially and completely edentulous applications; however, in a small percentage of cases, implant failure and morbidity have been reported. Implant failure due to surgically overheating bone has been minimized with the advent of slow-speed, high-torque internally, and often externally, irrigated drilling systems. After integration (either bio- or osseointegration), the major cause of implant failure is thought to be due to biomechanical (i.e., overload, heavy lateral interferences, lack of a passive prosthesis fit, etc.) or infectious (plaque-induced) etiology.

Complications can be eliminated or minimized if clinicians plan treatment adequately. Mounted study models with diagnostic waxups or tooth setups are mandatory to evaluate ridge relationships, occlusal schemes, and restorative goals. When taken with adequate radiographs and clinical examination, the implant team (restoring dentist, surgeon, and laboratory technician) can adequately plan for the location, number, and trajectory of implants to ensure the most healthy aesthetic and functional prosthesis. Often, additional implants may be proposed in order to satisfy the implant team and patient requirements (i.e., fixed vs removable prostheses). The final restoration should be one that is esthetic, adequately engineered (enough implants of sufficient length in sufficient quality and quantity of supporting bone), and gives the patient accessibility for adequate home care. When evaluating the ailing/failing implant, often one or more of the aforementioned criteria have not been met.

A. When referring to a dental implant as ailing, failing, or failed, one really is referring to the status of the peri-implant supporting tissues (unless the implant is fractured). The ailing implant is one that displays progressive bone loss and pocketing but no clinical mobility. The failing implant is one that displays similar features to the ailing implant but is refractory to therapy and continues to progress downhill. This implant is also immobile. The term *ailing* suggests a somewhat more favorable prognosis than the term *failing*.

B. A failed implant is one that is fractured, has been totally refractory to all methods of treatment, or demonstrates clinical mobility and/or circumferential peri-implant radiolucency. These implants must be removed immediately, because progressive destruction of surrounding osseous tissues may occur.

C. The etiology of peri-implant disease is often multifactorial. Many times the clinician must do his detective work in order to discover the potential etiology. Meffert has coined the terms the *traditional* and

retrograde pathways when differentiating bacterial versus biomechanical etiologies.

Although a hemidesmosomal attachment of soft tissues to titanium has been reported, it is doubtful that this histologic phenomenon has clinical relevance around titanium implant abutments. The peri-implant seal is thought to originate from a tight adaptation of mucosal tissues around the abutment via an intricate arrangement of circular gingival fibers and a tight junctional epithelium. Because this "attachment" is tenuous at best, it can be extrapolated that a plaque-induced (traditional pathway) peri-implant gingivitis may not truly exist and that plaque-induced inflammation of peri-implant tissues may directly extend to the underlying supporting osseous tissues.

The periodontal ligament acts as a "shock absorber" around the natural tooth when excessive occlusal or orthodontic forces are present. In the absence of bacterial plaque, occlusal trauma does not cause a loss of attachment to teeth; however, because implants lack a periodontal ligament, force can be transmitted to the implant/bone interface. If significant enough, microfractures of this interface can occur and allow for an ingress of soft tissues and secondary bacterial infection.

In fixed bridgework that does not fit passively and is cemented on natural teeth, orthodontic movement of abutments occurs owing to the presence of the periodontal ligament. In this scenario, little if any damage occurs around abutments due to this orthodontic movement. When this same phenomenon occurs on dental implant abutments (either screw-retained or cemented), one of a few complications can result. The restoration may become loose either as a result of cement failure, screws backing out, or fracture. Abutments can loosen or fracture, or the implant body may fracture or have bone loss due to progressive microfractures at the interface (retrograde pathway); therefore, it is imperative that frameworks fit precisely. Lateral interferences or excessive off-axis loading has led to greater stresses on components as well as implant—bone interface and should be minimized. Bruxism can be extremely destructive and should be addressed by modifying occlusal schemes to eliminate lateral contacts in function or parafunction; alternatively, the patient should commit to permanent splint/nightguard treatment before placement of the implant. In some instances, it is possible to plan a removable prosthesis to address this concern.

When evaluating the ailing/failing implant, clinical signs of peri-implant problems include increased probing depths, bleeding on probing, suppuration, erythema and flaccidity of tissues, and radiographic

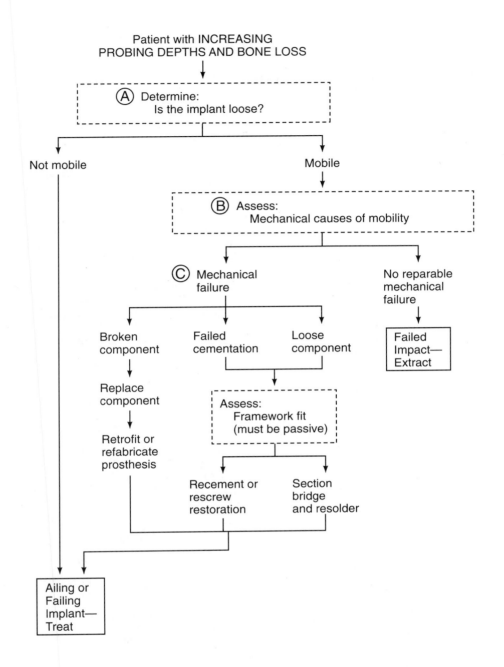

Patient with INCREASING
PROBING DEPTHS AND BONE LOSS

Ⓐ Determine:
Is the implant loose?

Not mobile

Mobile

Ⓑ Assess:
Mechanical causes of mobility

Ⓒ Mechanical
failure

No reparable
mechanical
failure

Broken
component

Failed
cementation

Loose
component

Failed
Impact—
Extract

Replace
component

Assess:
Framework fit
(must be passive)

Retrofit or
refabricate
prosthesis

Recement or
rescrew
restoration

Section
bridge
and resolder

Ailing or
Failing
Implant—
Treat

bone loss. Pain may be present, but usually it is a late symptom. If plaque is absent with minimally inflamed tissues, one must suspect occlusal etiology. Often this can be confirmed via culture and sensitivity testing. If bacteria associated with gingival health are present (i.e., *Streptococcus* sp. or *Actinomyces* sp.), then an occlusal component is strongly suggested. If, however, periodontal pathogens (i.e., *P. gingivalis, P. intermedius,* etc.) are present, one should have a high suspicion for peri-implant infection. This is not to say that there is not also an occlusal component. Inspect restorations for fit. If the restoration is loose, it is always bad news. Remove and evaluate each component until the loose or failed component is found. If the implant is loose, it is a failure and should be removed immediately. It will never reintegrate and be

functional. Replacement implants can be placed either at the time of implant removal or within 6 months of implant removal, as various regenerative techniques may be contemplated to maintain alveolar height and width.

References

Meffert R, Block M, Kent J. What is osseointegration? Int J Periodontol Restor Dent 1987; 11(2):88.

Newman M, Fleming T. Periodontal considerations of implants and implant associated microbiota. J Dent Ed 1988; 52(12):737.

Rosenberg E, Torosian J, Slots J. Microbial differences in 2 distinct types of failures of osseointegrated implants. Clin Oral Implant Res 1991; 2(3):135.

PERIMPLANTITIS: INITIAL THERAPY FOR THE AILING/FAILING DENTAL IMPLANT

Mark Zablotsky
John Kwan

A differential diagnosis should be made as early as possible in the initial stages of implant therapy, because information garnered may be critical in the follow-up and maintenance of the ailing/failing implant. If an accurate assessment of the etiology has not been established, then any interceptive therapy may be compromised.

A. Effective patient-performed plaque control is mandatory, and the patient must accept this responsibility. The therapist should customize a hygiene regimen for each implant patient. The use of conventional oral hygiene aids (i.e., brush, floss, etc.) can be augmented with any number of instruments (i.e., superfloss, yarn, plastic-coated proxibrushes, electric toothbrushes, etc.). If the patient's oral hygiene is suspect, the addition of a topical application of chemotherapeutics (i.e., chlorhexidine), either by rinsing or applying locally (via dipping brushes, etc.), may be very beneficial in maintenance. The restorative dentist must give the patient hygiene access to implant abutments circumferentially.

B. Evaluate occlusion, and eliminate centric/lateral prematurities and interferences via occlusal adjustment. Initiate nightguard/splint therapy if parafunctional activity is suspected. Often, the clinician can remove the prosthesis and place healing cuffs on the implants in hopes of getting a positive response by reducing the load if occlusal etiology is suspected. Single implants that are attached to mobile natural teeth may be overloaded as a result of the compression of the tooth and subsequent relative cantilevering of the prosthesis from the implant. If occlusal etiology is suspected in this case, contemplate the attachment of more implants to the existing weakened implant to support the cantilever of periodontally weak teeth. If one suspects bacterial etiology, initial conservative treatment may consist of subgingival irrigation with a blunt-tipped, side-port irrigating needle. Chlorhexidine is probably the irrigant of choice. Local application of tetracycline via monolithic fibers may be an effective adjunct.

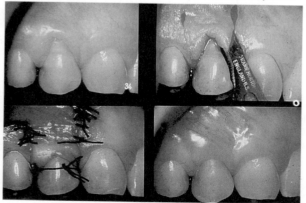

Figure 1. A shallow recession (4 mm) on a maxillary right first premolar is treated by a coronally positioned flap. Three millimeters of keratinized gingiva were available apical to the recession.

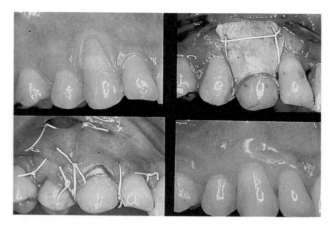

Figure 2. Guided tissue regeneration procedure on a maxillary right canine with a 6 mm recession.

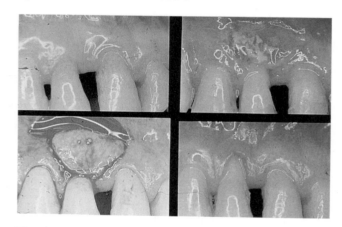

Figure 3. A recession associated with interdental bone resorption is treated by a free gingival graft. The final level of the gingival margin is consistent with the adjacent teeth.

C. Perform culture and sensitivity testing to guide therapy, if systemic antibiotics are contemplated. Consider debridement of hyperplastic peri-implant tissues utilizing hand or ultrasonic plastic (if the implant/abutment is going to be touched) instrumentation.

D. Ideally, the implant abutment should emerge through attached keratinized mucosa (Fig. 1). This will give the patient an ideal mucosa. It will also give the patient an ideal environment to perform home care, because moveable alveolar mucosal margins can be irritating and cause difficulty in effecting oral hygiene. Increased failures of implants and morbidity have been associated with areas that are deficient in attached keratinized gingival tissues (Fig. 2). Soft-tissue augmentation procedures can be performed either before implant placement, during integration, at uncovering (stage 2), or for repair procedures (Fig. 3).

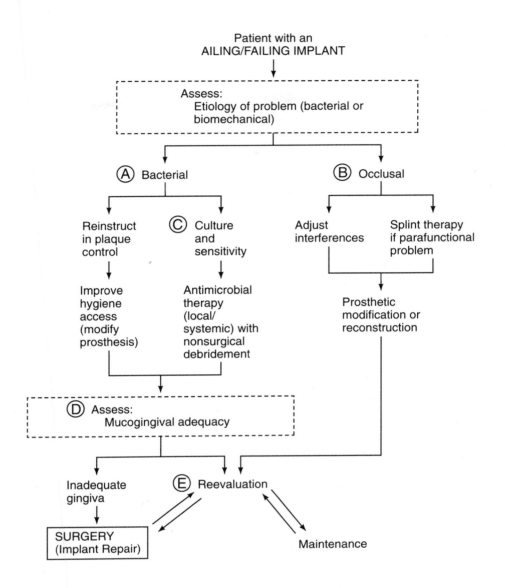

Patient with an
AILING/FAILING IMPLANT

Assess:
Etiology of problem (bacterial or
biomechanical)

Ⓐ Bacterial

Ⓑ Occlusal

Reinstruct
in plaque
control

Ⓒ Culture
and
sensitivity

Adjust
interferences

Splint therapy
if parafunctional
problem

Improve
hygiene
access
(modify
prosthesis)

Antimicrobial
therapy
(local/
systemic) with
nonsurgical
debridement

Prosthetic
modification or
reconstruction

Ⓓ Assess:
Mucogingival adequacy

Inadequate
gingiva

Ⓔ Reevaluation

SURGERY
(Implant Repair)

Maintenance

E. Consider reevaluation of peri-implant tissues 2 to 4 weeks after initial therapy. Probing depths should be reduced, and there should be no bleeding on probing or suppuration. The clinician must decide whether the improvement in clinical indices is a predictable long-term endpoint. One must remember that the success of periodontal therapy depends upon the therapist's ability to remove plaque, calculus, and other bacterial products from radicular surfaces. Because it is not possible or recommended to "root plane" the implant surfaces (due to the detrimental effects of conventional curettes or ultrasonics), one must consider that the titanium abutment or the hydroxylapatite-coated titanium implant surface is contaminated with bacteria and their products (i.e., endotoxin), therefore, one must conclude that the implant and peri-implant tissues would benefit from surgical intervention.

If the therapist feels that a successful endpoint has been attained, close maintenance with monitoring of clinical, radiographic, and microbiologic parameters is imperative. If prompt recurrence of problems occurs, one must question either the initial diagnosis (incorrect etiology) or the predictability of the more conservative nonsurgical therapy. In this instance, the clinician should strive to stabilize or arrest the active disease process (nonsurgically), then reevaluate to determine a clinical endpoint. Commonly, cases that are refractory to nonsurgical therapy do well after surgical intervention, because the contaminated implant surface can be addressed more adequately.

References

Gammage D, Bowman A, Meffert R. Clinical management of failing dental implants: Four case reports. J Oral Implants 1989; 15(2):124.

Kwan J, Zablotsky M. The ailing implant. J CDA 1991; 19(12):51.

Kwan J. Implant maintenance. J CDA 1991; 19(12):45.

Orton G, Steele D, Wolinsky L. The dental professional's role in monitoring and maintenance of tissue-integrated prostheses. Int J Oral Maxillofac Implants 1989; 4:305.

PERIMPLANTITIS: THE SURGICAL MANAGEMENT OF IMPLANT REPAIR

Mark Zablotsky
John Kwan

The surgical repair of the ailing/failing implant is dependent on an accurate diagnosis and effective nonsurgical intervention to stabilize or arrest the progression of the active peri-implant lesion.

A. It is important to assess the mucogingival status of peri-implant tissues before repair surgery. If only mucogingival defects exit around the ailing/failing implant, subsequent osseous repair surgery may not be necessary when soft-tissue augmentation is performed around the ailing/failing implant. If indicated, osseous repair surgery is less technically demanding when dealing with keratinized tissues.

B. Modifications of periodontal surgical procedures, either resective or regenerative, have been reported with some success. After making the initial incisions and degranulating the osseous defect (open debridement), one must evaluate the defect before selecting the appropriate surgical modality.

C. Peri-implant osseous defects that are predominantly horizontal in nature respond most predictably to resective procedures (i.e., definitive osseous surgery) with or without fixture modification.

D. Fixture modification is performed to remove macroscopic or microscopic features that interfere with subsequent plaque control in the supracrestal aspect of the defect. Fixture modification consists of smoothing with a series of rotary instruments in descending grit (i.e., fine diamond, white stone, rubber points) and using copious irrigation, because significant heat can be generated by these instruments. For those with concerns of contaminating implant surfaces or peri-implant tissues with rotary instruments, some have reported a healthy soft-tissue response against hydroxylapatite-coated or plasma-sprayed titanium implant surfaces. If the patient's oral hygiene is suspect, consider fixture modification for these microscopically rough surfaces.

E. Regenerative procedures (bone grafting with or without guided tissue regeneration [GTR]) has been reported for the repair of the ailing/failing implant. Regenerative procedures are most appropriate when the adjacent osseous crest is close to the rim of the implant (i.e., narrow two- or three-walled moat or dehiscence/fenestration defects). When these procedures are contemplated, fixture modification is not recommended.

F. Detoxification procedures to treat the infected implant surface are recommended before regenerative modalities. It appears that a 30-second to 1 minute application of a supersaturated solution of citric acid (pH 1) burnished with a cotton pledget may be very beneficial in detoxifying the infected hydroxylapatite-coated implant surface. If the coating appears pitted and altered, however, the coating should be removed either with ultrasonic or air/powder abrasives. A short application of an air/powder abrasive detoxifies the titanium implant surface. Extreme caution is recommended if the defect to be treated with the air/powder abrasive is a narrow intrabony defect, because pressurized air may enter the marrow spaces and there may be a risk of embolism.

G. Choice of bone-grafting materials should be based on the clinician's level of certainty that the site to be grafted is free of bacterial contaminants. If the clinician is certain that the defect is not contaminated, resorbable materials (i.e., autogenous bone, DFDBA, or resorbable hydroxylapatite, or GTR materials alone) may be considered. If the surface of the implant is suspect, nonresorbable materials (i.e., dense nonresorbable hydroxylapatite) should be considered. Use nonresorbable bone-grafting materials to obturate apical vents and basket holes, as osseous regeneration probably will not occur in these anatomically contaminated environments.

Contemplate combined therapies whenever defect combinations include horizontal bone loss and dehiscence or intrabony defects. Postoperative care is much like that for periodontal surgical procedures, with close follow-up and reevaluation prior to placing the patient back on a supportive maintenance schedule.

H. The goals of peri-implant surgical and nonsurgical therapies are to reestablish a healthy perimucosal seal and to regenerate a soft- or hard-tissue attachment to the implant/abutment. This requires a definitive diagnosis, comprehensive therapy, and effective maintenance. At this time, no prospective or retrospective studies exist when dealing with the short- or long-term results attained through implant repair procedures; therefore, close follow-up for recurrence of disease is warranted. Although the goals of therapy are clear, the clinician must be willing to accept and recognize failure when it occurs. The dental implant that is refractory to all attempts at treatment is a failure and should be removed as soon as this diagnosis is made.

References

Lozada J, James R, et al. Surgical repair of peri-implant defects. J Oral Implant 1990; 16(1):42.

Meffert R. How to treat ailing and failing implants. Implant Dent 1992; 1:25.

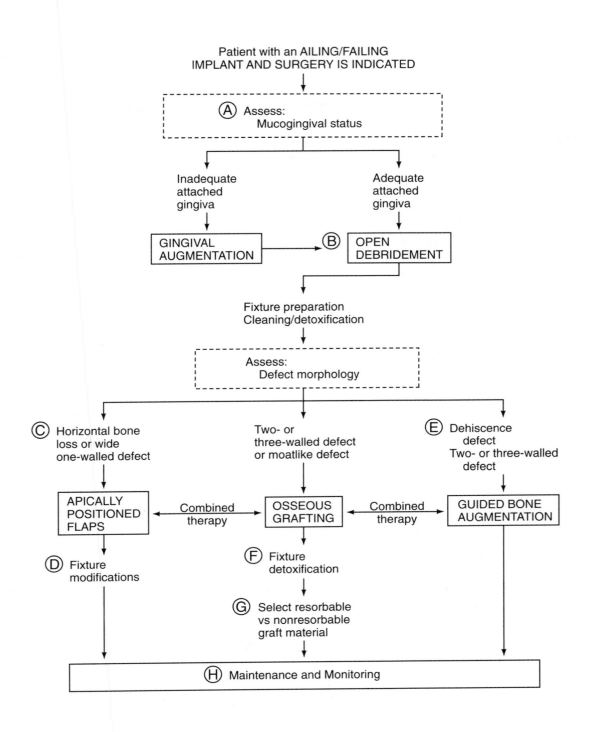

Patient with an AILING/FAILING
IMPLANT AND SURGERY IS INDICATED

(A) Assess:
Mucogingival status

Inadequate attached gingiva

Adequate attached gingiva

GINGIVAL AUGMENTATION

(B) OPEN DEBRIDEMENT

Fixture preparation
Cleaning/detoxification

Assess:
Defect morphology

(C) Horizontal bone loss or wide one-walled defect

Two- or three-walled defect or moatlike defect

(E) Dehiscence defect
Two- or three-walled defect

APICALLY POSITIONED FLAPS

Combined therapy

OSSEOUS GRAFTING

Combined therapy

GUIDED BONE AUGMENTATION

(D) Fixture modifications

(F) Fixture detoxification

(G) Select resorbable vs nonresorbable graft material

(H) Maintenance and Monitoring

Zablotsky M. The surgical management of osseous defects associated with endosteal hydroxylapatite-coated and titanium dental implants. Dent Clin North Am 1992; 36(1):117.

Zablotsky M, Diedrich D, Meffert R, Wittrig E. The ability of various chemotherapeutic agents to detoxify the endotoxin infected HA-coated implant surface. Int J Oral Maxillofac Implants 1991; 8(2):45.

Zablotsky M, Diedrich D, Meffert R. The ability of various chemotherapeutic agents to detoxify the endotoxin-contaminated titanium implant surface. Implant Dent (in press).

ROOT COVERAGE IN CASES OF LOCALIZED RECESSION

Carlo Clauser
Giovan Paolo Pini-Prato
Pierpaolo Cortellini

A. Miller has divided recession into four classes according to the prognosis for healing in terms of root coverage. Classes I and II (no loss of interdental bone or soft tissue) allow for complete root coverage; the reference point for measuring the recession is the cementoenamel junction. Classes III and IV (with interdental bone loss) do not guarantee 100% root coverage (see p 108).

B. Guided tissue regeneration (GTR) proved to be effective in the treatment of recession in animals (Cortellini et al, 1991) and in humans (Tinti and Vincenzi, 1990; Cortellini et al, 1991; Tinti et al, 1992). A comparative study was recently made on GTR in the treatment of gingival recession (Pini Prato et al). Mucogingival surgery (MGS) yielded better results in terms of root coverage when the recession was less than 4.98 mm, whereas greater root coverage was achieved with membranes when the recession was deeper than 4.98 mm. In either case, the membrane procedure resulted in a significantly greater gain in clinical attachment and a reduction in probing depth.

C. The 3-mm threshold was selected on the basis of the results obtained by Allen and Miller. These results showed an average 97.8% root coverage using coronally positioned flaps to treat shallow recessions, when at least 3 mm of keratinized gingiva (KG) was available apical to the exposed root.

D. A free gingival graft (FGG) may consist of connective tissue only or of both epithelial and connective tissue. No comparative study has been published to assess the appropriateness of either technique. Therefore, the choice of graft type is left to the discretion of the individual clinician.

E. GTR has been tested with no gingival augmentation, even when less than 1 mm of KG was present. The procedure requires designing a large and thick flap that can provide an abundant blood supply and be coronally positioned to cover the membrane entirely with no pulling. A slight increase in the amount of keratinized tissue is expected at the end of the treatment (Tinti et al, 1992; Pini Prato et al), although a shallow vestibule may result, therefore, a FGG before the regenerative procedure is advisable to prevent the reduction of the vestibule and to facilitate surgery.

F. In cases of interdental bone loss, we suggest using the adjacent teeth as reference points. The area to be covered may be measured as the distance between the gingival margin (GM) of the area to be treated and the line that connects the most apical levels of the gingival margins of the adjacent teeth. This may be considered the most coronal level able to be reached with a covering procedure.

References

Allen EP, Miller PD. Coronal positioning of existing gingiva: Short-term results in the treatment of shallow marginal tissue recession. J Periodontol 1989; 60:316.

Cortellini P, De Sanctis M, Pini Prato GP, et al. Guided tissue regeneration procedure in the treatment of a bone dehiscence associated with a gingival recession: A case report. Int J Periodont Restor Dent 1991; 11(6):472.

Cortellini P, De Sanctis M, Pini Prato GP, et al. Guided tissue regeneration procedure using a fibrin–fibronectin system in surgically induced recessions, in dogs. Int J Periodont Restor Dent 1991; 11:151.

Miller PD. A classification of marginal tissue recession. Int J Periodont Restor Dent 1985; 5:9.

Pini Prato GP, Tinti C, Vincenzi G, et al. Guided tissue regeneration versus mucogingival surgery in the treatment of human buccal recessions. Submitted to J Periodontol.

Tinti C, Vincenzi G. Il trattamento delle recessioni gengivali con la tecnica di "rigenerazione guidata dei tessuti" mediante membrana Gore-Tex (R). Variante clinica. Quintessence Int 1990; 6:465.

Tinti C, Vincenzi G, Cortellini P, et al. Guided tissue regeneration in the treatment of human facial recession: A twelve-case report. J Periodontol 1992; 63:554.

Patient with ROOT COVERAGE IN CASES OF LOCALIZED RECESSION

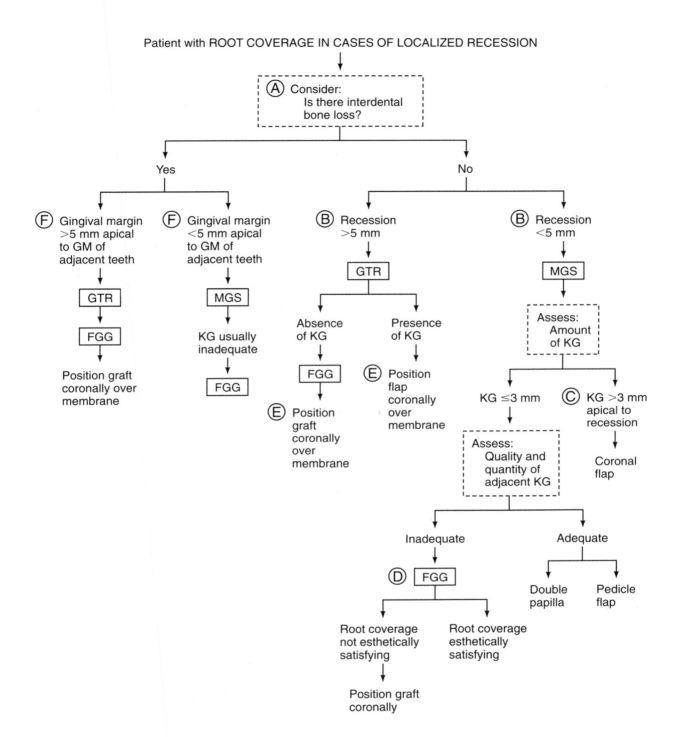

INDEX

and resection, 138
and two-walled osseous defects, 158–159
for vertical osseous defects, 152–153
"Gummy" smile, 102

H

Haemophilus actinomycetem comitans, 148
Hairy leukoplakia, 58, 59, 60
Handicapped
  decision tree for (diagram), 81
  and dental hygiene, 80
Health questionnaire, 2
Heart conditions, and treatment, 2
Hemangiomas, 134
Hemisection
  diagnosis and treatment (diagram), 139
  vs. root amputation, 138–139
Hemiseptal bone defect, 34
Hepatitis B, and treatment, 2
Herpes simplex, 48
Herpetic gingivostomatitis, 12, 46, 48–49, 58, 70
  diagnosis (diagram), 49
  and periodontal pain, 20
High lip line
  and esthetics, 102–103
  evaluation of (diagram), 103
HIV, 58
  and drug abusers, 60
HIV gingivitis, 12, 60
HIV periodontitis, 16, 60, 70
  and chemotherapy, 84
  and periodontal pain, 20
Hopeless tooth, 68–69
  assessment and procedure (diagram), 69
Horizontal bone loss, 30, 32
Human immunodeficiency virus. *See* HIV
Hyperparathyroidism, 134
Hyperplasias, 70

I

Implant(s)
  assessment and procedure for failing (diagram), 255
  failing, 252–253
  and indications for surgery (diagram), 257
  surgical management and repair, 256–257
Inadequate attached gingiva, 86
  assessment and procedure (diagram), 207
  diagnosis (diagram), 91–99
  estimating (diagram), 87
  and graft options (diagram), 105
  and recession, 98, 106
  and restoration procedure (diagram), 93
  and root exposure, 38
Infectious disease, and treatment, 2
Informed consent, 224–225
  problems requiring (diagram), 225
Infrabony crater, 34
Interdental papilla, and ulcerative gingivitis, 46
Interplak brush, 80
Interproximal brushes, 80
Isolated periodontal defects (IPD), 240–241
  assessment and procedure (diagram), 241

J

Juvenile periodontitis, 44–45
  examination and diagnosis (diagram), 45

K

Kaopectate, 48, 63
Kaposi's sarcoma, 134

L

Laboratory tests, 40–41
  and various diagnoses (diagram), 41
Leukemias, 132
  and treatment, 2
Leukoplakias, 12
Loose teeth
  and clenching and grinding, 126–127
  diagnosis and treatment (diagram), 125, 127
  and occlusal trauma, 50
Loss of attachment (LOA), 22
  in gingival enlargement, 52

M

Magenta (gingival color), 12
Mandible
  partially edentulous, 246–247
  potentially edentulous (diagram), 249
  procedure for posterior edentulous areas (diagram), 247
  totally edentulous, 248–249
"Material risk and objective standard," 224
Maxilla
  partially edentulous, 242–243
  totally edentulous, 244–245
  treatment of partially edentulous (diagram), 243
  treatment of totally edentulous (diagram), 245
Maxillary anterior teeth
  and diagnosis (diagram), 101
  and periodontal disease, 100
Medical history, 2–3, 42
Medical status (patient's), and periodontitis, 66
Medication
  postsurgical, 190–191
  and treatment, 3
Membrane selection, 150–151
Metallic taste, and diagnosis, 20
Metronidazole (Flagyl), 70, 80
Microbiologic investigation, and GTR, 148
Mobility
  differentiating degrees of, 26–27
  examination for (diagram), 27, 131
Molar furcation, status of, before surgery, 144
Molars
  furcation defects and diagnosis (diagram), 155
  furcation defects and GTR, 154–155
  and indications for resection, 138–139
  therapy evaluation (diagram), 145
Molar uprighting, 184
Mucocutaneous dermatoses, 62
Mucocutaneous disorders, 62
Mucogingival-osseous problems, 53–54
  assessment and treatment (diagram), 54

chemical control of, 84
and gingival enlargement, 52
history of control of, 6–7
and orthodontics, 96
and overhanging margins, 36
and probing, 22
and surgical therapy, 142, 172
Pocket elimination
assessment and treatment (diagram), 165
on the palate, 167
with flaps reflected treatment (diagram), 169
and Widman flap, 162
Pocket 5 mm or greater, and treatment (diagram), 173
Pocket formation, in gingival enlargement, 52
Pocket pain and tooth pain, assessment and procedure (diagram), 65
Polymorphonuclear leukocytes (PMNs), 44
Porous hydroxylapatite (PHA), 174
Porphyromonas, 148
Postsurgical evaluation, 220–221
Potassium salt of penicillin (Pen VK), 136
Pregnancy, and treatment, 2
Pregnancy gingivitis, 2
Pregnancy tumor, 134
Prepubertal juvenile periodontitis, 70
Prevotela, 148
Primary occlusal drama, 118–119
diagnosis and treatment (diagram), 119
Pritchard-type ATR, 182
Probing, 22–23
depths and bone loss (diagram), 253
periodontal (diagram), 23
pocket depths (diagram), 163
Prominent root, and missing bone cover assessment (diagram), 195
Prophylactic gingival grafting, 98
Prophylaxis
defined, 74
vs. root planing, 74–75
Pseudopockets, 23
Pulpitis, 56
Pure mucongingival problems
European view of, and orthodontics, 96–97
orthodontics assessement and procedures for (diagram), 95
Pure mucogingival surgery
afterwork (diagram), 217
dressing following, 216–217
restoration following, 218–219

R

Radiation therapy, and illness, 2
Radiography
and angular defects, 35
and bone loss, 32–33
and CGE, 134
for cracked tooth syndrome, 64
and dehiscence and fenestration, 194
and drug abuse, 60
and edentulous mandibles, 246
evaluation, 30–31
indications for, 10–11
interpreting (diagram), 33
and isolated periodontal defects, 240
and osseous defects, 176
and perimplantitis, 252
and periodontal etiology, 56
and periodontal pain, 18

procedure for (diagram), 11
procedure for evaluation of (diagram), 31
and reevaluation, 220
and ridgeplasty, 184
and root form, 82
and three-walled osseous defect, 180
and two-walled osseous defect, 158
Rapidly progressive periodontis (RPP), 44–45, 70
examination and diagnosis (diagram), 45
and testing, 40
Recall visits, behavioral approach to, 222–223
Recession
active vs. stability, 88
assessment (diagram), 89
assessment and procedure for localized (diagram), 259
classifying, 108–109
Class I, 110–111
Class II, 112–113
Classes III and IV, 114–115
diagnosis and treatment for Class I (diagram), 111
diagnosis and treatment for Class II (diagram), 113
diagnosis and treatment for Class III (diagram), 115
localized, 258–259
of marginal tissue (diagram), 109
and orthodontics, 98–99
prevention of, 98–99
and root coverage, 106–107, 108–109
and root coverage diagnosis (diagram), 107
Redness (gingival), 12
Reevaluation. *See* Postsurgical reevaluation
Refractory periodontitis, 84
Residual pocket depths, and therapy evaluation (diagram), 143
Restorations, and dental history, 4
Restorative margin location, assessment and procedure (diagram), 239
Rest-proximal plate-1 (RP1), 218
and gingival grafting, 92
Retrograde pathways, 252
''Reversed architecture,'' 168
Ridge area, procedure for improving edentulous (diagram), 215
Ridge augmentation, 214–215
Ridgeplasty, 184–185
Root amputation
diagnosis and treatment (diagram), 139
or hemisection, 138–139
Root coverage
assessment and procedure (diagram), 259
of localized recession, 258–259
and recession treatment, 106–107
Root exposure, 38–39
and pedicle graft assessement (diagram), 197
procedure for (diagram), 39
Root hypersensitivity, 228
Root planing
defined, 74
vs. prophylaxis, 74–75
repetitive, vs. surgery, 76–77
Root resection
assessment and treatment (diagram), 141
defined, 138
sequencing, 140–141
RUM position, 28

S

Scaling, defined, 74
Secondary occlusal trauma, 120–121